Sheila CARTER
1708 Meadowood Ct.
Edgewood, Md. 21040

3A

NUTRITION AND DIET THERAPY

NUTRITION AND DIET THERAPY

EDITION 3

VELMA L. KERSCHNER, RN, BS

Assistant Professor
Health Careers
St. Philip's College
San Antonio, Texas

F.A.DAVIS COMPANY Philadelphia

Printed in the United States of America

Library of Congress Cataloging in Publication Data

Kerschner, Velma L.
Nutrition and diet therapy.

Rev. ed. of: Nutrition and diet therapy for practical nurses. Ed. 2. c1976.
Bibliography: p.
Includes index.
1. Diet therapy. 2. Nutrition. 3. Nursing. I. Title. [DNLM: 1. Diet therapy—Nursing texts. 2. Nutrition—Nursing texts. WB 400 K41s]
RM216.K557 1983 615.8′54 82-22120
ISBN 0-8036-5302-6

TO MY HUSBAND,
HARRISON F. KERSCHNER, JR.,
WHO SPENT SO MANY HOURS
LOOKING FOR MY MISTAKES
IN TYPING!

TO THE STUDENT:

To use this book effectively, first read the text carefully. Ignore the questions and projects until the entire chapter has been read. Then reread the text, answering the questions mentally or on a separate sheet of paper. Check your answers. If they are correct, write them in your book; if incorrect, study the material again. You will find that reviewing the questions and answers at intervals during the year is helpful in studying for examinations.

PREFACE

The last decade has been a momentous one for those interested in nutrition. In 1972, a law was passed requiring that the nutrient content of foods be on the labels and now the percentage of the Recommended Daily Allowance must be given for certain nutrients. The National Nutrition Consortium Inc. was formed in 1974. The Federal Government has conducted many nutrition surveys and has provided more nutrition programs for the aged, children, and low-income families than ever before. In 1977, the Senate Select Committee on Nutrition and Human Needs published dietary goals for the people of the United States. The World Health Organization continues to try to elevate the standards of nutrition for the peoples of the world through its multiphased programs.

This new edition still incorporates the elements of a basic text and a workbook, which should assist the student in learning the principles of basic nutrition and diet therapy quickly and easily. Learners acquire knowledge through their own activities rather than the activities of others. Instructors may want to utilize educational material obtained from the list of sources in the Appendix.

There have been some changes to bring the text up-to-date and to include new material. Two new chapters cover concerns of today—weight control and drug and nutrient interactions. Several new tables have been added to the Appendix. Each chapter has learning objectives and activities that should enhance learning and make nutrition more interesting for students.

Section 1 deals with the basic principles of nutrition. Section 2 discusses the application of these principles in the treatment of medical and surgical conditions. Some schools may prefer to use Section 1 during the preclinical period and Section 2 during the clinical period of the student's training.

Each chapter is followed by questions or projects, or both, for the student to complete. These projects require no laboratory facilities that are not readily available to all schools. The optional activities given at the end of the chapter may be used for enrichment. At the end of each section, test questions are provided so that students can evaluate their comprehension of the material in that section.

VLK

CONTENTS

SECTION 1

FOODS AND NUTRITION

The nursing student may ask why the study of foods and nutrition is necessary. In the hospital, the nurse does not plan or prepare the patients' diets, and in the home, the doctor usually leaves a definite list of the foods the patient may have. However, the student should remember that often the nurse must explain the reasons for the diet to patients to win their acceptance and cooperation. The nurse must answer questions as to what foods are allowed, how they are to be prepared, and when they may be served. The doctor's dietary orders are easier to follow correctly if the nurse understands the reasons for the orders and anticipates the patients' reactions. Finally, the nurse is always a teacher, and understanding the basic principles of good nutrition enables the nurse to teach others and to set a good example.

1

INTRODUCTION TO NUTRITION

OBJECTIVES

Upon completion of this chapter the student should be able to:

- Describe at least six activities of the nurse when serving a meal.
- Describe a patient teaching session, listing at least five rules.
- Define: dietetics, diet therapy, health, malnutrition, nutrient, nutrition, nutritional deficiency (primary and secondary), and nutritional status.
- Discuss food habits, giving an explanation of their development and listing at least five that the nurse can observe and use in planning patient care.
- Given the ethnic background of a patient, give at least one food usually eaten by that person.
- Discuss the impact food fads and superstitions have upon nutrition of the individual, giving five reasons food misinformation exists.

ROLE OF THE NURSE

The nurse spends more time with the patient than anyone else involved in the patient's care. The nurse observes the condition, listens to the complaints, and fills most of the needs of the patient. The nurse works with doctors, nursing supervisors, and other health care personnel. Meeting the patient's nutritional needs is part of providing total care.

Some of the nursing activities involved in meeting the patient's nutritional needs may be receiving and implementing the doctor's orders, serving trays, feeding the patient, giving the patient explanations and instructions as required, and making observations. The doctor, other nurses, and the dietitian are resource persons that the nurse can consult when necessary.

The physician's dietary prescription is designed to provide the body with materials needed for maintenance, for overcoming specific nutritional problems, and for growth and development. In the hospital, the nurse communicates the dietary instructions to the department that prepares the food. If the patient is not hospitalized, the doctor may give the patient an instruction sheet or ask the nurse to explain the diet. Occasionally, the nurse providing home care may find that it is necessary to help prepare the food.

In some hospitals, personnel from the Food Service Department serve the food tray. In others, the tray is served by the nurse. Whoever serves the tray, the basic procedure is the same. First, the patient is prepared. The nurse assists the patient in cleaning the face and hands. Some like to brush their teeth before as well as after a meal. The bed is tidied and the overbed tray prepared. The patient's room is checked to be sure there are no objectionable sights, sounds, or odors. Some patients prefer to eat alone, others find that visitors stimulate the appetite.

Before bringing the tray to the bedside, the nurse checks the name on the tray, sees that the correct diet has been provided, and checks that the tray is complete and neatly and pleasingly arranged. On entering the patient's room, the nurse checks the name on the tray against the patient's identification. If the patient's condition permits, the head of the bed is elevated to a comfortable and convenient height and the overbed table is placed in position. The covers over the food are removed before the tray is placed on the overbed table as trapped odors may nauseate some patients if released directly under their noses. Further assistance such as opening milk cartons and plastic bags containing condiments and cutlery, buttering bread, and cutting meat may be required. Some patients must be fed.

While feeding patients, the nurse can get to know them and teach them about their diets. Mealtimes should be pleasant and unhurried, and the nurse should be prepared to discuss nondisturbing topics. The patient is given an opportunity to ask a blessing before the meal if so desired.

The bed and clothing should be protected with a towel. Food is presented in bite-size portions and in the order the patient prefers. The patient must be given time to chew and swallow and a napkin is used as necessary. The temperatures of all hot liquids are checked against the inside of the nurse's wrist before offering them to the patient.

The tray should be removed as quickly as possible after a meal. The nurse notes the amount eaten and charts it. If there has been any difficulty in eating or any food disliked, this too is recorded and brought to the attention of those in charge. The patient's face and hands are washed again and the patient is given the opportunity to brush the teeth. The patient is left comfortable and clean.

The nurse is often asked which foods the patient can eat and why a particular diet has been ordered. Sometimes the nurse will have to explain how to prepare a specific food, such as how to cook an egg without using grease.

The nurse must remember that telling is not teaching. A teaching session must be carefully planned with these rules in mind:

1. Teach one thing at a time. For example, a diabetic patient must learn to use the Food Exchange Lists, but at one teaching session all the nurse asks is that the patient learn to pick out the foods found in the Fat Exchange.
2. Use words the patient knows. If it is necessary to use an unfamiliar word, explain its meaning.
3. Use pictures or models when possible.
4. Repeat the lesson until the patient knows it. A patient may learn slowly because of fear, weakness, or the effect of drugs. The nurse must take this into account when setting goals.
5. Arrange for practice. For example, let patients select foods for their diets with supervision.
6. Give the patient a chance to ask questions and answer these questions as simply as possible. When you do not know the answer, go to the appropriate resource person and inform the patient of the answer.
7. Check learning by asking specific questions about the lesson or having the patient repeat the lesson. If teaching a procedure, such as preparing formulas, ask the patient to perform the procedure.

The nurse observes the amount and kind of food eaten, any difficulty with eating, and food likes and dislikes. Of equal importance is the observation of physical signs and symptoms that indicate nutritional problems. Conversations with patients or their relatives will often reveal food habits that relate to patients' problems. It is the nurse's responsibility to acquire the knowledge necessary to recognize important observations and the skill to communicate these observations to others.

Fill in the answers to the following:

1. What are the activities of the nurse in meeting the patient's nutritional needs?

Receiving & implementing the Doctor's orders, serving trays, feeding the patient, giving the patient explanations & instructions as required & making observations

2. List three reasons the doctor orders a diet.

1, Provide the body with materials needed for matinance
2, overcoming specific nutritional problems
3 Growth & developement

3. How would you prepare a patient to be served a meal?

Clean the patient's face & hands. Patient may wish to brush teeth, Bed is tidied & overbed tray prepared. Check room to be sure no objectionable sigths, sounds or odors are there.

4. When the food tray is received from Food Service, what does the nurse check it for? Checks the name & see's that correct diet has been provided. When she's in the room she checks the name on tray against identification badge. Before entering she checks to see if tray is complete & neatly & pleasingly arranged.

5. Why does the nurse check the name on the tray against the patient's identification? to be certain that the right diet is presented to correct patient.

6. List some of the ways the nurse may assist patients who are able to feed themselves. The head of the bed is elevated to comfortable & convient height. The overbed tray is placed in position. The covers over food are removed before placing food on table.

Are there some things the nurse can do to assist the patient that were not mentioned? Give examples.

7. If you were telling someone how to feed a patient, what would you tell them to do? Don't hurry meal. Protect clothing with a towel. Present food in bite size portions & in the order the patient prefers. Give patient time to chew & swallow & use napkin as necessary. Check temperatures of ~~food~~ hot liquids against inside of wrist before giving them to patients. Remove tray immediatly after meal. Note the amount eaten & write it down. Record also dislike food or that difficult to eat. Wash face & hands & give him the chance to brush teeth.

8. List seven rules the nurse follows in teaching patients.

(1) teach one thing at a time. (2) use words the patient knows. (3) use pictures or models when possible (4) repeat lessons till he knows them. (5) arrange for practice. (6) let him ask questions & answer as simple as possible. (7) check by asking questions or have him repeat lesson.

9. Why should the nurse have a knowledge of nutrition?

she is often asked which foods the patient can eat & why a particular diet is ordered. may have to explain how to prepare a specific food.

NUTRITION

NUTRITION. Nutrition is the combination of processes by which the body receives and uses food for growth, development, and maintenance.

NUTRIENTS. A **nutrient** is a substance that nourishes the body. The six classes of nutrients are: (1) fats, (2) carbohydrates, (3) proteins, (4) minerals, (5) vitamins, and (6) water.

NUTRITIONAL STATUS. Nutritional status is the condition of the body as a result of its receiving and using nutrients. When the body benefits from a well-balanced diet, good nutritional status is present. Enough essential nutrients are supplied and used to maintain the body and also to provide a reserve. Good nutrition is essential for:

1. Normal growth.
2. Normal development.
3. Normal maintenance.
4. Normal reproduction.
5. Normal resistance to disease.
6. Normal recovery from injury (repair).
7. Normal activity and working efficiency.

HEALTH. The World Health Organization defines **health** as "the state of complete physical, mental, and social well-being, and not merely the absence of disease or infirmity." Sufficient activity, rest, recreation, and sleep contribute to health. Eating the correct amount and variety of foods each day also contributes to health.

Well-nourished people are well developed with the correct weight for their height and bone structure. Their flesh is firm, muscles taut, and posture erect. Their skin is clear. Their eyes sparkle brightly, their expression is alert, and their hair is smooth and shining. They sleep soundly and awake refreshed and with a pleasant disposition. Their appetite is good and elimination is normal. In general, their health is good and they are able to resist most infections.

NUTRITIONAL DEFICIENCY. When the body is not supplied with the necessary amounts of nutrients, it suffers from **nutritional deficiency.** Nutritional deficiency is termed *primary* when it is the first cause of ill health. *Secondary* nutritional deficiency exists as a complication of another disease or condition.

Primary nutritional deficiency may be due to inability to obtain essential nutrients or to conditions that interfere with intake, absorption, or usage of nutrients. For example, the elderly who do not have necessary dentures may become deficient in those nutrients found in foods that require thorough chewing.

Secondary deficiency is caused by conditions that (1) increase the body's needs for nutrients, (2) destroy nutrients in the body, or (3) cause too rapid an excretion of nutrients from the body. An example of increased need for nutrients is the requirement of extra calcium, protein, and iron during pregnancy. In diarrhea, nutrients are excreted before the alimentary tract can digest and absorb them.

MALNUTRITION. Malnutrition is faulty or imperfect nutrition due to a dietary lack or an excess of one or more nutrients. An unbalanced diet leads to malnutrition.

Malnourished people are poorly developed, either underweight or overweight. Their skin is loose, pale, and prone to blemishes. Their eyes and facial expression are dull, and their hair is rough and without luster. Their posture is poor, with a tendency toward slumping. They sleep poorly and are irritable, nervous, and tired. They are often depressed and lacking in ambition. They complain of indigestion and constipation. Easily infected, they lack the energy of well-nourished people.

DIETETICS. Dietetics is the science of applying the principles of nutrition to the feeding of individuals or groups. A dietitian is responsible for the planning of diets.

DIET THERAPY. Treatment through prescription of a specific diet is known as **diet therapy.** The doctor prescribes the type of diet needed by the patient; the dietitian plans the patient's menus accordingly.

Supply the information necessary to complete the following:

1. The definition of nutrition is: the combination of processes by which the body receives & uses food for growth, developement & maintenance.

2. Foods that supply the essential nourishment of the body are called nutrients.

3. Anyone who does not get sufficient nourishment is suffering from Malnutrition.

If the patient has a severe case of diarrhea, the patient would have a nutritional deficiency.

4. The person who is too poor to buy sufficient food would be suffering from Malnutrition.

5. List the six classes of nutrients.

1) Fats
2) Carbohydrates
3) Proteins
4) Vitamins
5) Minerals
6) Water

6. Define "health."

the state of complete mental, physical, & social well being and not merely the absence of disease or infirmity.

7. Tell in your own words how nutrition and health are related.

when some one receives good nutrition there health is better. they sleep better, thier skin is clear, eyes are bright, better disposition, elimination is good, hair & skin are good, & thier resistance is better.

8. Using the description of the well-nourished persons given in the text as a guide, decide what your own nutritional status is.

Muscle tone:
Fair

Sleep pattern:
Rest well

Posture:
Fair

Appetite:
Good

Eyes:
Bright

Elimination:
Good

Hair:
Dull

Disposition:
Pleasant

Is your nutritional status good, fair, or poor?

Fair

FOOD HABITS

Food habits are characteristic attitudes and actions concerning food. Food habits are influenced by the availability of food, nationality, religion, social environment, and individual likes and dislikes.

Factors that lead to differences in food habits among the various ethnic groups include availability of foods, storage capabilities, and resources for preparing foods. People who live by lakes and seas use more fish in the diet. Where the terrain is unsuitable for cattle, milk used may be from goats. When refrigeration is lacking, foods are salted and pickled and then stored. Much of the food in Japan is prepared by "stir-fry" as this method conserves scarce cooking fuel. Thus, ethnic patterns of eating have developed over the centuries.

It is important for the nurse to be aware of ethnic food patterns. Table 1 shows some of the foods preferred by certain groups. In the blank column on the right side of the table check those foods that you regularly eat. In the blank at the bottom of the table list any foods that you eat that are not listed. Do your food habits fall into any specific ethnic group?

Within the United States, regional eating patterns have developed partly due to geographic situations and partly to the ethnicity of the settlers. However, because of the impact of mass media, advanced preservation and transportation methods, and the mobility of the people themselves, ethnic and regional eating patterns have become mixed, although certain foods are still associated with certain areas. New England is known for its clam chowder and codfish, Texas and the Southwest for Mexican food, and the Deep South for fried chicken, cornbread, and hot biscuits. New Orleans has its okra gumbo, crawfish, and French Creole cooking. Scrapple and shoofly pie come from Pennsylvania. Venison jerky was first prepared by American Indians. Economic factors led black Americans to develop an eating pattern that included wild game, greens, blackeyed peas, grits, and sweet potatoes.

Food habits include not only the types of food eaten but also family behavior at mealtime, seating arrangements, types of food containers, order of service, manner of eating, and buying habits. In some homes, the father fills everyone's plate, perhaps assisted by the mother. In other homes, food is placed on the plates in the kitchen, or each person may choose from a serving dish as it is passed around the table "family style." In some communities, men are served before women. It is sometimes the custom for children to have a separate dining area. Food can also be served in separate courses. Even the concept of good manners varies. In the United States, everyone is encouraged to eat as quietly as possible; in some countries a loud satisfied belch indicates enjoyment of a good meal.

Influence of a group and lack of will power can lead to the formation of bad food habits to the detriment of health. Teenage girls are especially prone

TABLE 1. FOOD PREFERENCES

	China	France	Greece	Hungary	Italy	Japan	Jewish	Mexico	Middle East	Poland	Portugal	Puerto Rico
Beans								*				*
Bean sprouts	*					*						
Beef	*	*				*	*	*			*	
Blintzes							*					
Blood, coagulated	*											
Borscht							*					
Bread, dark					*				*	*		
Butter		*						*	*			
Cabbage										*		
Cereals	*					*						
Cheeses		*			*			*	*			
Cheese, cottage										*		
Chicken		*				*	*	*			*	
Coffee, strong		*							*			
Corn and corn products								*				
Cream, sour		*		*						*		
Eggs	*	*		*	*	*			*			
Fish	*	*		*		*	*			*		*
Fish, pickled	*					*	*			*		
Fish, salted										*		*
Foods, highly seasoned				*				*				*
Fruits		*	*	*							*	*
Garlic					*			*				
Grains				*							*	
Gravies		*	*									
Lamb and mutton	*	*	*				*		*			
Meat, Kosher							*		*			
Meat, rich in fat			*									
Milk										*		
Milk, buffalo	*											
Milk, hot									*			
Milk, goat					*							
Olives and olive oil			*		*				*			
Onions				*				*				
Paprika				*								
Pasta					*							

TABLE 1. ***Continued***

	China	*France*	*Greece*	*Hungary*	*Italy*	*Japan*	*Jewish*	*Mexico*	*Middle East*	*Poland*	*Portugal*	*Puerto Rico*
Peppers, chili								*			*	
Peppers, green				*	*			*				
Peppers, red				*				*			*	
Potato		*		*			*			*		*
Potato, sweet	*						*					*
Pork	*	*		*				*		*		*
Rice	*					*		*	*		*	*
Sauce, tomato								*				*
Sauerkraut				*								
Sausage, highly seasoned								*		*		
Shellfish	*	*				*						
Shrimp		*		*		*						
Soup, vegetable		*			*		*					
Soup, chicken							*					
Spices		*						*			*	
Tomatoes								*				*
Vegetables	*	*				*	*		*	*	*	
Wines		*			*						*	
Yoghurt			*									

to skip breakfast. Adults often take too many "coffee breaks." Individuals seek relief from boredom and tension and anxiety in overeating.

Consider your (or your family's) food habits and complete the following:

1. Where do you obtain most of your food?

   DINNER

   Do you grow any of your food supplies?

   NO

   Do you usually buy supplies for one day, one week, or for a longer period?

   2 WEEKS

2. What national characteristics most closely describe the foods you choose and prepare? (e.g., Italian, English, German)

FRANCE

Is this characteristic of your community?

NO

3. Describe a typical mealtime in your home:

table is set for whole family. Dishes of food are set ~~for~~ on table. I usually place food on childrens plate & sometimes for my husband too.

4. Do others in your community follow this same mealtime pattern?

Yes

5. How does your religion affect your food habits?

my Religion doesn't but a prayer is said before meals.

6. What personal food habit do you think is your best?

Practice of not eating pork.

Why is this a good habit?

Pork can contribute to certain illnesses like high blood pressure.

7. Name several habits that may be detrimental to your health.

Skipping meals, over eating, too many coffee breaks,

8. How can you improve your habits?

Eat a piece of fruit for breakfast, take vitamins as a supplement.

9. At what age did you acquire your undesirable food habits?

I can't pinpoint exact date or age when parents started feeding me pork but I imagine around one.

It is important for parents to remember that habits acquired in childhood last a lifetime. The two crucial periods in establishing nutritional habits are (1) infancy and early childhood and (2) adolescence, when the individual begins to make decisions. The adolescent period need not be dangerous if training and discipline during the childhood period were adequate.

FOOD FADS. Food fads are customs followed for a time with exaggerated zeal. A food fad may be based upon a food fact or upon a food fallacy. For example, milk is an excellent food. However, if a faddist drank milk to the exclusion of all other foods, the diet would lack necessary bulk, iron, and vitamin C. There would be danger of malnutrition from an unbalanced diet.

Among the many food fallacies, one of the most common is that food grown with chemical fertilizers is not as nutritious as food grown in soil enriched "naturally." Science has shown that chemical fertilizers are safe and effective.

VEGETARIAN DIETS. For religious, health, or economic reasons, some people choose a **vegetarian diet**, which is composed of plant foods only. This can be an adequate diet for a normal adult if the foods chosen are carefully selected. Vegetables high in protein, such as soy beans, should be included. There is a tendency for persons on a vegetarian diet, especially pregnant women, to develop deficiencies of vitamin B_{12}, calcium, and iron. If milk and eggs are a part of the diet (lacto-ovovegetarian), it becomes a highly nutritious diet.

FOOD SUPERSTITIONS. There are also many food superstitions (irrational beliefs with no scientific basis), such as the idea that eating strawberries during pregnancy causes the baby to have a birthmark or that eating fish and milk together causes illness.

Food misinformation exists because:

1. During childhood, people accept their parents' beliefs and it is difficult to change these beliefs in later years.
2. Too few people understand the effects of various nutrients upon the body and how the body uses these nutrients.
3. Everyone wants the approval of their social peers and is influenced by the current beliefs of their peer group.
4. Unscrupulous advertisers use the ignorance of the public and the technique of fear to sell their products. Sometimes they distort the truth.
5. Many sick people reach out in desperation for anything that offers hope of a cure.

Supply answers to the following questions:

1. What is the danger in following a food fad?

AN UNBALANCED DIET.

2. Can you name some food fads being followed in your own community?

ALOT OF SANDWICH EATING WHICH LEAVES OUT NEEDED VEGETABLES IN A MEAL.

3. Why do food fads and fallacies exist?

MISINFORMATION

4. Under what condition is it possible to eat a strictly vegetarian diet and be adequately nourished?

EATING VEGETABLES HIGH IN POTEIN SUCH AS SOY BEANS.

A lacto-ovovegetarian diet also includes milk and eggs, providing a highly nutritious diet.

5. What are some of the food superstitions you have heard?

EATING A ORANGE WILL COUNTERACT THE DETRIMENTAL EFFECTS ABOUT CIGGERETS.

6. With your local newspaper or television and radio programs as your source, make a list of nutrition "untruths" or "half-truths" being used in advertising.

Why is this type of advertising dangerous and deplored by responsible advertisers and nutritionists?

OPTIONAL ACTIVITIES TO ENHANCE LEARNING

ACTIVITY 1

Divide the class into small groups and assign each group to a geographic area within the community in such a way that all social strata are represented. Have each group interview four families in the assigned area. Topics to cover in the interview should include:

1. Where and how food is obtained, including who does the shopping.
2. Who prepares the food and when it is prepared.
3. Number and types of meals per day.
4. Types of food containers used.
5. Description of mealtime behavior and religious observances.
6. Special diets required by family members.
7. Beliefs about food (food fads and superstitions).

Have each group prepare a report to be given during discussion in class.

ACTIVITY 2

Plan a luncheon, asking each class member to bring a food typical of the ethnic background of their families. At the luncheon, have everyone take a taste of each dish. Afterward, have class members discuss how they feel about different foods, and the similarities and differences that were noted.

BIBLIOGRAPHY

BALLENTINE, R: *Diet and Nutrition: A Holistic Approach.* The Himalayan International Institute, Honesdale, Pennsylvania, 1978. Chapter 1, *Eating patterns—Ancient and modern.*

BRIGGS, GM AND CALLOWAY, DH: *Bogert's Nutrition and Physical Fitness,* ed 10. WB Saunders, Philadelphia, 1979. Chapter 16, *Food habits and beliefs.*

BUCHAN, JW: *America's health: Fallacies, beliefs, practices.* FDA Consumer Memo, October, 1972.

CALIENDO, MA: *Nutrition and Preventative Health Care.* Macmillan, New York, 1981. Chapter 1, *Introduction—Nutrition and health promotion.* Chapter 4, *Dietary and nutritional status of the general United States population.* Chapter 12, *Nutritional education in perspective—Influences on North American eating habits.*

CHOATE, RB AND ENGLE, PC: *Edible TV: Your child and food commercials.* US Government Printing Office, Washington, DC, September, 1977.

DWYER, J: *Vegetarianism.* Contemporary Nutrition 4(6), June, 1979.

HODGES, RE: *Nutrition in Medical Practice.* WB Saunders, Philadelphia, 1980. Chapter 1, *Evaluation of the nutritional status of patients.* Chapter 13, *Food fads and "megavitamins."*

HOFMAN, L: *The Great American Nutrition Hassle.* Mayfield, Palo Alto, California, 1978. Chapter 1, *The psychology and physiology of eating.* Chapter 5, *How nutritious are fast food meals?*

KRAUSE, MV AND MAHAN, LK: *Food, Nutrition and Diet Therapy,* ed 6. WB Saunders, Philadelphia, 1979. Chapter 1, *Introduction—Nutrition in the health of individuals and populations.* Chapter 17, *Geographical and cultural dietary variations.*

LOWENBERG, ME ET AL: *Food and People,* ed 3. John Wiley & Sons, New York, 1979. Chapter 2, *Food patterns—Origins and development.* Chapter 3, *Food patterns—Origins and development from medieval times through 19th century.* Chapter 4, *Food patterns and foodways.* Chapter 6, *Food, people and religion.*

MAYER, J: *10 nutritional myths.* Family Health, vol 11, May, 1979.

ROBINSON, CH: *Basic Nutrition and Diet Therapy,* ed 4. Macmillan, New York, 1980. Chapter 1, *Food, nutrition, and health.* Chapter 15, *Food acceptance, cultural food patterns, and food habits.*

SUITOR, CW AND HUNTER, MF: *Nutrition: Principles and Application in Health Promotion.* JB Lippincott, Philadelphia, 1980. Chapter 1, *Overview of nutrition and nutritional concerns.* Chapter 3, *Meeting nutrient needs by means of vegetarian diets.* Chapter 6, *Promoting sound eating habits in different sociocultural situations.*

WHITE, PL: *Food faddism.* Contemporary Nutrition 4(2), February, 1979.

WILLIAMS, SR: *Mowry's Basic Nutrition and Diet Therapy,* ed 6. CV Mosby, St Louis, 1980. Chapter 13, *Food habits and national food patterns.*

WORTHINGTON-ROBERTS, BS: *Contemporary Developments in Nutrition.* CV Mosby, St Louis, 1981. Chapter 15, *Vegetarianism as a way of life.*

2

THE DAILY DIET

OBJECTIVES

Upon completion of this chapter the student should be able to:

- Define the term "food" and give the functions of food in the body.
- Name the four food groups that provide essential nutrients for the daily diet, list the foods included in each group, and give the number of servings recommended per day for a normal adult.
- Apply the four food groups to an eating pattern selected by the student.

Food includes all the substances, both solid and liquid, taken into the body through the digestive tract for use in growth, maintenance, and repair of the body (Fig. 1). The functions of food are:

1. To give energy and heat,
2. To act as building material in growth and repair, and
3. To regulate the life processes.

The daily diet is said to be adequate when it supplies enough of the essential nutrients to perform the functions of food. An adequate diet furnishes the proper amount of each of the six classes of nutrients—fats, proteins, carbohydrates, minerals, vitamins, and water.

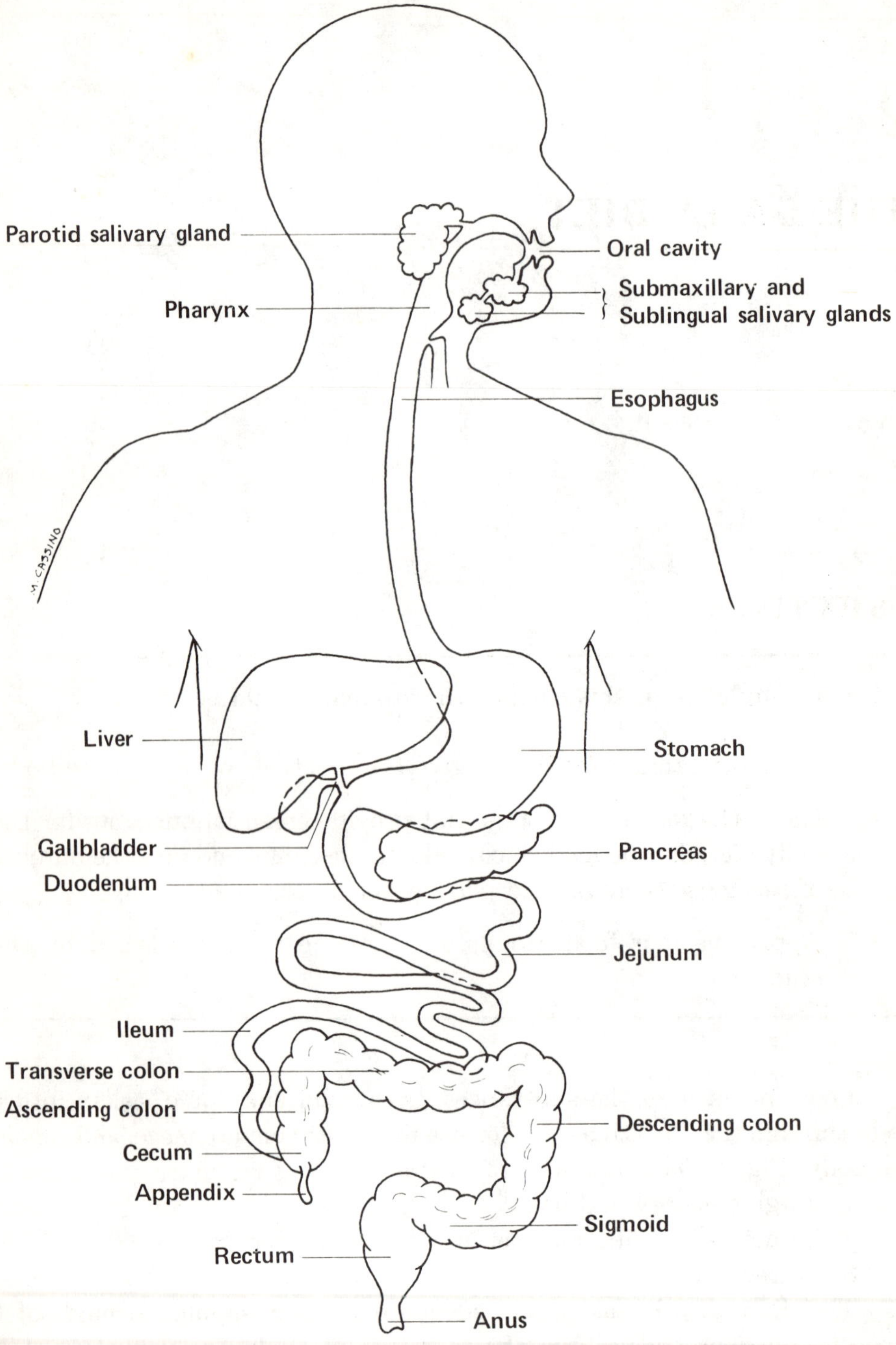

FIGURE 1. Digestive tract.

Proteins are obtained from meat, fish, eggs, milk and milk products, and certain vegetables, such as legumes and grains. Carbohydrates are abundant in grains, fruits, and vegetables. Fats come from butter, oils, and creams. Other foods with some fat content are meats, eggs, nuts, and avocados. Minerals and vitamins are found in almost all foods with some foods being richer than others in certain minerals or vitamins. Cellulose is found in the skin, peelings, and pulp of many fruits and vegetables. Many fruits and vegetables have a high water content, but the most common source of water is water itself.

ESSENTIAL NUTRIENTS

To provide the essential nutrients, the daily diet should include:

Milk	1 pint or more for the normal adult. 1 quart (3 to 4 cups, depending upon age) for a child. 1 quart for a teenager.
Meat, poultry, fish, eggs	Two or more servings. (Bacon is classified as a fat. Eggs should be eaten at least three times a week.)
Vegetables and fruits	Four or more servings. One serving of citrus fruit or vegetable high in vitamin C, and one serving of dark green or deep yellow vegetable.
Bread and cereals	Four or more servings of whole grain, enriched, or restored bread or cereal.

These dietary allowances are based upon the Basic Four Food Groups recommended by the Institute of Home Economics, United States Department of Agriculture (Fig. 2). Nutrition science is now in a growth phase. The USDA now recognizes a fifth food group, fats-sweets-alcohol. This fifth group provides mainly calories and little in the way of nutrients.

In addition to the Basic Four Food Groups, certain foods should be included in the daily diet. A minimum of four teaspoons of butter (or fortified margarine) daily is recommended. As butter is used in the preparation of various foods, a separate group was not felt to be necessary. Water is also an essential nutrient, and six or more glasses should be taken each day. In addition to the essential daily foods, one or more times per week the individual should have dried beans, liver, and saltwater fish.

Molasses, syrup, honey, jellies, jams, sugar, and candy only provide energy, and they should not be included in the daily diet until the essential nutrient-carrying foods have been chosen.

Answer the following questions in the space provided.

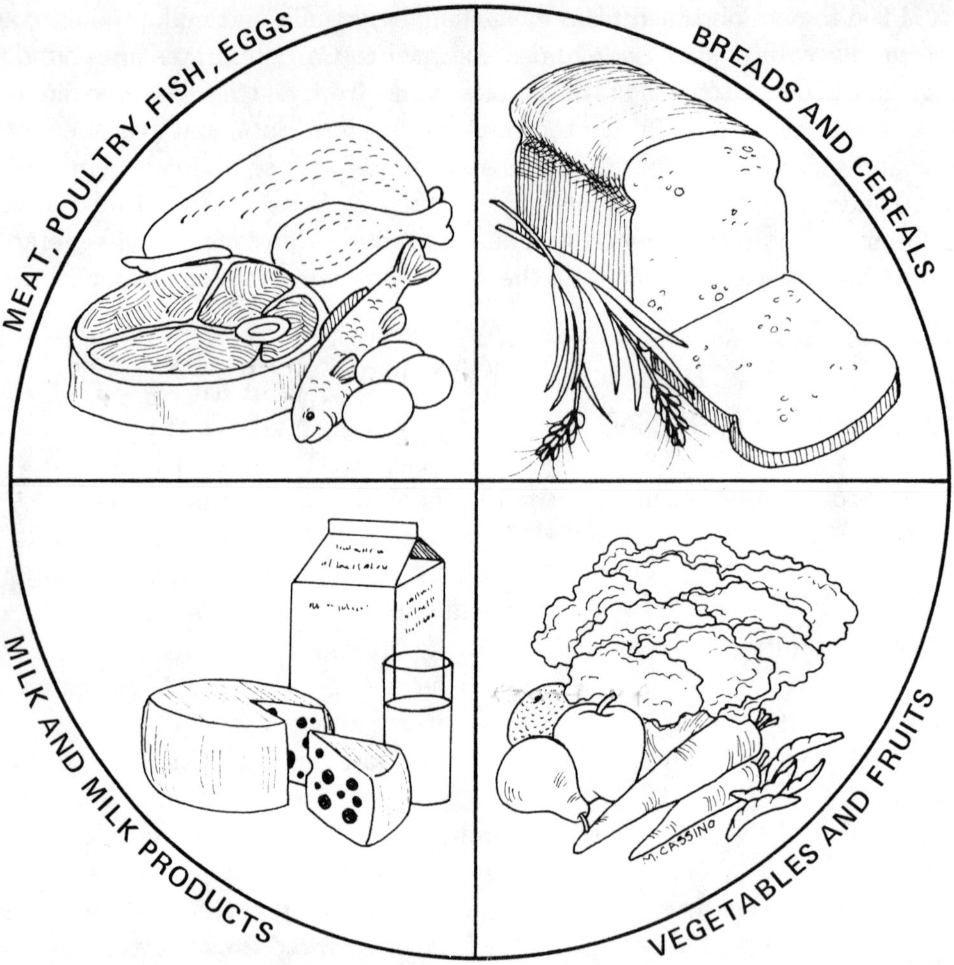

FIGURE 2. Basic four food groups—essential for good nutrition. Nutrition science is now in a growth phase. The USDA now recognizes a fifth food group, fats-sweets-alcohol. This fifth group provides mainly calories and little in the way of nutrients.

1. What are the functions of food in the body?

   TO GIVE HEAT & ENERGY
   to ACT AS building MATERIAL IN growth & REPAIR
   to REGULATE the LIFE PROCESS

2. Name the groups of food essential for an adequate daily diet and give the recommended daily amount.

   MILK = ATLEAST 1PINT FOR NORMAL ADULT, 1 QUART FOR TEEN AGER
   (3 to 4 cups depending on AGE OF child)
   MEAT, POUTRY, FISH & EGGS = 2 OR MORE SERVINGS
   VEGETABLES & FRUITS = 4 OR MORE SERVINGS
   BREADS & CEREALS = 4 OR MORE SERVINGS.

3. What is the minimum number of eggs recommended per week? If an individual does not like the taste of egg, can you name some ways to include eggs in the diet so that the individual is unaware of taking it?

Eggs should be eaten 3 times a week. You could give him his eggs through French toast, pancakes, foods that must be dipped in eggs before cooking.

4. What is the purpose of the daily diet?

to supply enough essential nutrients to perform the functions of food, to furnish the proper amounts of minerals, vitamins, water, protein, carbohydrates & fats.

5. How is water obtained in the daily diet?

through many fruits & vegetables with a high water content & through water itself.

6. Which food groups give us minerals and vitamins?

Almost all foods.

7. What essential nutrient is found in the milk, meat, and egg group?

Protein

8. From which food group is the major portion of dietary cellulose obtained?

Fruits & vegetables

9. If butter were omitted from the daily diet, would it be fat-free? Why?

Because meat, eggs, nuts & avacodo's have fat.

10. How often should liver be served?

2 or more times

11. How often should saltwater fish be served?

2 or more times

12. How much sugar and other sweets should be served daily?

Not necessary. No nutritional content.

13. Use the chart below to determine if you are taking an adequate diet. Keep a detailed list of the foods you eat or drink during a 24-hour period. If you carry a small card or paper in your pocket, you can record what you consume immediately and your record will be more accurate. List everything except water. Then classify the food as to group. Using the tables in the back of the text or in one of your dietary resource references, compute the number of calories consumed during the 24 hours.

DAILY INTAKE CHART

Time	*Food*	*Group*	*Amount Eaten*	*Calories in Serving*
Example:				
7:00	*Orange juice*	*Fruit-vegetable*	*1 cup*	*135*
6:30	Apple	Fruit-vegetable	whole	70
12:00	Balogna ~~Sandwich Bread & meat~~	Meats	1 slice	150
	Bread	Breads	2 slices	150
5:00	Fishsticks	Meats/Fish	4	210
				70
	corn on cob	Veg.	1	70
	Butter	Fats	1 tea	
	String beans	Veg	1 cup	28

~~688~~ 758

14. How many servings of leafy green or yellow vegetables did you eat? ________ Citrus fruits? ________ Other fruits or vegetables? __3__

15. How much milk did you drink? __None__ Did you use milk in your diet other than as a drink? No

16. Did you eat an egg? __No__ If not, have you eaten three this week? No

17. How much butter or fortified margarine did you have?
1 teaspoon

18. How many servings of meat, poultry, or fish did you have?

2 servings

19. Study your answers. Was your diet adequate?

NO

20. What was your diet deficient in?

Eggs, leafy vegetables, milk

21. What foods could you add to your diet to make it adequate?

~~Salad, B~~ Salad w/ Boiled eggs
milk

22. Foods such as candy and soda do not contribute any of the essential nutrients. The calories they contain are sometimes called "empty calories." How many "empty calories" did you have for the 24-hour period?

None

PLANNING THE DAILY DIET

Food is the most expensive item in the budget of many families. The amount of money a family needs depends upon the number of family members, their ages, the activities of individuals in the family, and any special dietary problems.

Many factors must be considered when planning the daily diet:

1. The diet must be planned around available foods. For example, fresh green vegetables are more abundant in the spring than in the fall and winter. The Asian diet includes more rice than potatoes because it is easier to grow there.
2. The amount of money budgeted for food must be considered. Lobster and tuna are equally good saltwater proteins. But lobster is too expensive to serve often or to large groups.
3. The ages of the family members determine what foods are purchased. When there are many children in the family, a larger proportion of the food budget will be needed for milk. If the family includes adult men, hearty meals must be planned.
4. The taste preferences of the family members must be considered—not only as to types of food but also as to method of preparation.

5. The facilities for storing and preparing food must be kept in mind. To prepare custard dishes without having adequate refrigeration space is to invite gastrointestinal upsets.
6. Cooking skills must be considered. The simplest dishes are often the most difficult to cook well. Few women will attempt crepe suzettes (French pancakes with a flaming sauce), although they may be very skilled in making the American flapjack.

EATING PATTERNS

The body's energy output must be matched by intake. Dividing the day's requirement into three portions, or meals, prevents complete depletion without necessitating constant eating throughout the day. (Less energy is needed during sleep.)

Certain persons, such as small children and the aged, may require five or more meals a day. The energy output of small children is great due to their rapid growth and the elderly often eat small amounts at mealtimes. These groups may need to replenish their energy at frequent intervals.

Breakfast literally means "to break the fast." Because the body has been without food for eight or more hours, it needs nourishment; however, the first meal of the day is usually the most neglected. Starting the day without breakfast is like starting an automobile trip with only part of a tank of gasoline. The automobile will go only a short way; a human body begins to rebel before noon. Without an adequate breakfast, fatigue sets in earlier, irritability is increased, work output is reduced, and reaction time is slowed.

The noon meal may be called "lunch" or "dinner," the evening meal "supper" or "dinner." Dinner is the heaviest meal of the day, regardless of the time it is eaten. The time an individual habitually has dinner depends upon the individual's social environment, the amount of time allotted to the noon meal, and the availability of food at midday.

Although there are a number of menu patterns, the following suggested pattern provides the minimum amount of all essential nutrients:

Breakfast:

- One serving from the fruit and vegetable group.
- One serving from the cereal and bread group.
- One serving from the milk group.

Lunch or supper:

- One serving from the meat, poultry, fish, and egg group.
- One serving from the fruit and vegetable group.
- One serving from the milk and milk products group.
- One serving from the bread and cereal group.

Dinner includes:

One serving from the meat, poultry, fish, and egg group.

Two servings from the fruit and vegetable group.

Two servings from the cereal and bread group.

Each day one of the servings from the fruit and vegetable group should be a citrus fruit (or another fruit or vegetable high in vitamin C) and one serving should be a dark green or deep yellow vegetable. Milk can be added to each meal to provide the amount needed by children.

The meal pattern can be changed to suit individual preference. For example, citrus fruit might be served at lunch instead of breakfast. Or fruit may be served as dessert for dinner. Or one of the servings of meat could be eaten at breakfast rather than lunch or dinner. However, an effort should be made to include all of the groups furnishing the essential nutrients at some time during the day. Many nutrients are not stored by the body and must be taken daily.

If the three-meals-a-day pattern does not suit an individual's needs, the essential nutrient groups must still be considered. During periods of great energy output, such as when a child is growing rapidly, a snack between meals may be necessary. Snack foods should contain the essential nutrients. A candy bar is less desirable than an orange or a glass of milk and a peanut butter sandwich. Snacks should not interfere with regular mealtimes but should supply quick energy to combat midmorning or midafternoon fatigue.

Complete the following:

1. When a family budgets money for food, what four factors must be considered?

   Number of family members, thier age, activities of individuals in family & special dietary problems.

2. When a daily menu is being planned, the six factors to be remembered are: (1) plan about available food (2) Amount of money available (3) Ages of family members (4) taste preference of family members (5) facilities for storing & preparing. (6) cooking skills

3. Plan a midmorning snack for yourself.

   Orange

   Is this your usual snack?

   ~~I u~~ NO

What factors influenced your choice of snack foods?

Where I am & how hungry I am.

4. Plan a midafternoon snack for yourself.

~~PB~~ Peanut Butter & Jelly Sandwich

OPTIONAL ACTIVITIES TO ENHANCE LEARNING

ACTIVITY 1

Prepare a visual aid (e.g., poster, model) to teach the planning of the daily diet using the Basic Four Food Groups. Identify the person you are teaching and prepare the visual aid so that it is appropriate for that person.

ACTIVITY 2

Conduct a survey of the students using the school cafeteria to find out their breakfast habits. Ask the following questions:

(Check whether the person being interviewed is male ____ or female ____.

Do you eat breakfast every day?

Do you eat breakfast *before* coming to school?

If you do not eat breakfast or do not eat before coming to school, is it because you are not hungry ____, on a diet ____, do not have time ____, or for another reason ____ (specify ____________________).

If you eat breakfast, what do you *usually* have?

After the survey, discuss the implications of the findings in class. Who had the poorest breakfast habits? Were the foods eaten for breakfast nutritional? What were the most usual reasons for not eating breakfast? What influence on grades do breakfast habits have? What other problems did the survey indicate?

ACTIVITY 3

Conduct a survey of 100 persons (not students). Prepare a set of questions based on the Basic Four Food Groups that will indicate how much these people know about a balanced diet. Use the survey report for a discussion in class on the need to teach nutrition to the general public. Indicate ways the nurse can help.

BIBLIOGRAPHY

BELOIAN, A AND SCHRAYER, D: *What consumers know about nutrition.* FDA Consumer Memo, July/August, 1974.

BRIGGS, GM AND CALLOWAY, DH: *Bogert's Nutrition and Physical Fitness,* ed 10. WB Saunders, Philadelphia, 1979. Chapter 19, *Adequate diets for healthy people.*

HALPERN, SL ET AL: *Quick Reference to Clinical Nutrition: A Guide for Physicians.* JB Lippincott, Philadelphia, 1979. Chapter 2, *Nutritional advice to the healthy patient.*

HARPER, AE: *Uses and misuses of recommended dietary allowances.* Contemporary Nutrition, 3(7), July, 1978.

HOFMANN, L: *The Great American Nutrition Hassle.* Mayfield, Palo Alto, California, 1978. Chapter 2, *The requirements of human nutrition.*

KRAUSE, MV AND MAHAN, LK: *Food, Nutrition and Diet Therapy,* ed 6. WB Saunders, Philadelphia, 1979. Chapter 10, *Recommended dietary allowances and the adequate diet.*

NUTRITION DEPARTMENT: *A Status Report on the American Diet and Health—1980.* General Mills, Minneapolis, 1980.

ROBINSON, CH: *Basic Nutrition and Diet Therapy,* ed 4. Macmillan, New York, 1980. Chapter 4, *Guide for nutritional planning.* Chapter 13, *Meal planning for adults.*

SUITOR, CW AND HUNTER, MF: *Nutrition: Principles and Application in Health Promotion.* JB Lippincott, Philadelphia, 1980. Chapter 2, *Meeting nutrient needs by following a "daily food guide."* Chapter 11, *Menu planning and the purchase of food.*

WATT, BK: *Tables of food composition: Uses and limitations.* Contemporary Nutrition 5(2), February, 1980.

WILLIAMS, SR: *Mowry's Basic Nutrition and Diet Therapy,* ed 6. CV Mosby, St Louis, 1980. Chapter 1, *The importance of a balanced diet.* Chapter 10, *Planning menus for the whole family.*

3

FOOD ECONOMICS AND PUBLIC HEALTH

OBJECTIVES

Upon completion of this chapter the student should be able to:

- Discuss ways to stretch the food dollar, applying this to the student's own situation.
- Plan a shopping list, within a stated food budget, that provides an adequate diet for four normal adults for one week.
- Read labels on foods and select those that have the most value for the cost.
- Read labels on foods and compare the nutritive value of several foods, selecting the one that has the most nutritive value.
- Describe what happens to foods that have been adulterated, mislabeled, dehydrated, enriched, or fortified.
- Discuss food additives, giving at least 10 examples and their functions, and some of the problems additives can cause.
- Given the age and situation of an individual, to select a nutrition program where an individual can receive assistance.
- Give the mode of entry into the body, the symptoms produced, and the prevention for: ptomaine poisoning, bacterial poisoning, staphylococcal poisoning, botulism, ameba, trichinosis, tapeworm, tularemia, tuberculosis, and typhoid fever.

There are many ways to make the food dollar purchase more. The wise homemaker constantly studies the market and frequently re-evaluates the family's needs. The following suggestions have proved helpful to many homemakers.

1. Plan menus for a week at a time. By planning ahead one food item may be used for several dishes and leftovers incorporated into other meals.
2. Make a list of foods needed after the menus for the week have been planned. Shopping with a list helps eliminate impulse buying of expensive or unneeded items.
3. Watch newspaper advertisements for "specials." Compare the various stores to be sure that an advertised bargain is really a bargain. Check the usual price also.
4. Buy in quantity if storage is no problem. Price per unit is lower when more units are bought.
5. Read labels carefully and do comparison buying. Purchase two cans or packages containing the same amount by volume or weight but prepared by different companies. Compare the two items to determine which has the most pulp or meat of the fruit or vegetable and which includes the most liquid or waste material. Often a large package contains no more edible food than a smaller package.
6. Try to pay cash for food. The store that grants credit must add the cost of keeping charge accounts to the price of its groceries.
7. Buy foods in season. This saves money and provides a refreshing change.
8. Remember that whole or half pieces of fruits and vegetables take up more room in a can than sliced, cubed, diced, or mashed. A can of the smaller pieces provides more servings.
9. Store foods properly and plan for their use while they are still nutritious and flavorsome.
10. Cook only the amount needed. Most cans and packages specify the number of average servings they contain.
11. If there is sufficient freezer or refrigerator space, prepare foods such as meats in quantity to save on fuel. They need only be heated for a subsequent meal.
12. Learn to prepare a wide variety of dishes utilizing the cheaper cuts of meat, meat substitutes, and powdered milk.
13. Watch for sales of dairy products, day-old bread, and farm produce. In some areas, farmers sell vegetables and fruits in the field at a fraction of the grocery store's price. This is a bargain if the homemaker knows how to can or freeze foods. Many bakeries have retail outlets for day-old bread, cakes, and cookies and most dairies will sell quarts of milk several cents cheaper if the purchaser comes to the dairy.

14. Use all edible parts of food purchased. When buying fresh beets, for example, pick those with crisp green tops as well as properly filled out bottoms. The tops make a good addition to salads or can be served like spinach.
15. Select cooking methods that require the least energy output. If baking, plan to prepare several dishes in the oven. As fuel costs have risen sharply in recent years, more people have turned to alternatives to the conventional stove. Some prepare "sun tea." Many utilize microwave ovens to save time and money. Vegetables are cooked in a minimum of water in the microwave, which also saves vitamins, and it is an excellent method of reheating leftovers.

The use of already prepared foods must be considered carefully. Certain fresh foods that must be pared or cored prior to cooking lose a large portion of the purchase weight. During seasonal shortages, the prepared food may cost less than the fresh product. A homemaker considering a cake or bread mix should estimate the cost of a homemade cake or loaf of bread before deciding to use the mix.

In recent years, frozen TV dinners have become popular. Easy to store and prepare, they offer the homemaker a wide variety of foods. However, investigators have expressed concern that food processing methods leave the vitamin content of the finished product in question. Many of the low-priced dinners are composed predominately of carbohydrate foods. The homemaker should consider the Basic Four Food Groups when choosing TV dinners, making sure the family receives a balanced diet.

The homemaker who has a garden or access to a wholesale market can save by canning or freezing fruits and vegetables during the growing season. With today's large freezers a wider variety of meats can be had by purchasing in quantity. Meat (beef, pork, mutton) can be obtained by half or whole carcass. These purchases should be for cash as the interest rate on the installment plan eliminates any saving.

Answer the following questions:

1. Almost everyone has found ways to save money on food. What are some of the ways you have found or observed? List them below for class discussion later.

Food co-op

Buying larger quantities with family members & splitting

Check your pantry, local newspaper, or grocer's shelves for the answers to the following questions:

2. How many servings in a #303 (1 pound) can of sliced carrots? ________ How much does the can cost? ________ How many serv-

ings are in a package of frozen carrots? ________ How much does one package cost? ________ How many bunches of carrots would you have to purchase to get an equal number of servings? ________ What is the cost? ________

3. How many servings in a #303 (1 pound) can of sliced peaches? ________ How much does the can cost? ________ How many servings in a package of frozen peaches? ________ How much does one package cost? ________ How many pounds of fresh peaches would provide an equal number of servings? ________ What would be the cost? ________

4. How much does a pound of butter cost? ________ A pound of fortified margarine? ________

5. If an adult woman should have approximately 3 pounds of potatoes per week, or one serving per day, what is the cost if fresh potatoes are used? ________ Instant potatoes? ________ Frozen potatoes? ________

6. How much does one gallon of homogenized milk cost? ________ How much does one gallon of homogenized milk cost if purchased by the quart? ________ In pint bottles? ________ What does a package of dried skim milk, which makes two gallons of milk, cost? ________

7. What is the price of one dozen large grade A eggs? __109¢__ Medium size grade B eggs? __89¢__ Is there a difference in price for white shelled and brown shelled eggs? __NO__ (Brown and white eggs do not differ in nutritive value.)

8. Which is cheaper, aged beef or veal? ________ Fryers or hen?________

9. How much does a one-pound loaf of bread cost? ________ A one and one-half pound loaf of bread? ________

10. How much does round steak cost per pound? ________ Sirloin steak? ________ Which has the most lean meat per pound? ____________

11. How much does a 5-pound bag of enriched flour cost per pound? ________ How much does a 25-pound bag of enriched flour cost per pound? ________

12. TV dinners save time. What will four of your favorite TV dinners cost? ________ What would it cost to prepare the same foods for four persons in the usual way? ________

Condiments, pickles, sauces, relishes, and snack foods such as potato chips add variety and flavor to a meal, but add greatly to the cost if not well chosen. A few basic spices, oils, and vinegars can be made into tasty dressings. Sour and dill pickles are less expensive than sweet pickles. Canapés and dips made from simple ingredients are less expensive than prepared ones.

LABELS

In 1966, the Fair Packaging and Labeling Act was passed, which made labeling mandatory. The Act has been updated several times and now includes the following regulations.

1. Foods with two or more ingredients must have all ingredients listed. The ingredient that is in the greatest amount in the food must be listed first.
2. The percentage of the characterizing ingredient must be given. For example, a fruit drink must state what percentage of the drink is real fruit juice.
3. All foods must have open date coding. This shows the date a food must be pulled from the shelf and not be offered as food acceptable to humans.
4. Dietary claims on labels or in advertisements must be substantiated.
5. It must state on the label what must be added to complete the preparation of the dish. For example, a cake mix that requires the addition of milk and eggs must state so on the label.
6. Nutritional quality guidelines for frozen dinners, cereals, and other pre-prepared foods were established and labels must give the percentage of nutrients.

7. The source of fats and oils must be given.
8. All nutrients and other substances added to a food must be listed.
9. US Recommended Daily Allowances (RDA) were established and nutrients in foods must be listed as a percentage of RDA.
10. The number of servings in the container must be shown in some familiar household measure. The serving should be of a size suitable for an adult man doing light physical activity.
11. There is a standard format for giving nutrient content on a label.

Label Format

Labels will read "Nutrition Information per Serving" and must be located to the right of the primary display panel on the package. If the package is too small for the amount of information given, it can be put on an insert or attachment, or the information can be displayed next to the item at the store.

If the food is combined with other foods when used (cereal with milk, rice with meat) there must be two columns. One must show the nutritive value before the addition; the other must show the nutritive value of the combined foods.

The amount of protein in a serving must be given in amount by weight (grams) and as a percentage of the RDA. Carbohydrates and fats are given by weight. Whether or not fats are designated as saturated or unsaturated is optional. Minerals and vitamins are expressed as percentages of RDA. It is required that the label list the minerals calcium and iron and the vitamins A, C, D, thiamin, niacin, and riboflavin.

Cholesterol and sodium are optional listings and are given in milligrams per serving. Because there has been so much concern over cholesterol and sodium in the diet in recent years, many companies have voluntarily added them to the label. The American diet is especially heavy in sodium and some legislators are attempting to make the listing of sodium compulsory.

A part of the label today is the Universal Product Code which is the thirty-one parallel lines used on an electronic scanner. The first five numbers at the bottom of the Code indicate the company that makes the product; the last five numbers give information, such as size and weight and about the product itself.

In addition to regulating labels, the government requires grocers to put prices on the shelf facing, usually below the item. It is also necessary to put the price on each item.

Complete the following:

1. List 11 labeling regulations:

A. Foods with 2 or more ingredients must have all ingredients listed, the larger amount is listed first,

B. the percentage of the characterizing ingredient must be given.

C. All Food must be date coded.

D. Dietary claims on labels or advertisment must be substantiated.

E. must be stated what must be added to complete the preparation of the dish

F. Labels must give the percentage of nutrients

G. Source of fats & oils must be given.

H. All nutrients & other substances added to food must be listed

I. nutrients in foods must be listed as a percentage of US Reccommended Daily Allowances.

J. NUMBER OF SERVINGS IN CONTAINER MUST BE SHOWN IN FAMILIAR HOUSEHOLD MEASUREMENT SUITABLE FOR AN ADULT MAN DOING LIGHT PHYSICAL WORK.

K. STANDARD FORMAT FOR GIVING NUTRIENT CONTENT ON A LABEL.

Fruit Drink #1

CONTAINS WATER, SUGAR AND CORN SWEETENERS, CONCENTRATED ORANGE JUICE, CONCENTRATED PINEAPPLE JUICE, NATURAL FLAVORS, CITRIC AND MALIC ACIDS (PROVIDE TARTNESS), VITAMIN C, ARTIFICIAL COLORS, ETHYL MALTOL.
Contains 10% fruit juices

Serving size	6 Fl. Oz.
Servings per container	7 2/3
Calories	90
Protein	0 Gms.
Carbohydrate	23 Gms.
Fat	0 Gms.
Percentage RDA:	
Vitamin C	100%

Less than 2% of RDA for protein, Vitamin A, thiamin, riboflavin, niacin, calcium, and iron.

Fruit Drink #2

CONTAINS PINEAPPLE JUICE AND VITAMIN C

Serving size	(6 Fl. Oz.)	3/4 cup
Servings per container		1
Calories		100
Protein		0 Gms.
Carbohydrates		25 Gms.
Fats		0 Gms.
Percentage U.S. RDA:		
Protein		*
Vitamin A		*
Vitamin C		100%
Thiamin		6%
Riboflavin		2%
Niacin		2%
Calcium		2%
Iron		2%

*Contains less than 2% of RDA.

2. Which of the fruit drinks is the most nutritious? Why?

   #2 BECAUSE IT DOESN'T CONTAIN ARTIFICIAL ADDITIVES & GIVES THE SAME OR MORE RDA.

3. What ingredient does #1 have the most of?

   Additives

4. What ingredient does #2 have the most of?

   PINEAPPLE JUICE

5. If #1 costs 89¢ per container and #2 costs $1.45 for a pack of six, which one would supply the daily vitamin C most economically?

   #2

Evaporated Milk	
Serving size	1/2 cup
Servings per container	3 1/4
Calories	170
Protein	8 Gms.
Carbohydrates	12 Gms.
Fats	10 Gms.
Percentage U.S. RDA:	
Protein	20%
Vitamin A	4%
Vitamin C	*
Thiamin	2%
Riboflavin	20%
Niacin	*
Calcium	30%
Iron	*
Vitamin D	25%
Phosphorus	25%
*Contains less than 2% RDA.	
Sodium	60 mg.

Instant Nonfat Dry Milk	
Serving size	8 Oz.
Servings per container	80
Calories	80
Protein	8 Gms.
Carbohydrates	12 Gms.
Fats (Less than 1 Gm.)	
Percentage U.S. RDA:	
Protein	20%
Vitamin A	10%
Vitamin C	2%
Thiamin	6%
Riboflavin	25%
Niacin	*
Calcium	30%
Iron	*
Vitamin D	25%
Vitamin B_6	4%
Vitamin B_{12}	20%
Phosphorus	25%
Pantothenic Acid	8%
*Contains less than 2% of RDA.	

6. Which of the milks has the most calories?

INSTANT NONFAT DRY MILK

7. If you needed to restrict the amount of fat in your diet, which one would you choose?

EVAPORATED MILK

8. Which milk would you choose if you needed more protein?

INSTANT NON FAT DRY MILK

9. Which would you choose if you had to increase your calcium intake?

either

10. Which has the most vitamin A?

INSTANT NON FAT MILK

Instant Pudding

Serving size: 1/2 cup Servings per package: 4	Mix Before Preparation	Prepared Serving
Calories	100	180
Protein	0	4 Gms.
Carbohydrates	25 Gms.	31 Gms.
Fats	0	5 Gms.
Percentages of U.S. Recommended Daily Allowances (U.S. RDA)		
Protein	*	10%
Vitamin A	*	4%
Vitamin C	*	2%
Thiamin	*	2%
Riboflavin	*	10%
Niacin	*	*
Calcium	*	15%
Iron	*	*
Phosphorus	20%	30%

*Contains less than 2% of U.S. RDA

Ingredients: Sugar, dextrose (corn sugar), modified starches (tapioca and corn), sodium phosphates (for proper set), hydrogenated soybean oil with BHA (a preservative), di- and monoglycerides (emulsifier–for uniform dispersion of oil), nonfat dry milk, natural and artificial flavors, artificial color.

11. What ingredient is there the most of in this product before milk was added?

    ~~Carbo~~

12. What is the difference when milk is added?
    Calories? 80
    Protein? 4 gms.
    Carbohydrates? 6 gms.
    Fat? 5 gms.
    Vitamins? 6
    Minerals? 57

13. What would be the difference in nutritive value of this dessert if water were used to prepare the pudding?

    No Protein, Vit. A & C, Thiamin, Riboflavin, Niacin, Calcium, Iron, 10% less phosphorus, ~~less 5 gms. Fats, less 6 gms~~

Within a food budget of $100.00 a week, plan a week's menus for four adults. Prepare a shopping list for the week. (Be sure to include all essential food groups each day.)

	Mon.	Tues.	Wed.	Thurs.	Fri.	Sat.	Sun.
Breakfast:	~~Eggs Milk toast & butter Bacon~~ Grapefruit toast Butter milk	Orange juice oatmeal @ m toast Butter	G/J T @ melted cheese	Applesauce English muff. scrambled eggs			
Lunch:	tuna fish crackers milk apple	orange egg salad bread milk	club sand. banana	fish sticks coleslaw milk			
Dinner:	~~Fried chicken~~ Fish stringbeans cornbread sliced pineapples	Quiche t/s OJ	spinach BBQ chic. hot rolls ice cream	apple pie spa. @ meat garlic bread tossed salad			

SHOPPING LIST

Item	*Amount*	*Cost*
Eggs	1 Doz	
milk		
Bread		
Grapefruit		
Butter		
apple sauce		
english muffin		
Noodles		
Ground beef		
sliced pineapples		
		Total Cost ______

TERMS

The homemaker should know the following terms used in discussing foods:

ADULTERATED. A substance has been added, intentionally or unintentionally, to the food.

MISLABELED. The contents of the container are not as listed on the label.

DEHYDRATED. Water has been removed from the food.

ENRICHED. Minerals and vitamins have been added to the final product. This term is usually applied to cereal and grain products. Minerals and vitamins are added to the final products of the milling process, as both are lost when the grain is refined. More may be added than were in the original grain.

RESTORED. The minerals or vitamins lost in processing food are replaced so that the proportion of mineral or vitamin is the same as in the unprocessed food.

FORTIFIED. Minerals or vitamins not present in the food before processing have been added so that the end product is more nutritious than the original.

ADDITIVE. A chemical substance added to the food to preserve it or to make it more appealing. Nearly three thousand substances may be added to food to perform over three dozen functions. These include flavoring, coloring, preserving, texturizing, emulsifying (most common type of additive), extending shelf life, and protecting the nutritive value of foods. Many foods, especially the so-called convenience foods, could not be shipped and sold unless some preservative was used. Some foods, such as soybean "steak" would have no taste appeal without special flavoring. Ascorbic acid is added to fruits so that they do not turn brown when frozen. Of course, for centuries salt has been added to meats to preserve them.

Not all additives are essential and any can cause problems to persons with a hypersensitivity. MSG (monosodium glutamate) used to enhance flavor, especially in Chinese foods, not only adds excess sodium to the diet but can cause headache, nausea, and dizzyness (Chinese restaurant syndrome) in persons allergic to it. Preservatives, artificial flavors, and colors are thought to be a cause of hyperkinesis in children. Sodium nitrite, cyclomates and, possibly, saccharin are carcinogenic.

Everyone should read labels carefully, especially those persons with allergies or physical conditions requiring special diets.

Complete the following:

1. Look at the labels on the previous pages. Which of the foods had additives?

Instant Pudding
Fruit Drink

2. In your own words answer the question "Should additives be prohibited?"

Not if they arn't harmful to people

PUBLIC HEALTH

The World Food Conference in 1974 dealt with malnutrition and food supply as a world problem. Many countries lack the technology to develop available resources, but malnutrition can be present even in well-developed countries with a good food supply. Malnutrition can be the result of insufficient money to buy food, inability to obtain and prepare foods, incompetent agricultural methods, and, of primary importance, ignorance about foods and nutrition.

In 1977, The National Nutrition Consortium, composed of representatives of all the major professional societies in food, nutrition, and dietetics, urged the United States government to establish a National Nutrition Policy to assure food supply at a reasonable cost, to maintain a food supply for emergency and world needs, to develop public knowledge of nutrition, to maintain a system of quality and safety control, and to support food and nutrition research.

Also in 1977, the US Senate Select Committee on Nutrition and Human Needs prepared the following dietary goals for the people of the United States.

1. To avoid overweight.
2. To reduce consumption of refined sugar.
3. To increase intake of starches and natural sugars.
4. To reduce fat intake.
5. To reduce intake of saturated fats.
6. To reduce cholesterol intake.
7. To limit sodium intake.

All of the above goals can be incorporated into the dietary pattern of anyone without hardship or extra cost.

There are a number of Federal programs designed to help overcome malnutrition at this time. The nurse should know what resources are available.

1. National Nutrition Program for the Elderly—Provides inexpensive balanced meals at a central location.
2. Special Supplemental Program for Women, Infants, and Children—Provides nutrition education and supplemental food for pregnant women, infants, and children in low-income families.
3. Head Start Program—Provides meals that give 1/3 of the essential nutrients for a day to children attending Head Start Programs for part of the day and 2/3 for children attending a full day.

4. Child Nutrition Programs—include the following:
   Direct Food Assistance—Low-cost or free lunches.
   School Breakfast Program.
   Special Milk Program—Low-cost or free milk.
   Summer Feeding Program—Meals in recreation centers and camps.
   Child Care Food Program—Reimbursement for meals in preschool child care centers.
   Special Food Service Program—Reimbursement of school.
5. Food Stamps—For the low-income family to help with the cost of food.
6. Food Distribution Program—Distribution of food to schools and in emergency situations.

Complete the following:

1. What are some of the reasons for malnutrition?

   INSUFFICIENT MONEY TO BUY FOOD
   INABILITY TO OBTAIN & PREPARE FOOD
   IGNORANCE ABOUT FOOD & NUTRITION.

2. What do you think is the most common reason for malnutrition in the United States?

   IGNORANCE ABOUT FOOD & NUTRITION

3. Dietary goals suggested by the Select Committee on Nutrition and Human Needs include:

   1. TO AVOID OVERWEIGHT
   2. TO REDUCE CONSUMPTION OF REFINED SUGAR
   3. TO REDUCE FAT INTAKE
   4. TO INCREASE INTAKES OF STARCHS & NATURAL SUGARS
   5. TO REDUCE INTAKE OF SATURATED FAT

6. to REDUCE cholESTORAL INTAKE

7. to limit sodium INTAKE

4. What foods would you have to give up to meet these goals?
JUNK Foods, ~~SUGAR~~ SWEETS, Butter, cookin oil, Some Eggs

5. What foods would you have to add to your diet to meet these goals?
BREAD, CORN, RICE, FRUITS

6. Name nutrition resources (Federal programs) for:
Elderly: NATIONAL NUTRITIONAL PROGRAMS FOR THE ELDERLY

Woman who is pregnant: SPECIAL SUPPLEMENTARY PROGRAM FOR WOMAN, INFANTS & CHILDREN

Infant: ↙

Preschool child: HEAD START PROGRAM

School child: child NUTRITION PROGRAMS.

The United States government is vitally concerned with health and nutrition. Federal, state, and municipal laws free the consumer from worry about contamination, falsification, or adulteration of food. In addition, the Public Health Services try to help the consumer by teaching sanitation, basic nutrition, and food economics. Food samples are tested to see that the food offered for sale meets government standards. Processing plants, wholesale and retail outlets, and food preparation areas such as cafes must pass rigid inspections in order to do business. Food handlers must pass physical examinations to see that they are free of communicable disease.

However, much food related illness is caused by homemakers who ignore the principles of good hygiene in handling, preparing, and storing food. Knowing the causes of food illnesses and how they are transmitted helps conscientious homemakers prevent sickness in their families.

FOOD POISONING

Food poisoning is an illness caused by bacteria, chemicals, or foods that are poisonous in themselves. (For example, certain mushrooms are poisonous.)

PTOMAINE "POISONING." Ptomaine poisoning only occurs if obviously decayed food is consumed. Most illnesses called ptomaine poisoning are in actuality due to other causes.

BACTERIAL POISONING. Bacterial poisoning is usually caused by organisms belonging to either the genus Salmonella or the genus Shigella. They are spread through contaminated meats, milk, eggs, and vegetables. Symptoms of gastroenteritis caused by these organisms occur within one to three days after the individual has ingested the causative organism. Contamination is prevented by washing vegetables thoroughly under running water prior to preparation, and handling milk and meat under the most sanitary conditions. Chicken eggs should not be eaten raw as the porous egg shells can admit organisms.

ENTEROTOXIC POISONING

Enterotoxic poisoning is caused by the toxins produced by the bacteria rather than by the organism itself.

STAPHYLOCOCCAL POISONING. About 75 percent of all gastrointestinal upsets are due to food organisms belonging to the genus Staphylococcus. The food is usually contaminated during processing from a skin lesion or throat infection of the food handler. As the toxin produced by the staphylococci is destroyed only by prolonged heat, any dish that does not require high temperatures for a period of time makes an excellent "garden" for the growth of this organism. Milk, egg dishes, and salads are frequent offenders. The onset of gastroenteritis is usually within one to six hours after eating contaminated food.

BOTULISM. Botulism is a poisoning caused by the botulinus toxin. It can be fatal. Fruits and vegetables are contaminated with the bacillus as they grow. As the organism is a spore-former and grows well without oxygen, improperly canned foods of low acid content make excellent breeding grounds. For this reason, all home-canned vegetables should be boiled for 5 to 10 minutes as heat destroys the toxin. Because some authorities feel that as small a dose as $^{1}/_{100}$ mg of toxin can be fatal, this precaution should be observed. The symptoms of botulism may be mistaken for other conditions as the toxin affects the nervous system. In addition to severe abdominal cramps, nausea, vomiting, and diarrhea, the victim may complain of headache, distorted vision, and difficulty in swallowing. There may be some paralysis. In three to seven days, if the cause of the shock and collapse is not recognized and treated, death occurs.

PARASITES

Parasites are small animals that "live off" other organisms and cause diseases in the human body. Certain parasites cause disease only when ingested with food.

AMEBA. The presence of amebas initially causes dysentery. After the initial stage, the infecting organism can remain in the human intestinal system without causing apparent distress. As long as the ameba is present, the host can contaminate food during handling. Amebas can also be spread through contaminated water, improperly washed raw food, and partially cooked meats.

TRICHINELLA. In trichinosis, a small worm of the genus Trichinella works its way from the intestinal tract to the muscles of its host. There it proceeds to burrow, damaging the muscle. The most commonly contaminated food is pork. A simple preventive measure is to cook all pork thoroughly. Freezing pork at 0°F for 72 hours will also destroy the worm.

TAPEWORM. Flat segmented worms known as tapeworms are sometimes found in pork, beef, and fish. The worm attaches its head to the intestines of its host and there grows to great lengths. The symptoms resemble those of malnutrition and anemia, with distention of the abdomen. The feces of the infected individual contain segments of the worm, which have broken from the parent worm. Cooking of pork, beef, and fish prevents transmission of tapeworms.

OTHER INFECTIONS

Other infections that can be transmitted to man by food include:

TULAREMIA. Tularemia is transmitted by the bite of a tick commonly found on wild rabbits. Three days after the bite, an ulcer forms on the site of infection. The victim complains of headache, chilliness, fever, and swollen lymph glands. Because some authorities feel that the lymph or tissue serum of an infected animal is also capable of transmitting the disease, rabbits should never be handled with the bare hands.

TUBERCULOSIS. Drinking milk obtained from tuberculous cows can transmit tuberculosis. Prevention entails purchasing milk from dairies whose cows have been tested and certified free of the disease.

TYPHOID FEVER. This disease is transmitted through contaminated water or milk. The preventive measure is to purchase milk only from dairies inspected by the Public Health Department and found free of contamination. Water should come from wells that have been tested and found free of infectious organisms.

Complete the following:

1. Define the following terms:

   A. Adulterated: A substance that has been Added, intentionally or unintentionally to the Food

   B. Additive: A chemical substance added to the Food to preserve it or make it more appealing. (coloring, preserving, texturizing, emulsifying, extend shelf life, protect nutritional value of Food)

   C. Dehydration: WATER has been removed from Food

   D. Enriched: Minerals & vitamins have been added to final product more may be added then were orgginally there.

   E. Fortified: minerals or vitamins not present in the food before processing have been added so the end product is more nutricous than original.

2. Is the margarine at your grocery enriched or fortified?

3. Is flour at your grocery enriched or fortified?

ENRiched

4. Jane went to a lunch counter at noon and had a ham sandwich, a cream puff, and coffee. Within an hour, she developed abdominal cramps with nausea and vomiting. What organism most likely was the cause of her distress and which food was most likely contaminated?

5. Amanda is proud of her canned string beans. She plans to serve some for dinner as a chilled green bean salad. How should she prepare them for salad and why?

Should bE boiled FOR 5-10 minutes As heat destroys all toxins

6. Robert is going to the country to visit his grandparents' farm. As it is the time of year that they butcher pigs, Robert is looking forward to the fresh pork sausage Grandma makes. He also wants to hunt rabbits. What food health hazards might Robert encounter on his visit?

PARASITE INFECTION

OPTIONAL ACTIVITIES TO ENHANCE LEARNING

ACTIVITY 1

Obtain copies of all local newspapers and compare advertisements of food items that are "on special." Select three items advertised by most stores. Visit at least three stores and compare these items. For example, if ground beef has been advertised, does one store offer a better quality (e.g., fresher, less fat, no additives) than the others? Are the canned vegetables offered by the stores of equal value with the solid vegetables in greater quantity than the fluids in the cans? While doing the comparison shopping, an estimation should be made of the time and cost of transportation involved in getting to the store offering the most for the food dollar. Make a decision as to where it would be most economical to obtain the items. Give reasons for the decisions.

ACTIVITY 2

Consult the local public health unit and find out what food diseases are endemic to the local area. Ask about measures instituted to prevent the spread of these diseases.

ACTIVITY 3

Divide into small groups. Each group selects a food class such as cereals, canned and frozen vegetables, or citrus fruits. The small group then obtains nutrition labels from as many items within the food class as possible. The labels are arranged or copied on a visual aid so that comparisons can be easily made. After comparing the nutrition labels with the RDA chart, each group selects the most nutritious and the least nutritious items among the foods for which there are labels.

BIBLIOGRAPHY

A Summary Report on US Consumers' Knowledge, Attitudes and Practices About Nutrition. General Mills, Minneapolis, 1980.

ALSTON, E: *How to build your frozen assets.* Family Health, July, 1972.

BRIGGS, GM AND CALLOWAY, DH: *Bogert's Nutrition and Physical Fitness,* ed 10. WB Saunders, Philadelphia, 1979. Chapter 18, *Food: Nonnutrients, enrichment and labels.*

CHANEY, MS, ROSS, ML, AND WITSCHI, JC: *Nutrition*, ed 9. Houghton-Mifflin, Boston, 1979. Chapter 1, *Nutrition, food, and health.*

Facts About Food Poisoning. FDA Consumer Memo, April, 1974.

HOFMANN, L: *The Great American Nutrition Hassle.* Mayfield, Palo Alto, California, 1978. Chapter 7, *Food additives—Food for thought.*

HUTCHENS, C: *Subtracting additives.* Journal of Practical Nursing, Vol 28, July, 1979.

HUTT, PB AND SLOAN, AE: *Important public hearings on food labeling and nutrition.* Nutrition Policy Issues, July, 1978.

HUTT, PB AND SLOAN, AE: *Final FDA regulations governing label statements for foods represented as useful in reducing or maintaining caloric intake or body weight.* Nutrition Policy Issues, November, 1978.

HUTT, PB AND SLOAN, AE: *NAS issues saccharin report.* Nutrition Policy Issues, March, 1979.

HUTT, PB AND SLOAN, AE: *National Academy of Sciences issues food safety report.* Nutrition Policy Issues, April, 1979.

HUTT, PB AND SLOAN, AE: *Proposed new legislation on food labeling and nutrition.* Nutrition Policy Issues, November, 1979.

HUTT, PB AND SLOAN, AE: *FDA issues tentative positions on food labeling and nutrition issues.* Nutrition Policy Issues, February, 1980.

JANSSEN, WF: *America's first food and drug laws.* FDA Consumer Memo, June, 1975.

KERMODE, GO: *Human Nutrition: Readings from Scientific American.* WH Freeman & Company, San Francisco, 1978, pp 107–113. *Food additives.*

KRAUSE, MV AND MAHAN, LK: *Food, Nutrition and Diet Therapy,* ed 6. WB Saunders, Philadelphia, 1979. Chapter 16, *Agencies dealing with nutrition-related issues.* Chapter 17, *Federal food and nutrition programs.*

LARKIN, T: *Natural poisons in food.* FDA Consumer Memo, October, 1975.

LOWENBERG, ME ET AL: *Food & People,* ed 3. John Wiley & Sons, New York, 1979. Chapter 7, *Food, people, and the influence of business.* Chapter 10, *Programs to improve nutrition.*

MALBIN, I: *Computerizing supermarket checkout.* FDA Consumer Memo, November, 1975.

MAYER, J: *US nutrition policies in the seventies.* WH Freeman & Company, San Francisco, 1973.

MAYER, J: *Food fortification: How much is enough?* Family Health, Vol 11, February, 1979.

Nutrition Labeling: How It Can Work for You. The National Nutrition Consortium, Inc, Washington, DC, 1975.

Nutrition Labeling—Terms you should know. FDA Consumer Memo, February, 1976.

Nutrition Labeling—Tools for Its Use. Agriculture Information Bulletin No 382. US Government Printing Office, Washington, DC, April, 1975.

ROBINSON, CH: *Basic Nutrition and Diet Therapy,* ed 4, Macmillan, New York, 1980. Chapter 16, *Safeguarding the food supply.* Chapter 17, *Food legislation, labeling and selection.*

ROEUCHE, B: *Eleven Blue Men and Other Narratives of Medical Detection.* Little, Brown & Company, Boston, 1953.

SELECT COMMITTEE ON NUTRITION AND HUMAN NEEDS, US SENATE: *World Food and Nutrition Study—Report of Study Team 9 (Nutrition).* US Government Printing Office, Washington, DC, 1977.

STEPHENSON, MG: Making food labels more informative. FDA Consumer Memo, October, 1975.

STEPHENSON, MG: *The changing food supply.* FDA Consumer Memo, October, 1974.

SUITOR, CW AND HUNTER, MF: *Nutrition: Principles and Application in Health Promotion.* JB Lippincott, Philadelphia, 1980. Chapter 10, *The changing nutritional scene.*

Toward a national nutrition policy. Nutrition Policy Issues, December, 1980.

WILLIAMS, SR: *Mowry's Basic Nutrition and Diet Therapy,* ed 6. CV Mosby, St Louis, 1980. Chapter 12, *The community food supply and its relation to health.*

WINIKOFF, B: *Nutrition and National Policy.* MIT Press, Cambridge, Massachusetts, 1978. Chapter 11, *Nutrition and government policy in the United States.*

ZOTTOLA, EA: *Food-borne disease I.* Contemporary Nutrition 2(9), September, 1977.

ZOTTOLA, EA: *Food-borne disease II.* Contemporary Nutrition 3(1), January, 1978.

4

METABOLISM

OBJECTIVES

Upon completion of this chapter the student should be able to:

- Define metabolism, anabolism, and catabolism and list the factors that influence each.
- Define basal metabolism and list the factors that influence it.
- Compute the caloric needs of an adult, given that individual's desired weight.

Metabolism is the total of all physical and chemical changes that occur within the body. The two processes of metabolism are: **anabolism,** the building up of tissue as in growth, maintenance, and repair; and **catabolism,** the breaking down of tissue into simpler chemical units known as wastes. During metabolism, heat and energy are produced.

When anabolism exceeds catabolism, growth and development occur. Anabolism is increased by an increase in food supplied to the body, rest, and hormones such as insulin, epinephrine (Adrenalin), and sex hormones.

When catabolism exceeds anabolism, the body loses weight and tissue. Catabolism is increased by fever, bacterial toxins, fractures, burns, and certain hormones such as thyroxine.

BASAL METABOLISM

Basal metabolism is the amount of metabolic processes that take place in the body at rest and fasting and which are necessary to keep the body alive and functioning. Even while the body is relaxed and fasting, certain activities still take place—the heart continues to beat, the respiratory organs continue to function—and the body must produce the energy for these to continue. Any other activity would require additional metabolism to produce the energy needed for that activity.

The basal metabolic rate differs with each individual and depends upon the following factors:

BODY SURFACE. The greater the body surface, the more heat is lost from the body.

BODY COMPOSITION. Muscular tissue produces the most heat and energy; fat produces the least.

SEX. Because women have more fatty tissue than men, their basal metabolic rate is less than that of men. However, during menstruation, pregnancy, and lactation, the basal metabolic rate increases.

AGE. During periods of rapid growth, the metabolic rate is increased.

GLANDULAR ACTIVITY. The amount of activity of the thyroid gland and the adrenal glands has a marked effect upon the metabolic rate.

NUTRITIONAL STATUS. A body depleted by starvation has less tissue to enter into the process of metabolism.

ENERGY REQUIREMENTS

As metabolism takes place, *heat* and *energy* are produced. Calories are used to measure energy. A **calorie** is the amount of heat required to raise the temperature of one kilogram of water one degree centigrade.

The number of calories required for energy each day varies from individual to individual. The factors affecting energy requirement are as follows:

BASAL ENERGY REQUIREMENT. The basal energy requirement of an individual is the number of calories required to keep that person alive in an inactive state. A 1-year-old infant needs 100 calories per kilogram of body weight. As the child grows, the basal requirement decreases until adulthood when the standard requirement is 24 calories per kilogram of body weight. To determine the basal energy requirements of an adult, first convert the number of pounds that person weighs to kilograms. Then multiply the number of kilograms the person weighs by 24. The result equals the number of calories needed by that individual to stay alive *but not if the individual is active or growing.*

AGE. The greatest need for calories is during periods of greatest growth. Fewer calories are needed during old age.

DESIRED WEIGHT. The desirable weight of an individual depends upon height and type of bone structure.

SEX. Women require fewer calories than men.

STATE OF HEALTH. Physical and emotional conditions can alter energy requirements.

CLIMATE. When body heat is lost to the exterior environment, as in cold climates, energy requirements increase.

ACTIVITY. The kind and amount of physical activity are the biggest factors in determining energy requirements. Unless the body receives enough food to provide energy expended in work (Table 2), it must use its own tissues (usually adipose tissue). If more food is provided than is necessary for energy, the excess is stored (usually as adipose tissue).

The person who digs ditches needs many more calories than the individual who works at a desk all day, even though all other factors (e.g., age, sex) are the same. It has been estimated that nursing duties require 50 percent more than basal requirement. In other words, the nurse needs the determined basal requirement plus 50 percent of the requirement in order to perform nursing duties without becoming deficient in energy or losing weight.

For example, suppose a nurse weighing 132 pounds wishes to maintain this weight; the caloric needs would be computed as follows:

1. Convert pounds to kilograms. Approximately 2.2 pounds equal one kilogram.

$$\frac{132}{2.2} = 60 \text{ kg}$$

2. Multiply the number of kilograms by 24 calories to find the daily basal need.

$$60 \text{ kg} \times 24 \text{ calories} = 1440 \text{ calories}$$

3. Nursing duties require approximately 50 percent increase over basal need. Take 50 percent of 1440 calories.

$$0.50 \times 1440 \text{ calories} = 720 \text{ calories}$$

TABLE 2. Calories per Hour For 132 Lb (60 Kg) Person

Activity	*Calories Expended*
Bicycling	150
Boxing	684
Dancing	228
Dishwashing	60
Exercise, moderate	186
Football	408
Golf	90
Ironing	60
Making beds	180
Mopping	72
Office work	36
Rowing	588
Skating	210
Skiing	618
Sweeping	84
Swimming	474
Tennis	300
Typing	60
Walking	120

4. Basal calories plus the 50 percent for nursing duties equals the number of calories required by the nurse each day. 1440 basal calories plus 720 calories allowed for nursing activities equal 2160 calories per day.

On the basis of what you have read, answer the following questions:

1. What is a calorie?

2. Define metabolism:

3. List six factors that affect basal metabolism.
   A.

   B.

   C.

   D.

   E.

   F.

4. Energy is the power to work. Where does the body get its energy?

5. List seven factors that influence the body's energy requirement.
   A.

   B.

   C.

   D.

   E.

F.

G.

6. If you use 3,000 calories a day, you must take in food that supplies ________ calories. If you use 3,000 calories a day and you take in food that supplies 1200 calories, where does the body get the 1800 extra calories it needs?

7. If you use 2200 calories a day and take in 3600 calories a day, what does the body do with the extra calories?

Calculate your own daily caloric requirements as a nurse by answering the following:

1. Your weight in pounds is ________ .

2. If there are 2.2 pounds in each kilogram, how many kilograms do you weight?

3. If the basal requirement is 24 calories per kilogram, how many calories do you need for basal requirement?

4. Allowing a 50 percent increase for nursing activities, how many calories should you get to maintain your present body weight?

5. Looking back to the chart you kept on your own food intake for one day, how do total calories actually consumed and the number of calories actually required for you compare?

6. If you take in 1000 calories more than required for your nursing duties, what happens to those calories?

7. What happens if you take in less calories than you require?

OPTIONAL ACTIVITIES TO ENHANCE LEARNING

ACTIVITY 1

Each student measures height and weight. Compare the actual weights with the suggested weights. (See the chart in the Appendix.) Compute the number of calories needed in the daily diet to bring the actual weight to the desired weight.

ACTIVITY 2

Keep a record of time spent in physical activities per day. Compute the number of calories expended in these activities.

BIBLIOGRAPHY

ALBANESE, AA: *Nutritional and metabolic effects of physical exercise.* Food and Nutrition News, May, 1967.

BRIGGS, GM AND CALLOWAY, DH: *Bogert's Nutrition and Physical Fitness,* ed 10. WB Saunders, Philadelphia, 1979. Chapter 2, *The need for energy.*

KRAUSE, MV AND MAHAN, LK: *Food, Nutrition and Diet Therapy,* ed 6. WB Saunders, Philadelphia, 1979. Chapter 2, *Energy.*

ROBINSON, CH: *Basic Nutrition and Diet Therapy,* ed 4. Macmillan, New York, 1980. Chapter 8, *Energy metabolism.*

WILLIAMS, SR: *Mowry's Basic Nutrition and Diet Therapy,* ed 6. CV Mosby, St Louis, 1980. Chapter 5, *Energy requirements.*

5

CARBOHYDRATES

OBJECTIVES

Upon completion of this chapter the student should be able to:

- Classify the carbohydrates, giving the source of each.
- List the functions of carbohydrates in the body.
- Describe carbohydrate digestion and metabolism, given the carbohydrate ingested.
- Compute the number of calories in a carbohydrate food, given the total weight of sugars and starches in the food.

Carbohydrates are the major source of food for all peoples of the world. Carbohydrates are the cheapest, the most easily obtained, and the most readily digested of all nutrients. The chief sources of carbohydrates are cereals, vegetables, fruits, and syrups and sugars. Carbohydrates are formed from the chemical elements carbon, hydrogen, and oxygen. Plants use these elements to form carbohydrates through the process of photosynthesis.

CARBOHYDRATE CLASSIFICATION

Monosaccharides (Simple Sugars)

GLUCOSE. Found in fruits and vegetables, glucose is the form in which the body uses carbohydrates. It can be converted into **glycogen** and stored in the muscles and liver.

FRUCTOSE. Fructose is found in fruits, honey, and vegetables.

GALACTOSE. Produced by the digestion of *lactose* (milk sugar), galactose is never found free in nature.

Disaccharides (Double Sugars)

SUCROSE. Known as table sugar, sucrose is found in sugar cane, sugar beets, and maple sap.

MALTOSE. Known as malt sugar, maltose is found in malt and malt products produced from grain.

LACTOSE. Known as milk sugar, lactose is found in all mammalian milk. It is an expensive form of sugar and is less soluble and sweet than the others. Its laxative action can cause diarrhea if taken in excessive amounts.

Polysaccharides (Starches, Cellulose, Glycogen)

STARCHES. Starches are found encased in the cellulose walls of grains and vegetables. To make starches available for digestion, the cellulose must be broken down by grinding or cooking. Because starch is abundant over all the earth, it is the cheapest form of body fuel and usually constitutes the largest portion of a menu.

CELLULOSE. The framework of plants is formed of cellulose. The terms plant fiber, roughage, and bulk denote cellulose. A polysaccharide, or carbohydrate of a very complex nature, cellulose is insoluble in hot or cold water and resists digestion. By furnishing bulk in the digestive tract, cellulose stimulates peristaltic action.

The amount of cellulose required per day varies with the individual and with the type of fiber consumed. Cellulose from fruits, vegetables, and whole-grain cereals is less irritating to the digestive tract than cellulose in the form of bran.

The polysaccharides agar-agar and pectin are very similar to cellulose in their action. When cooked, they absorb water to form a bulky gel. Agar-agar may be used in cases where cellulose fibers are too irritating to the intestinal tract. Pectin is used to make fruit juices jell.

GLYCOGEN. Carbohydrates are stored in the muscles and liver in the form of glycogen or "animal starch." In an emergency, glycogen is a source of quick energy. Glycogen in animal muscles has little dietary significance. When the animal dies, it is converted to another compound.

Polyols (Alcohols Derived from Sugar)

For those who cannot metabolize sugars properly, polyols can provide the sweet taste in foods. Polyols do not leave a bitter taste in the mouth (as saccharin does) and requires little insulin to metabolize. Some of the polyols are Sorbitol, Xylitol, Mannitol, and Maltitol. They are used in diabetic foods and sugar-free candy and gum.

Excessive ingestion of polyols can cause diarrhea because they are absorbed so slowly from the digestive tract.

FUNCTIONS OF CARBOHYDRATES

The functions of carbohydrates in the body are:

1. Provision of heat and energy. This is the most important function.
2. "Sparing of protein." Because protein is the only nutrient for building tissue, it should never be used for energy alone.
3. Assisting in metabolism of fat. Without carbohydrates, fat metabolism cannot be completed.

Carbohydrates not needed by the body as immediate energy or for glycogen storage are converted and stored as adipose tissue. One gram of carbohydrate will provide 4 calories. The daily requirement of carbohydrates in the adult diet is 40 to 50 percent of the daily calories allowed.

CARBOHYDRATE DIGESTION

Carbohydrate digestion begins in the mouth where the enzyme **ptyalin** starts turning starch into maltose. A weak enzyme ptyalin usually has very little time to work on the starch. Carbohydrates receive no digestive action in the stomach. In the small intestine the enzyme **amylase** from the pancreatic juice changes starch to maltose. Three enzymes from the intestinal juices act upon the double sugars to change them to simple sugars. **Sucrase** acts upon sucrose; **lactase** acts upon lactose; **maltase** acts upon maltose. The final product of this enzymatic action is **glucose,** which is absorbed into the body through the intestinal capillaries.

The body takes longer to digest starch than any other carbohydrate, but the simple sugar, glucose, does not have to be digested at all. Therefore, glucose provides energy the quickest after ingestion. Glucose can be utilized in three ways:

1. It can be used (oxidized) immediately for energy.
2. It can be converted to *glycogen* and stored in the muscles and liver for later use.
3. It can be distributed to the body fluids. For instance, there are 70 to 120 milligrams of glucose in 100 centimeters of whole fasting blood in the normal adult.

One of the most important regulators of blood sugar is *insulin,* produced in the islands of Langerhans in the pancreas. Insulin helps to increase the oxidation and the storage of sugar, thus reducing the amount of sugar in the blood.

Complete the following exercises:

1. Carbohydrates are compounds composed of CARBON, OXYGEN, and HYDROGEN.

2. The biggest portion of carbohydrates in the diet is furnished in the form of ______________.

3. The five chief sources of carbohydrates are SYRUPS, CEREALS, FRUITS, SUGAR, and VEGETABLES.

4. Carbohydrates are classified as ______________, ______________, and ______________.

5. Sugars are divided into simple sugars and double sugars. The three simple sugars are FRUCTOSE, GALACTOSE, and GLUCOSE.

6. Glucose is found in FRUITS and VEGETABLES.

7. Fructose is found in Honey, FRUITS, and vegetable.

8. Galactose is produced by the digestion of lactose.

9. The double sugars are SUCROSE, MALTOSE, and LACTOSE.

10. Another name for sucrose is table sugar, for maltose is malt sugar, and for lactose is milk sugar.

11. The best form of sugar to give when an immediate supply of energy is needed is Glucose. Why?

Does not have to be digested

12. Lactose has a laxative action on the digestive tract and an excessive amount may cause diarrhea.

13. If the nurse needs to add more calories with sugar without making food too sweet, which sugar should be used?

LACTOSE

14. Which sugar is the most expensive?

15. Starch is found in grains and vegetable.

16. Glycogen is sugar stored in muscles and liver.

17. Because it is found in abundance over all the world, Carbohydrates is the cheapest form of body fuel.

18. To receive full value from starches, what must be done to the starch food? the cellulose must be broken down by grinding or cooking.

Why?

19. One gram of carbohydrates contains ______ calories. Ten grams of carbohydrates contain ______ calories. One-half gram of carbohydrates contains ______ calories.

20. The primary function of carbohydrate in the diet is:
Provision of heat & Energy

21. Normal fasting blood sugar level in the adult is ______________ .

22. To what class of carbohydrate does each of the following belong?

Bread Starch
Potato Starch
Honey ______________
Rice Starch
Malted milk Maltose
Maple syrup Sucrose
Table sugar Sucrose

23. The daily requirement of carbohydrate in the diet is 40-50% .

24. Fill in completely the following chart.

DIGESTION OF CARBOHYDRATES

Area	*Enzyme*	*Acts on:*	*To Produce:*
	SUCRASE	SUCROSE	
	MALTASE	MALTOSE	
	GLUCOSE		

25. In what form are carbohydrates absorbed into the blood?

26. How are carbohydrates used by the body?

ASSISTING IN METABOLISM OF FAT
SPARING OF PROTEIN
PROVISION OF HEAT & ENERGY

27. Chew an unsalted cracker for five minutes. How did it taste when you started chewing?

At the end of five minutes?

What action has taken place?

28. What part of the plant is cellulose?

the FRAMEWORK

29. What are the characteristics of cellulose?

plant fiber, bulk, Roughage

30. Why is cellulose important in the diet?

stimulates peristaltic action

31. Why is agar-agar sometimes given to treat constipation?

when cellulose fiber irritates the intestinal tract

32. Check those of the following foods that have a high cellulose content.

______ Egg custard	✓ Rhubarb
✓ Celery stalks	✓ Apple
✓ Lettuce	

33. What is frequently used to sweeten diabetic foods?

Polyols

OPTIONAL ACTIVITIES TO ENHANCE LEARNING

ACTIVITY 1

Obtain one teaspoon of honey, table sugar, lactose, fructose, and glucose. (It may be necessary to obtain some of these from the pharmacy.) Dissolve each sugar in one cup of water. Ask some of the members of the class to taste the solutions while blindfolded. Give each person a small amount of the solution and have them keep it in the mouth for several minutes before swallowing. Which sugar solution is the sweetest? Did the honey and fructose taste the same? Were all the tasters of the same opinion? If not, why?

ACTIVITY 2

Blindfold three members of the class. Then give each a food to chew, taste, and identify. Give one a piece of unsalted cracker; the second, a small piece of unsalted bread; and the third student a piece of unsalted baked potato. Ask them to chew until the food has a sweet taste. Then ask each to identify the food. It makes it more difficult if all pieces of food have been pulverized before putting into the students' mouths.

BIBLIOGRAPHY

BRIGGS, GM AND CALLOWAY, DH: *Bogert's Nutrition and Physical Fitness,* ed 10. WB Saunders, Philadelphia, 1979.

CARBARY, LJ: *Fiber is a factor.* Journal of Practical Nursing, Vol 30, April, 1980.

CHANEY, MS, ROSS, ML, WITSCHI, JC: *Nutrition,* ed 9. Houghton Mifflin, Boston, 1979. Chapter 6, *Carbohydrates.*

DAMON, GE: *A primer on four nutrients: Proteins, carbohydrates, fats, and fiber.* FDA Consumer Memo, February, 1975.

DANOWSKI, TS: *Sugar and Disease.* Contemporary Nutrition 3(12), December, 1978.

Dietary Fiber. Contemporary Nutrition 4(9), September, 1979.

KRAUSE, MV AND MAHAN, LK: *Food, Nutrition and Diet Therapy,* ed 6. WB Saunders, Philadelphia, 1979. Chapter 3, *Carbohydrates.*

ROBINSON, CH: *Basic Nutrition and Diet Therapy,* ed 4. Macmillan, New York, 1980. Chapter 7, *Carbohydrates.*

WILLIAMS, SR: *Mowry's Basic Nutrition and Diet Therapy,* ed 6. CV Mosby, St Louis, 1980. Chapter 5, *Carbohydrates.*

WORTHINGTON-ROBERTS, BS: *Contemporary Developments in Nutrition.* CV Mosby, St Louis, 1981. Chapter 1, *Carbohydrates in health and disease.* Chapter 2, *Dietary fiber.*

6

FATS

OBJECTIVES

Upon completion of this chapter the student should be able to:

- Classify fats, giving the sources of each class.
- State the differences between saturated and unsaturated fats and give some examples of each.
- Discuss cholesterol, giving its sources, uses in the body, and the problems encountered in excessive cholesterol intake.
- List the functions of fats in the body.
- Describe the digestion and absorption of fats.
- Compute the number of calories in a given amount of fat.
- List some of the best sources of essential fatty acids.

Fats are the most concentrated source of heat and energy, yielding 9 calories from each gram of fat. The recommended daily allowance is one fifth, or 20 percent, of the daily caloric allotment.

Today, Americans consume approximately 40 percent of their total calories in the form of fat—a level of consumption made possible by American prosperity. Fats are "status foods," costing more than ordinary carbohydrate foods, and also give food a better taste. In very cold countries, the diet contains more fat to provide additional body heat. The most common fatty foods in the American diet are butter and cream. In some other countries, these items are too expensive for the majority of the population.

Fats belong to a group of chemicals called **lipids.** *True fats* are composed of the chemical elements carbon, hydrogen, and oxygen, but in a different chemical arrangement and ratio from carbohydrates. True fats are known as **fatty acids.**

FAT CLASSIFICATION

Fats can be classified in several ways—by their source, by their chemical composition, and by whether or not they are visible in the food. Animal fats are found in cream, milk, meat, eggs, and fish. Vegetable fats are found in corn, nuts, olives, avocados, and cottonseed. The fat content of butter is obvious, but the fat content of egg is not; in egg, the fat is said to be invisible.

SATURATED FATS. Saturated fats are those fatty acids that contain all the hydrogen possible in their molecules. Saturated fats are solid at room temperature. Examples are tallow, lard, animal fat, butter, and hydrogenated shortenings.

UNSATURATED FATS. Fatty acids that can take on more hydrogen under certain conditions are termed **unsaturated fats.** Some fats are partially unsaturated and others are highly unsaturated. The latter are called **polyunsaturated fats.** Unsaturated fats are soft or liquid at room temperature. Oils from animals, fish, corn, cottonseed, olives, peanuts, and safflower are unsaturated fats.

Some researchers seeking the causes of heart disease recommend the use of polyunsaturated fats because they induce lower blood cholesterol levels than saturated fats. However, when the diet contains an excessive number of calories and is high in carbohydrates, the body converts this to fat and the cholesterol level remains high. It is not advisable to make drastic changes in the fat content of the diet without consulting a physician.

Many of the shortenings on the market are unsaturated fats that have been **hydrogenated;** that is, hydrogen was added to the unsaturated fat. After it is hydrogenated, the unsaturated fat has the characteristics and properties of saturated fat. Margarine is an example. Margarine fortified with vitamins A and D is the same as butter in food value.

ESSENTIAL FATTY ACIDS. Essential fatty acids cannot be constructed in the body from other materials and are necessary for growth and metabolism.

The essential fatty acids, ~~linolenic~~, linoleic, and ~~arachidonic acid~~, are polyunsaturated. One to three percent of the fat calories in the daily diet should come from essential fatty acids. The best sources are butter, egg yolk, and meats.

FALSE FATS. False fats are hydrocarbons, such as motor oil, and are of no value nutritionally. The most commonly used "false fat" is mineral oil. Mineral oil is used as a laxative and a lubricant, but it also disturbs the absorption of certain vitamins and caution should be exercised when it is prescribed. It should not be taken too near mealtime or for extended periods.

CHOLESTEROL

Although **cholesterol** is associated with fats, chemically it is a sterol. Normally found in all body cells and fluids, cholesterol is stored in the liver and can be made by the body. Normally, there are 100 to 150 milligrams of cholesterol in 100 milliliters of whole blood. Abnormally high blood cholesterol levels may result in deposits on blood vessel walls or in the liver or in gallstones. Cholesterol is also associated with hypertension, nephrosis, and diabetes, and in these cases the physician may prescribe a low cholesterol diet.

Cholesterol in the blood not only comes from food; it is also produced by the liver. A high-fat diet increases the fat in the liver, which apparently stimulates cholesterol production. Because fats instead of carbohydrates are used for energy in uncontrolled diabetes, the cholesterol level is increased in that condition.

Although excessive blood cholesterol can cause problems, cholesterol has important functions in the body. It is a necessary part of brain and nerve tissue and is the starting chemical compound in production of the sex hormones, certain adrenal hormones, bile, and the chemical in the skin that becomes vitamin D when exposed to sunlight. Cholesterol in the skin prevents water evaporation and makes the skin resistant to chemicals.

Foods high in cholesterol are egg yolk, liver, kidney, sweetbreads, brains, fish roe, oysters, fat of meats, and fat in milk products. Foods low in cholesterol include fruits, vegetables, cereals, syrups, egg white, lean meat, low-fat fish, and skim milk.

FUNCTIONS OF FAT

The functions of fat in the body are:

1. Fat serves as a concentrated source of heat and energy.
2. Fat carries the fat-soluble vitamins A, D, E, and K.
3. Fat gives a feeling of satiety because it is digested more slowly in the stomach than carbohydrates and proteins.

4. Fat aids in normal tissue function.
5. Stored fat can be used as reserve supply of body fuel.
6. Stored fat helps to maintain body temperature by acting as insulation.
7. Stored fat helps to hold organs in place and protects them from injury.

Fat is stored in the body as adipose tissue. Too much adipose tissue is harmful as the extra weight requires the heart to work harder and the life span is shortened. Obesity is not only unsightly but is also a forerunner of arteriosclerosis.

Fatty foods react to oxygen and light by becoming **rancid** with destruction of the vitamin content. Even at low temperatures, the storage time for fatty foods should be limited. Fats are slower to digest, and cooking at high temperature makes them less digestible.

The digestion of fats begins in the stomach where emulsified fats (fats in which the droplets are tiny and evenly distributed throughout the substance) are acted upon by the enzyme **gastric lipase,** which is secreted by the gastric mucosa. In the small intestine, **bile** from the liver and the gallbladder emulsifies all other fats. This product is then acted upon by *lipase* from the pancreas to produce fatty acids and glycerol. Lymph vessels in the intestinal walls absorb fatty acids and glycerol into the body for use in metabolism.

Complete the following:

1. Excess fat is stored as ____________________ .

2. Fats are composed of the chemical elements ____________________ , ____________________ , and ____________________ .

3. Seven functions of fat in the body are:

   A.

   B.

   C.

   D.

   E.

F.

G.

4. A visible fat is ______________________________ . An example is ____________________ .

5. Two sources of animal fat are ____________________________ and ____________________ . Two good sources of vegetable fats are ____________________ and ____________________ .

6. How can you tell by looking that a fat is saturated?

7. How can you tell by looking that a fat is unsaturated?

8. Give two examples of saturated fat:

9. Give two examples of unsaturated fat:

10. What are "essential fatty acids"?

11. What are the three best sources of essential fatty acids?

12. Mineral oil is not a true fat. It is dangerous to use it indiscriminately because:

13. The normal level of cholesterol in 100 milliliters of whole fasting blood is ______________________ to ______________________ .

14. The functions of cholesterol are:

15. Cholesterol is produced in the body by the ______________________ .

16. Low cholesterol foods include ______________________ , ______________________ , ______________________ , ______________________ , and ______________________ .

17. High cholesterol foods include ______________________ , ______________________ , ______________________ , ______________________ , and ______________________ .

18. Vitamins found in fat foods are ______________________ , ______________________ , ______________________ , and ______________________ .

19. A fat that has been subjected to light, heat, and air becomes ______________________ .

20. Fats are not hard to digest; they are ______________________ to digest. They should be cooked at ______________________ temperatures.

21. Are fats a cheap or an expensive source of energy?

22. One gram of fat will give ____________________ calories of heat.

23. Fats are known as "status foods." Why?

24. Fats add to the palatability of foods because they give it ____________________.

25. ____________________ percent of the daily caloric intake should be fats.

26. ____________________ percent of the daily fat intake should be essential fatty acids.

27. Fill in completely the following chart.

DIGESTION OF FATS

Area	*Enzyme or chemical*	*Acts on*	*To Produce*

28. Fats are absorbed into the ____________________ vessels in the small intestines in the form of ____________________ and ____________________.

OPTIONAL ACTIVITIES TO ENHANCE LEARNING

ACTIVITY 1

Divide into nine groups. Each group is to choose one food below and find as many brands as possible and the price of each. During class discussion, a comparison is to be made of the various forms of fat foods and the cost of each.

Shortening
Lard
Butter
Olive oil
Cottonseed oil
Saturated and polyunsaturated margarine
Coffee and whipping cream
Safflower oil
Peanut oil

ACTIVITY 2

Invisible fats can add greatly to the caloric content of a diet. Obtain a week's menu from the school cafeteria. Identify the dishes that contain invisible fats or cholesterol. Identify the dishes that have fats added during cooking.

ACTIVITY 3

Ask 10 students in your school what fast foods or snacks they have eaten in the past 24 hours. Identify the foods that contain cholesterol or fats, classifying the fats as saturated or unsaturated. Discuss in class the impact of these foods on the nutritional status of the individuals questioned.

BIBLIOGRAPHY

BRIGGS, GM AND CALLOWAY, DH: *Bogert's Nutrition and Physical Fitness,* ed 10. WB Saunders, Philadelphia, 1979. Chapter 4, *Fats and other lipids.*

CHANEY, MS, ROSS, ML, AND WITSCHI, JC: *Nutrition,* ed 9. Houghton Mifflin, Boston, 1979. Chapter 5, *The lipids.*

DAMON, GE: *A primer on four nutrients: Proteins, carbohydrates, fats, and fiber.* FDA Consumer Memo, February, 1975.

ERDMAN, JW, JR.: *Bioavailability of nutrients from foods.* Contemporary Nutrition 3(11), November, 1978.

Fats in Food and Diet. Agriculture Bulletin No 361, US Government Printing Office, Washington, DC, 1977.

FLYNN, MA: *The cholesterol controversy.* Contemporary Nutrition, 3(3), March, 1978.

GOLUB, S: *Can mamma's food be bad?* American Journal of Nursing, 65(8), August, 1965.

KRAUSE, MV AND MAHAN, LK: *Food, Nutrition and Diet Therapy,* ed 6. WB Saunders, Philadelphia, 1979. Chapter 4, *Lipids.*

KRITCHEVSKY, D AND CZARNECKI, SK: Lipiproteins. Contemporary Nutrition, 5(5), May, 1980.

ROBINSON, CH: *Basic Nutrition and Diet Therapy,* ed 4. Macmillan, New York, 1980. Chapter 6, *Fats.*

WILLIAMS, SR: *Mowry's Basic Nutrition and Diet Therapy,* ed 6. CV Mosby, St Louis, 1980. Chapter 4, *Fats.*

WORTHINGTON-ROBERTS, BS: *Contemporary Developments in Nutrition.* CV Mosby, St Louis, 1981. Chapter 3, *Questions related to dietary fats.*

7

PROTEIN

OBJECTIVES

Upon completion of this chapter the student should be able to:

- Classify proteins, giving the sources of each class.
- State the differences between complete and incomplete protein foods.
- List the functions of protein, identifying the one that only protein can perform.
- Describe the digestion and absorption of protein.
- Compute the calories in a given amount of a protein food.
- Choose foods that are complete protein foods containing all the essential amino acids.

Protein was one of the first substances recognized as a vital part of living tissue. The word, protein, means "of first importance." Eighteen percent of the body is some form of protein. Living cells are all protein.

Proteins are composed of carbon, hydrogen, oxygen, and nitrogen. Although other elements, such as sulfur and phosphorus, may be present, the nitrogen distinguishes the protein molecule from all others.

Protein molecules are very complex. They are made up of units known as **amino acids,** sometimes called the "building blocks" of the body. Of the 23 different amino acids, eight are classed as essential for adults because the body must be supplied with them daily. Nine or ten are essential for children.

PROTEIN CLASSIFICATION

Proteins may be classified according to:

1. The amount of amino acids they contain. *High-protein* foods include eggs, milk, meat, fish, nuts, and legumes. *Low-protein* foods include fruits and vegetables other than legumes.
2. The source. *Animal proteins* include milk, meat, fish, and eggs. *Plant proteins* include peas, beans, and other legumes, as well as nuts, fruits, and vegetables.
3. Completeness. *Complete proteins* contain all the essential amino acids in sufficient quantity to maintain nitrogen equilibrium in adults and growth in children. All animal proteins except gelatin are complete proteins. *Incomplete proteins* do not supply all the essential amino acids. Most plant proteins are incomplete. However, soybeans are the exception and they are currently used to supplement meat products, or as a "filler" in a dish. Efforts are being made to introduce the use of soybean flour in undeveloped nations.

PROTEIN FUNCTIONS

The functions of proteins in the body are:

1. To build and repair body tissue. *(No other nutrient can do this.)*
2. To aid the body to resist diseases.
3. To provide heat and energy.
4. To contribute to body secretions and fluids.

One gram of protein yields 4 calories. An adult requires approximately 0.8 gram of protein per kilogram of body weight daily. This is approximately 10 percent of the daily caloric requirement. In times of growth, the need is greater. A child requires 2 to 3 grams of protein per kilogram of body weight and an adolescent needs 1 to 2 grams. Many authorities feel that the elderly have increased protein needs because their bodies do not always utilize the nutrient efficiently. Many conditions, such as pregnancy, fever, hyperthyroidism, and burns, also require additional protein intake.

Recent studies have shown that the amount of protein needed daily by an individual is dependent upon its quality. If complete protein foods, such as milk and eggs, are ingested, less protein is needed. But protein intake should be increased if the foods contain incomplete proteins. The protein content of foods is listed in Table 3.

Protein loss or deficiency is serious. Sudden protein loss, as in hemorrhage, surgery, and burns, results in shock. Gradual loss, usually due to dietary deficiency, may cause the following symptoms: loss of weight, nutritional edema, dry and scaly skin, and impaired healing and low resistance to infections.

PROTEIN DIGESTION

Proteins should be cooked at a temperature of 300°F. A higher cooking temperature results in an unappetizing, tough product that is difficult to digest.

Protein digestion begins in the stomach where the enzyme **rennin** acts upon milk protein to make curds of it. The milk curds and other proteins are then partially digested by the enzyme **pepsin,** aided by *hydrochloric acid.* In the small intestine **trypsin,** from the pancreas, and **erepsin,** from the intestinal mucosa, finish the digestive process. The resulting product is *amino acid,* which is absorbed into the blood vessels for distribution throughout the body.

There is practically no storage of amino acids in the body. Most absorbed amino acids are used to build or repair the body tissue. If enough carbohydrates are not available in the diet, some of the protein can be converted to glucose and fatty acids for use as heat and energy. Because protein is so important for body tissue, carbohydrates should be ingested "to spare the protein."

Complete the following:

1. Proteins are composed of ___Oxygen___, ___Carbon___, ___Hydrogen___, and ___Nitrogen___. These elements make up units called ___Amino Acids___.

2. Proteins that contain all the essential amino acids in sufficient quantity to maintain nitrogen balance in adults and growth in children are known as ___Complete___ proteins.

3. Good plant sources of protein would be ___Meat___, ___Eggs___, and ___Milk___.

TABLE 3. PROTEIN CONTENT OF FOODS*

Food	*Amount*	*Grams*	*Protein (grams)*
Bacon	2 slices	15	5
Beef, hamburger	3 oz patty	85	21
roast	3 oz	85	17
steak	3 oz	85	20
Beans, lima (dry and cooked)	1 cup	190	16
navy (dry and cooked)	1 cup	190	14
Biscuit	1	28	2
Bread, white	1 slice	25	2
whole wheat	1 slice	28	3
Cheese, Cheddar	1 inch cube	17	4
cottage	1 cup	245	33
Chicken (flesh only)	3 oz	85	20
Cocoa, homemade	1 cup	250	10
Corn flakes	1 cup	25	2
Corn muffins	1	40	3
Custard, baked	1 cup	265	14
Egg	1	50	6
Frankfurter	1	56	7
Gelatin dessert	1 cup	240	4
Ham	3 oz	85	18
Ice cream	1 cup	133	7
Lamb chop	4 oz	137	25
Liver, beef	2 oz	57	15
Macaroni	1 cup	130	6
Milk, whole	1 cup	244	9
Noodles	1 cup	160	7
Oatmeal	1 cup	240	5
Ocean perch	3 oz	85	16
Oysters	1 cup	240	20
Peanuts, roasted	1 cup	144	37
Peanut butter	1 tbsp	16	4
Peas, black-eyed (dry and cooked)	1 cup	248	13
Pecans	1 cup	108	10
Pork links	2	26	5
Rice	1 cup	185	4
Salmon, pink, canned	3 oz	85	17
Shrimp	3 oz	85	21
Spaghetti	1 cup	140	5
Walnuts	1 cup	126	26

*From: *Nutritive value of foods.* US Department of Agriculture, Home and Gardens Bulletin No 72, 1970.

4. Functions of protein in the body include:
   A. Build & repair tissue

   B. Provide heat & energy

   C. Aid the body to resist disease

   D. Contribute to body secretions & fluids

5. The daily adult requirement of dietary protein is ___1670___ or approximately 10 percent of the total daily calories. How much protein should you have in your own daily diet? (Refer to Chapter 4 on Metabolism and your own determination of your caloric requirement.)

6. During periods of growth, the need for protein is greater. Children need ___2___ to ___3___ grams of protein per kilogram of body weight daily. Adolescents need ___1___ to ___2___ grams of protein per kilogram of body weight daily.

7. Check the appropriate answer. During old age, the need for protein is:
   Higher than for normal adult. ___✓___
   Lower than for normal adult. ______

8. Signs of protein deficiency include:
   A. Dry & scaly skin

   B. weight loss

C. NUTRITIONAL EDEMA

D. LOW RESISTANCE

9. The best sources of animal protein are Egg, MEAT, and Fish.

10. Animal proteins are the best protein foods because:

they ARE COMPLETE

11. The one animal protein that is incomplete is Gelatan.

12. Most incomplete proteins are plant in origin. The exception is soybean.

13. The amount of heat used in cooking and the manner of its application may destroy or alter amino acids so that the protein becomes resistant to digestive enzymes. In general, a temperature of 300F° is best.

14. Although protein can be used for energy, the main function of protein in the body is:

Build + Repair Body tissue.

15. One gram of protein equals 4 calories.

16. Eggs are protein but they are also important because they contain other essential nutrients. What is another essential nutrient in egg?

How many eggs are recommended for the daily diet?

17. Liver is also an excellent complete protein that is recommended because it contains other nutrients. How much liver is suggested per week?

18. How often should dried beans and peas be added to the diet?

19. Fill in completely the following chart.

DIGESTION OF PROTEINS

Area	*Enzyme or Chemical*	*Acts on*	*To Produce*

20. The end product of the process of digestion of protein is AMINO ACId.

21. The form in which proteins are absorbed and utilized by the body is AMINO ACId

OPTIONAL ACTIVITY TO ENHANCE LEARNING

ACTIVITY 1

Divide into seven groups.

Group 1 is to go to a health food store and make a list of all the meat substitutes sold there and their prices, note the amount of protein in each, and identify the source of the protein.

Group 2 is to go to a supermarket and make a list of all the meats and meat substitute packages that have had soybean products added. Obtain the prices of the items.

Group 3 is to consult cookbooks and make a list of ways to include plant proteins in the diet as meat substitutes.

Group 4 is to consult cookbooks for ways to prepare liver and other variety meats as the main dish in a menu.

Group 5 is to price liver and other variety meats at the supermarket. Include canned varieties.

Group 6 is to find out what fish or shellfish is sold in the community and the prices that are asked for them.

Group 7 is to locate sources of eggs in the community other than the grocery or convenience stores. Compare the prices of eggs at the grocery or convenience store and the prices elsewhere.

Discuss in class the findings of each group. Relate these findings to protein nutritional needs of a family, possible acceptance or nonacceptance of these foods by family members, and the cost of using them in meal planning in place of the traditional steak, hamburger, or roast.

BIBLIOGRAPHY

BRIGGS, GM AND CALLOWAY, DH: *Bogert's Nutrition and Physical Fitness,* ed 10. WB Saunders, Philadelphia, 1979. Chapter 5, *Protein and amino acids.*

CHANEY, MS, ROSS, ML, WITSCHI, JC: *Nutrition,* ed 9. Houghton Mifflin, Boston, 1979. Chapter 6, *Protein.*

DAMON, GE: *A primer on four nutrients: Proteins, carbohydrates, fats, and fiber.* FDA Consumer Memo, February, 1975.

ERDMAN, JW, JR: *Bioavailability of nutrients from foods.* Contemporary Nutrition 3(11), November, 1978.

HUTT, PB AND SLOAN, AE: *FDA regulation of vegetable protein products.* Nutrition Policy Issues, No 3, January, 1979.

KRAUSE, MV AND MAHAN, LK: *Food, Nutrition and Diet Therapy,* ed 6. WB Saunders, Philadelphia, 1979, Chapter 5, *Proteins.*

KRITCHEVSKY, D AND CZARNECKI, SK: *Lipoproteins.* Contemporary Nutrition 5(5), May, 1980.

MAYER, J: *The ABC's of proteins.* Family Health, May, 1973, pp 24, 25.

PALOMBO, JD AND BLACKBURN, GL: *Human protein requirements.* Contemporary Nutrition 5(1), January, 1980.

PATTON, S: *Human Nutrition: Readings from Scientific American.* WH Freeman & Company, San Francisco, 1978, pp 89–97.

ROBINSON, CH: *Basic Nutrition and Diet Therapy,* ed 4. Macmillan, New York, 1980. Chapter 5, *Proteins and amino acids.*

WILLIAMS, SR: *Mowry's Basic Nutrition and Diet Therapy,* ed 6. CV Mosby, St Louis, 1980. Chapter 3, *Proteins.*

WINICK, M: *Nutrition and aging.* Contemporary Nutrition 2(6), June, 1977.

WORTHINGTON-ROBERTS, BS: *Contemporary Developments in Nutrition.* CV Mosby, St Louis, 1981. Chapter 4, *Proteins and amino acids.*

8

MINERALS

OBJECTIVES

Upon completion of this chapter the student should be able to:

- List the functions and sources of calcium, phosphorus, iron, iodine, magnesium, zinc, and copper, and discuss some of the problems encountered with deficient or excessive intake of each.
- Discuss the digestion and absorption of calcium and iron.
- Explain how the body conserves iron.
- List the uses and sources of potassium, sodium, and chlorine, and discuss some of the problems encountered in deficient or excessive intake.
- List the functions and sources of sulfur, selenium, manganese, molybdenum, cobalt, and fluorine.

Minerals are simple chemical elements. Of the 19 or more different minerals used by the body, approximately 17 are essential. Almost 4 percent of the body weight is mineral, with calcium and phosphorus in the bones accounting for the major portion.

The general functions of minerals in the body are to:

1. Compose a necessary part of all cells and body fluids.
2. Form the structural framework of the body as a part of the bones and teeth.
3. Assist in regulating vital life processes, such as maintenance of acid-base balance and osmotic pressures.
4. Regulate metabolism of enzymes.
5. Aid in transmission of nerve impulses.

CALCIUM

Of all the minerals, a dietary deficiency of calcium is most frequent. Calcium is needed throughout life, but the greatest need occurs during childhood, pregnancy, and lactation.

Approximately 2 percent of body weight is calcium; 99 percent of the calcium in the body is found in bones, cartilage, and teeth.

The functions of calcium in the body include:

1. Skeletal formation, giving it rigidity and strength.
2. Assistance in coagulation of blood.
3. Formation and maintenance of teeth.
4. Enabling normal activity of muscles, including the heart muscle.
5. Keeping the nervous system healthy and active.
6. Enabling growth in height.
7. Activation of many body processes such as the absorption of vitamin B_{12} and the reaction of pancreatic lipase on fat.

Calcium deficiency results in:

1. **Rickets** in the young, manifested by retarded growth and abnormal development of the bones.
2. **Osteomalacia** or **osteoporosis** in the adult and the elderly.
3. Poor tooth formation.
4. Delayed blood clotting and prolonged bleeding.
5. Irritability of nerve fibers resulting in muscle spasm.

Only 30 percent of the calcium taken in the diet is absorbed by the intestine. The remaining 70 percent is excreted in the feces. To aid in calcium absorption, four things should be present *at the time of ingestion:* lactose, an acid environment, vitamin D, and certain amino acids. Although foods such as spinach, chard, and oatmeal contain organic acids that prevent absorption of calcium, the amount is too small to be significant. Laxatives and bulky foods increase peristalsis, thereby decreasing the time allowed for absorption. Individuals on prolonged bed rest do not absorb calcium efficiently. Instead, they lose calcium from bones because of the lack of stress, or weight, on the bones. This calcium loss frequently leads to the formation of renal calculi.

Some foods give up their calcium more easily than others. The very best sources of calcium are milk and milk products. (In milk that has been fortified with vitamin D, three aids to absorption are present.) Clams, oysters, and green leafy vegetables such as kale, turnip greens, mustard greens, and broccoli are also good sources of calcium. In recent years, experiments have been made with flour made from fish meal to try to find an economical source of calcium and protein for use in underdeveloped countries. Fish flour is extremely rich in calcium but its undesirable flavor has prevented its wide acceptance. Table 4 lists foods that are high in calcium.

Calcium needs should be met as follows: children should have 1 quart of milk a day, adults should have 1 pint of milk a day, pregnant women need 1 quart of milk a day, and lactating women need 1½ quarts of milk a day. For those individuals who do not tolerate milk well, aged cheese, fermented buttermilk, and yoghurt can be substituted.

TABLE 4. FOODS HIGH IN CALCIUM

	Grams	*Calcium (mg)*
Powdered skim milk, dry, ¼ cup	30	367
Evaporated milk, whole, ½ cup	120	302
Skim milk, 1 cup	240	298
Buttermilk, 1 cup	240	296
Whole milk, 1 cup	240	288
Powdered milk, whole, ½ cup	30	252
Cheese, Cheddar, 1 oz	30	218
Collards, cooked, ½ cup	100	188
Kale, cooked, ½ cup	100	187
Turnip greens, cooked, ½ cup	100	184
Cheese spread, 1 oz	30	158
Dandelion greens, cooked, ½ cup	100	140
Mustard greens, cooked, ½ cup	100	138
Ice milk, ½ cup	75	120
Pie, cream, ⅙ of 9″ pie	160	120
Pudding, ½ cup	100	117
Sardines, 1 oz	30	115
Custard, baked, ⅓ cup	100	112
Ice cream, ½ cup	75	110
Salmon, with bones, 1 oz	30	51
Shrimp, 1 oz	30	35
Oysters, 1 oz	30	31
Clams, 1 oz	30	29

The RDA for calcium is 1 gram for adults, 0.6 gram for infants, and 0.8 gram for children under age 4. Pregnant and lactating women need 1.3 grams.

Complete the following:

1. 1 percent of the body weight is composed of mineral. The greatest portion of this is Calcium and phosphorus.

2. The mineral most frequently found to be lacking in the diet is Calcium.

3. The three periods of greatest need for calcium are:
childhood
pregnency
lactation

4. The functions of calcium are:
A. Skeletal formation, giving it strength & rigidity
B. Assistance in coagulation of blood
C. Formation & matinance of teeth
D. Enabling normal activities of muscles
E. Keeping the nervous system healthy & active
F. Enabling growth in height
G. Activation of many body processes such as absorption of Vit. B12.

5. Calcium deficiency is manifested by:

A. Rickets

B. Poor Tooth formation

C. Osteomalacia or osteoporosis in the adult & elderly

D. Delayed blood clotting & prolonged bleeding

E. Irritability of nerve fibers resulting in muscle spasms

6. Why is milk the best source of calcium?

Gives up its calcium more easily than other foods

7. Why is vitamin D added to milk to fortify it?

Aids in Absorption

8. How much milk should you have each day?

Children = 1 qt. Pregnant women = 1 qt.
Adults = 1 pt.
Lactating women = 1 1/2 qt.

Referring to your records kept for the 24-hour period, do you get this much?

9. Name some ways to include milk in the diet for those who do not like to drink milk.

Aged cheese
Yogurt
Fermented butter milk.

10. In Mary Jones' family there are 2 children, 1 elderly person, and 2 adults. Mary is nursing her baby. How much milk is needed by this family each day?

What would be an economical form of milk to buy?

11. Adults should get at least 1 pt milk each day, and children should have at least 1 qt.

12. If Mary wants to serve foods other than milk that are good sources of calcium, what dishes could she prepare?

Greens, Cream pie

13. What four factors aid in the absorption of calcium?

14. The daily requirement for calcium is 800 milligrams each day. Pregnant women and lactating women should have extra calcium. It is recommended that pregnant women have 1 qt milk per day and women nursing should have 1 1/2 qt milk per day.

PHOSPHORUS

Phosphorus works very closely with calcium in the body. About 80 percent of bodily phosphorus is found in the bones and teeth. The remainder is found in all the other cells of the body, where it is a very essential part of the cell.

The functions of phosphorus are:

1. Aids in the formation of bones and teeth.
2. Aids in the absorption and transportation of nutrients.
3. Necessary for the metabolism of fat, protein, and carbohydrate, and for the release of energy from these nutrients.

Absorption of phosphorus is increased when vitamin D is present and when calcium and phosphorus are present in equal amounts.

Although the daily intake of phosphorus should be about the same as that of calcium, there is little chance of a deficiency because phosphorus is found in a variety of protein foods. The best sources of phosphorus are milk and milk products, but other good sources are cereals, legumes, eggs, fish, meat, and nuts. Phosphorus deficiency would result in rickets and osteomalacia.

Approximately 1 gram of phosphorus is required per day.

Complete the following:

1. Phosphorus is found mostly in bones & teeth and other cells in the body.

2. The functions of phosphorus are:

   A. Aids in formation of bones & teeth

   B. Aids in the absorption & transportation of nutrients

   C. Necessary for the metabolism of fat, protein, & carbohydrates, & for the release of energy from these nutrients.

3. Why is phosphorus deficiency so rare?

   Because it is found in a variety of protein foods

4. Milk and Milk products are the best sources of phosphorus. Other good sources are:

   cereals, legumes, eggs, fish, meat & nuts.

5. The daily intake of phosphorus should be 1/2 gram that of calcium.

6. The same factors that influence calcium absorption also aid in phosphorus. What are they?

   lactose, acid environment, vit. D. & certain amino acid.

7. Phosphorus deficiency would result in Rickets for children and Osteomalcia for adults.

IRON

Iron is present in small amounts in the body but that small amount has the important function of carrying oxygen to the tissues. Over 70 percent of the iron in the body performs this function by combining with protein to become hemoglobin in the red blood cell. Much of the remainder is stored in the liver, spleen, and bone. A deficiency of iron results in iron deficiency anemia.

The body absorbs only as much iron as it needs; dietary excess is excreted through the feces. When a red blood cell dies, the iron in the hemoglobin is not excreted but is used over and over again. This is why the normal adult man needs only 10 milligrams a day and the adult woman needs 18 milligrams a day during her reproductive years. Pregnant or lactating women should also receive 18 milligrams per day. Iron is especially important in the diet of women and babies. The monthly loss of hemoglobin depletes the woman's supply of iron. Babies are born with a small reserve of iron, but because milk is deficient in iron, the pediatrician starts the baby on egg yolk or pureed liver and beef as soon as possible.

Absorption of iron is retarded by:

1. Lack of vitamin C in the diet.
2. Lack of hydrochloric acid in the stomach.
3. Lack of the intrinsic factor in the stomach.
4. Excessive ingestion of alkalies.

The very best source of dietary iron is liver. The next best sources are oysters and lean beef. Other good sources are leafy green vegetables, egg yolk, beans, peas, dried fruits, and whole grain cereals (Table 5).

Complete the following:

1. Although iron is present only in small amounts in the body, it is of great importance. The function of iron is:

   carrying oxygen to the tissues

2. 70% percent of the body's iron is found in hemoglobin.

3. The body will absorb only as much iron as needed. Factors that prevent the proper absorption of needed iron are:

   1) Lack of Vit. C in diet
   2) " " hydrochloric acid in stom

TABLE 5. FOODS HIGH IN IRON

	Grams	*Iron (mg)*
Kidneys, beef, 2 oz	60	4.7
Liver, beef, 2 oz	60	4.7
Clams, 2 oz	60	4.2
Oysters, raw, 2 oz	60	3.4
Heart, beef, 2 oz	60	2.8
Yeast, dried, brewer's, 2 T	15	2.7
Beef, corned, medium fat, 2 oz	60	2.6
Beet greens, cooked, 1/2 cup	75	2.4
Dandelion greens, cooked, 1/2 cup	75	2.3
Turkey, 2 oz	60	2.3
Lentils, dry, cooked, 1/2 cup	30 (dry)	2.2
Veal roast, cooked, 2 oz	60	2.2

A. LACK OF VIT. C in diet

B. " " hydrochloric Acid in stomack

C. " " intrinsic FACTOR in the stomach

D. Excessive ingestion of Alkalies

4. The best source of iron is Liver. How much is recommended in the weekly diet?

10 milligrams

5. Egg yolk and pureed liver are added to the infant's diet because:

Milk is deficient in Iron

6. A deficiency of iron results in Anemia.

7. Why is iron so important in a woman's diet?

~~Monthly~~ Month loss of blood

8. What foods other than liver are the best sources of iron?

oysters, lean beef

What foods are good sources of iron?

Kidneys, oysters, clams

9. Each of the following foods in the amount specified below would provide one day's iron requirement. Which do you think is the most logical choice? Why?

1/3 pound beef liver	20 slices whole wheat bread
1 cup oysters	4 1/2 cups cooked spinach
10 egg yolks	2 cups raisins
3 cups cooked dried beans	

1/3 pound beef liver because its portion size is small

10. Plan a meal for yourself that will provide your daily requirement of iron.

IODINE

Iodine aids in the formation of the thyroid gland hormone, thyroxine. No other function is known, although iodine is found in all cells. Lack of iodine causes enlargement of the thyroid gland called **simple goiter.** Goiter is found more often in women, and menarche, pregnancy, and menopause increase susceptibility. Severe iodine deficiency during early childhood may result in **cretinism,** with physical and mental retardation.

The National Research Council recommends that 100 to 150 micrograms of iodine be taken daily. Pregnant and lactating women need an additional amount.

Seafoods such as clams, lobster, oysters, and sardines are rich in iodine. Foods grown along the seacoast contain varying amounts of iodine. Away from the coast, daily use of iodized salt will meet the minimum daily requirement for iodine. Three grams of iodized table salt available in the United States will provide 250 micrograms of iodine.

Complete the following:

1. Iodine is used by the body only in the Formation to form ~~thyroid~~ ~~Gland~~ ~~hormo~~ thyroxine.

2. Absorption of iodine takes place easily, and for most people in the United States the best source is ____________ . Other sources are:

3. A deficiency of iodine results in:

   Enlargement of the thyroid gland – simple goiter

4. How often should saltwater fish and other saltwater foods be included in the diet?

5. Who would be most likely to develop a simple goiter, someone living in Kansas or someone living in San Francisco?

   Kansas

   Why?

   Lack of seafood

6. The three periods in a woman's life when she is most susceptible to goiter are: pregnancy, menopause, and menarche.

POTASSIUM

Sodium, potassium, and chlorides are elements that form the "salts" in the diet. Potassium is an electrolyte and an important component of intercellular fluid. It helps maintain normal water balance and osmotic pressures, is necessary in maintaining a normal acid-base balance, and acts upon enzymes involved in protein and carbohydrate metabolism. It is required before glycogen can be produced.

Potassium deficiency causes muscular weakness (including muscles of the intestinal tract and respiratory system) and cardiac symptoms. Causes of potassium deficiency are diarrhea, prolonged vomiting, the administration of diuretics, postoperative conditions, or complications of conditions such as diabetic coma, chronic lung disease, and adrenal cortex malfunction.

Cereals, fruits, and vegetables are rich sources of potassium (Table 6). The usual intake of potassium is two to four grams per day.

Complete the following:

1. The functions of potassium are:

   A. help maintain normal water balance & osmotic pressures

   B. necessary in maintaining normal acid-base balance

   C. acts upon enzymes involved in protein & carbohydrate metabolism

   D. required before glycogen can be produced

   E.

2. Potassium deficiency causes muscular weakness and cardiac symptoms.

3. Potassium deficiency may occur when an individual has diarrhea, prolonged vomiting, adm. of diuretics, postoperative conditions, adrenal cortex malfunction, diabetic coma, or chronic lung disease.

4. The usual intake of potassium is 2 to 4 grams.

TABLE 6. FOODS HIGH IN POTASSIUM

	Grams	*Potassium (mg)*
Apricots, fresh, 2–3 medium	100	280
Apricot nectar, canned, 1/2 cup	125	190
Avocado, 1/2 fruit, 4″ long	125	680
Banana, raw, 1 medium	175	440
Celery, raw, 2 large stalks	80	270
Cherries, raw, sweet, 10	75	130
Cucumber, raw, peeled, 1/2 small	80	125
Grapefruit, raw, 1/2	175	128
Grapefruit juice, canned, 3/4 cup	180	300
Melons:		
Cantaloupe, 1/2 melon or 1 cup cubed	160	400
Honeydew, 1/8 melon, or 1 cup cubed	170	425
Watermelon, 1/16 melon, or 2 pounds with rind	425	425
Milk, whole, 1 cup	245	370
Molasses, blackstrap, 1 T	20	585
Orange, raw, 1 medium	140	270
Orange juice, fresh or frozen, 3/4 cup	185	370
Papaya, raw, 1/2 papaya or 1 cup cubed	225	355
Prunes, dried, raw, 5	50	355
Pumpkin, canned, 1 cup	245	560
Raisins, 1/4 cup	35	275
Scallops, steamed, 3 1/2 oz	95	455
Sprouts, Mung bean, raw, 1 cup	100	235
Squash, winter, baked, 1/2 cup	100	470
Strawberries, fresh, 2/3 cup	100	165
Sweet potato, baked, 1 potato, 2″ diameter × 5″	145	340
Tomato, raw, 1 medium	135	300
Tomato juice, canned, 3/4 cup	180	415

Note: Many prepared foods are high in potassium. The above foods can be used to increase potassium content in the diet while not adding a large number of calories.

5. Potassium deficiency has a dietary cause only in cases of actual starvation. Although most foods contain potassium, the richest sources are ~~Apricots~~ Avacado, Pumpkin, and Molasses.

SODIUM

The need of animals and humans for sodium chloride (table salt) has been known for centuries. Salt was so highly valued at one time that it was used for money.

Sodium is also an electrolyte. Approximately half of the sodium in the body is found in extracellular fluids; most of the remainder is in the bones. Daily sodium chloride intake ranges from 7 to 15 grams according to the amount of table salt used. An adult should have only one to three grams in the daily diet. (One teaspoon of table salt contains two grams of sodium.) Salts are readily absorbed and are excreted through urine, feces, and sweat.

The functions of sodium include:

1. Helps in maintaining water balance and osmotic pressures in the body.
2. Helps in maintaining acid-base balance in the body.
3. Aids in the absorption of glucose.
4. Necessary for normal nerve activity.

In general, foods from animal sources are higher in sodium than those from plant sources. In some areas, the water contains sodium; "softened" water has a very high sodium content. Preservatives found in canned and processed foods are also high in sodium.

A deficiency of sodium results in dehydration and, in the severest form, in shock. Deficiency occurs during prolonged vomiting, severe diarrhea, profuse sweating, and adrenal insufficiency. Excessive sodium in the diet causes water retention.

Complete the following:

1. The functions of sodium include:
   A. helps in maintaining water balance & osmotic pressures in the body
   B. helps in maintaining acid-base balance
   C. Aids in absorption of glucose
   D. Necessary for normal nerve activity

TABLE 7. FOODS HIGH IN SODIUM

	Grams	*Sodium (mg)*
Soy sauce, 2 T	35	2665
Pickle, dill, 1 large	135	1930
Beef, dried, 1 oz	28	1219
Sauerkraut, 2/3 cup	100	1170
Frankfurter, 1	50	627
Rice, cooked, salt added, 2/3 cup	135	515
Cheese spreads, 2 T	30	456
Cold cuts, 1 slice	45	369
Buttermilk, 1 cup	240	319
Olives, green, 3 medium	30	308
Potato chips, 1 oz	30	300
Peas, canned, 1/2 cup	100	294
Asparagus, canned, 1/2 cup	100	282
Beans, green, canned, 1/2 cup	100	282
Sausage, pork, 2 links	40	250
Bacon, cooked, 2 slices	15	245
Ham, 1 oz	30	212
Crackers, Rye Krisp, 3 wafers	30	191
Cheese, Cheddar, 1 slice	30	147
Sardines, 1 oz	28	145
Celery, 2 large stalks	80	100
Cornbread, 1 1/2″ cube	35	98

Note: Processed foods usually contain large amounts of sodium and this list is not complete.

2. Foods from animals sources are usually higher in sodium than foods from plant sources.

3. A deficiency of sodium results in dehydration and shock.

4. Excessive ingestion of sodium can cause water retention.

5. Deficiency of sodium may occur during prolonged vomiting, severe diarrhea, profuse sweating, and adrenal insufficiency.

6. Salts are excreted through urine, feces, and sweat.

7. Plan a day's menu that will provide a high sodium intake.

CHLORINE

Closely associated with sodium in the diet, chlorine is necessary for maintaining acid-base balance and aids in maintaining osmotic pressures. It is essential as a part of hydrochloric acid in the stomach.

Most bodily chlorine is found in the spinal fluid and the gastric and pancreatic juices. Deficiencies result from sodium loss during diarrhea, vomiting, and sweating.

The best dietary source of chlorine is table salt. Other good sources are seafoods, milk, meat, and eggs.

Complete the following:

1. The functions of chlorine are:

   A. maintaining acid-base balance

   B. maintaing osmotic pressures

   C. part of hydrocloric acid in the stomach

2. Chlorine deficiency occurs after diarrhea, vomiting, and sweating.

3. The best source of chlorine is table salt.

4. Other good sources are:

   seafood, milk, meat & eggs

SULFUR

Sulfur is found in every cell, but the highest concentrations are in hair, skin, and nails.

Sulfur is essential in the formation of blood clots. It is a part of heparin, thiamin, and biotin. It is a part of compounds used by the body to convert toxic substances to harmless substances.

If there is adequate protein in the diet, the body's need for sulfur is met.

Complete the following:

1. Most of the sulfur in the body is found in the hair, skin, and nails.

2. The functions of sulfur are:

   A. Essential in formation of blood clots

   B. Part of heparin, thiamin & biotin

   C. Part of compounds used by body to convert toxic substances to harmless substances

3. Sulfur is found in ____________ foods.

MAGNESIUM

Over half of the magnesium in the body is found in bone. It activates many enzymes, promotes conduction of nerve impulses, and preserves tooth enamel.

Magnesium deficiency causes tremors and convulsions. Alcoholism, severe protein deficiency (kwashiorkor), and prolonged intravenous therapy of magnesium-deficient fluids can lead to magnesium deficiency.

The best sources of magnesium are soybeans, whole grain cereals, nuts, and cocoa. The RDA for magnesium is 400 milligrams per day for an adult.

Complete the following:

1. Magnesium is necessary for:

   A. Activation of many enzymes

B. Promotes conduction of of nerve impulses

C. Preserves teeth enamel

2. Magnesium deficiency results in tremors and convulsions.

3. The three conditions most commonly leading to magnesium deficiency are Alcoholism, prolonged intravenous treatment, and severe protein deficiency.

4. The best sources of magnesium are soybeans, cocoa, nuts, and whole grain cereal.

OTHER MINERALS

The minerals described below are sometimes called trace elements because they are needed in minute quantities by the body. Deficiencies of these minerals are seldom found as a balanced diet provides the necessary amounts.

SELENIUM. This mineral can replace vitamin E in some reactions and promotes normal growth. The bran and germ part of cereal grain, organ meat, and seafoods are the richest sources. Excessive ingestion of selenium is toxic, but this occurs only in areas where it is used industrially.

MANGANESE. Manganese is essential for enzyme activity and is a part of the enzyme necessary for urea formation. Whole grain cereals and green vegetables are the best sources. Excessive ingestion of manganese interferes with the absorption of iron and the formation of hemoglobin.

COPPER. Copper is associated with hemoglobin formation although it is not a part of hemoglobin and apparently aids in iron absorption. Good sources of copper are organ meats, oysters, nuts, dried beans and peas, cocoa, mushrooms, cherries, and whole grain cereals. The RDA is two milligrams per day.

MOLYBDENUM. This mineral is an essential component of an enzyme involved in uric acid formation and an enzyme that moves iron out of the liver as the body needs it. Peas, beans, and leafy green vegetables are good sources of molybdenum.

COBALT. Cobalt is an essential part of vitamin B_{12}, which aids in the maturing of the red blood cells. Liver, kidney, oysters, and clams are high in cobalt.

FLUORINE. Fluorine, in sufficient amount, reduces the incidence of dental caries and possibly prevents bone loss. Some communities add fluorine to drinking water to prevent dental caries. Excessive fluorine can lead to mottling of the teeth.

ZINC. Zinc is found in many enzymes and may be necessary for the contraction and relaxation of muscles. It is a component of insulin and is essential for growth and for development of the sex glands. The best sources of zinc are meats, milk, egg yolk, oyster, and whole grain cereals. The RDA is 10 milligrams per day for children and 15 milligrams per day for adults. Children, during periods of rapid growth, and pregnant and lactating women are more apt to become marginally deficient in zinc.

OPTIONAL ACTIVITIES TO ENHANCE LEARNING

ACTIVITY 1

Obtain a week's menus from the school cafeteria. Assuming that normal portions of each dish are consumed, compute the amount of calcium that has most likely been *absorbed* during the week. Discuss findings in class and decide whether or not calcium requirements were met.

ACTIVITY 2

Obtain a week's menus from the school cafeteria. Assuming that normal portions of each dish are consumed, compute the amount of iron available during the week. Discuss findings in class and decide whether or not necessary conditions for absorption were present.

ACTIVITY 3

During extremely hot weather when perspiring has been profuse or in conditions when sodium is depleted, it may be necessary to increase sodium intake. Prepare a day's menu that increases sodium intake and is palatable.

BIBLIOGRAPHY

BLOCH, MR: *Human Nutrition: Readings from Scientific American.* WH Freeman & Company, San Francisco, 1978. *The social influence of salt,* pp 13–129.

BRIGGS, GM AND CALLOWAY, DH: *Bogert's Nutrition and Physical Fitness,* ed 10. WB Saunders, Philadelphia, 1979. Chapter 9, *Mineral elements.* Chapter 10, *Water and minerals: The electrolytes (sodium, potassium, and chlorine).* Chapter 11, *Calcium, phosphorus, and magnesium.* Chapter 12, *Trace elements (iron, iodine, copper, manganese, zinc, fluorine, and others).*

CHANEY, MS, ROSS, ML, AND WITSCHI, JC: *Nutrition,* ed 9. Houghton Mifflin, Boston, 1979. Chapter 7, *Calcium, phosphorus, and magnesium.* Chapter 8, *Iron.* Chapter 9, *Iodine.* Chapter 10, *Other mineral elements.* Chapter 13, *Water and electrolyte balance.*

COLLIER, DR: *Fluorine: An essential element for good dental health.* Contemporary Nutrition 4(10), October, 1979.

DAMON, GE: *A primer on dietary minerals.* FDA Consumer Memo, September, 1974.

DARBY, WJ: *Why salt? How much?* Contemporary Nutrition 5(6), June, 1980.

FELVER, L: *Understanding the electrolyte maze.* American Journal of Nursing, 80(9), September, 1980.

GREELEY, S AND SANDSTEAD, HH: *Zinc in human nutrition.* Contemporary Nutrition 5(4), April, 1980.

KRAUSE, MV AND MAHAN, LK: *Food, Nutrition and Diet Therapy,* ed 6. WB Saunders, Philadelphia, 1979. Chapter 7, *Minerals.* Chapter 9, *Water and electrolytes.*

LEVANDER, OA: *Selenium and human nutrition.* Contemporary Nutrition 5(11), November, 1980.

LINKSWILER, HM AND ZEMEL, MB: *Calcium to phosphorus ratios.* Contemporary Nutrition 4(5), May, 1979.

MARSH, AC, KLIPPSTEIN, RN, AND KAPLAN, SD: *The Sodium Content of Your Food.* Home and Garden Bulletin No 233, US Government Printing Office, Washington, DC, August, 1980.

MERTZ, W: *Trace elements.* Contemporary Nutrition 3(2), February, 1978.

ROBINSON, CH: *Basic Nutrition and Diet Therapy,* ed 4. Macmillan, New York, 1980. Chapter 10, *Fluid and electrolyte balance.*

SUITOR, CW AND HUNTER, MF: *Nutrition: Principles and Application in Health Promotion.* JB Lippincott, Philadelphia, 1980. Chapter 28, *Alteration in fluid and electrolyte balance.*

WILLIAMS, SR: *Mowry's Basic Nutrition and Diet Therapy,* ed 6. CV Mosby, St Louis, 1980. Chapter 6, *Minerals.*

WORTHINGTON-ROBERTS, BS: *Contemporary Developments in Nutrition.* CV Mosby, St Louis, 1981. Chapter 8, *Calcium and sodium.* Chapter 9, *Trace element nutrition.* Chapter 10, *Iron: A case study in nutrient availability.*

9

VITAMINS

OBJECTIVES

Upon completion of this chapter the student should be able to:

- Define: vitamin, avitaminosis, hypervitaminosis.
- Give the functions, sources, and absorption of the fat-soluble vitamins, and discuss the conditions caused by deficient and excessive intake of each.
- Give the functions, sources, and absorption of the water-soluble vitamins, and discuss the conditions caused by deficient and excessive intake of each.

Vitamins are organic food substances needed only in minute quantities by the body but they are essential for proper growth and maintenance. Many of the more than 500 enzymes require the presence of vitamins as catalysts in metabolic processes.

The general functions of vitamins are to:

1. Promote growth.
2. Aid in producing healthy infants.
3. Resist infections.
4. Aid in vital body processes.

New vitamins are still being discovered, and many of the previously identified vitamins have been found to actually consist of several vitamins. Vitamins used to be named by letters of the alphabet. Now they are named by their chemical formula or function.

AVITAMINOSIS. Avitaminosis means "without vitamins" and is the term for vitamin deficiency. The diet must supply vitamins as the body is unable to synthesize most of them. Vitamin deficiency may be due to a dietary lack, to a problem in absorbing the vitamin, or to a condition increasing need for the vitamin. Usually several vitamins are deficient at one time. Because vitamins work closely together, deficiency of one vitamin affects the use of other vitamins.

HYPERVITAMINOSIS. An excessive amount of vitamins results in **hypervitaminosis.** The most common cause is the use of excessive amounts of vitamin supplements. As overdosage of some vitamins causes toxicity, supplements should only be given with a physician's supervision.

PRECURSORS. Some foods supply vitamins in *precursor* form. Precursors can be changed to the vitamin by the body; for example, the body can change *carotene* to vitamin A.

ANTIVITAMINS. Substances that prevent normal use of a vitamin are called antivitamins.

FAT-SOLUBLE VITAMINS

Vitamins are classified as either fat soluble or water soluble. The fat-soluble vitamins are A, D, E, and K. All others are water soluble.

Vitamin A (Retinol)

The first vitamin discovered, vitamin A is essential for growth and development and is especially necessary for the health of epithelial cells. Vitamin A helps the body to resist infections and increases longevity. It is important for good vision, especially night vision; is necessary for proper formation and maintenance of tooth enamel; and is needed by the adrenal glands for the production of corticosterone. Most vitamin A is stored in the liver, but a small amount is stored in fatty tissue. An adult should receive 5,000 international units (IU) of vitamin A daily; pregnant and lactating women, 8,000 IU daily. Generally, children need 2,500 IU of vitamin A per day but this varies with age and size.

One serving of any type of liver provides three to six times the daily requirement of vitamin A. Other good sources of vitamin A are yellow vegetables. Table 8 gives a more detailed list.

Vitamin A and its **precursors** are absorbed into the lymphatic system in the intestinal tract. Absorption of vitamin A is poor when the diet is deficient in fat or protein and is slow during extreme youth and extreme old age.

A deficiency of vitamin A results in night blindness, keratosis, paralysis of the lungs, defective tooth enamel, and increased susceptibility to infection.

Hypervitaminosis A causes bone fragility, enlargement of the spleen, pruritis, nausea, menstrual disorders, and loss of hair. Deficiency is much more common than hypervitaminosis A.

Complete the following statements:

1. Vitamins are organic food substances needed only in minute quantities but they are necessary for:
   A.

   B.

   C.

   D.

2. Vitamins act as **catalysts.** Consult a dictionary and write the definition here.

3. The fat-soluble vitamins are ______________, ______________, ______________, and ______________. All other vitamins are ____________________.

4. Supply definitions for the following:
   Avitaminosis:

TABLE 8. FOODS HIGH IN VITAMIN A

	Grams	*Vitamin A (IU)*
Apricots, 2–3 medium	100	2700
Broccoli, fresh or frozen, boiled, 1/2 cup	85	1900
Carrots, raw, 1 carrot, 71/2″ × 1/8″	80	7900
Chard, Swiss, boiled, 1/2 cup	70	3900
Collards, cooked, 1/2 cup	70	3900
Crab meat, 1/2 cup, packed	100	2300
Dandelion greens, cooked, 1/2 cup	50	6100
Swordfish, broiled, 3 oz	100	2000
Kale, cooked, 1/2 cup	55	4600
Kidney, beef, braised, 31/2 oz	100	1100
Liver:		
Beef, fried, 3 oz	85	45,400
Calf, fried, 3 oz	85	27,800
Chicken, simmered, 1/2 cup, chopped	70	8600
Mangos, raw, 1 cup, diced	165	7900
Melons:		
Cantaloupe, 1/2 melon, or 1 cup, cubed	160	5400
Watermelon, 1/16 of a melon, 2 pounds with rind	425	2500
Mustard greens, cooked, 1/2 cup	70	4100
Pokchoy, raw, 2/3 cup	100	3000
Papaya, raw, 1/2 papaya, or 1 cup, cubed	225	2700
Peaches, peeled, raw, yellow, 1 medium	115	1300
Peppers, sweet, red, raw, 1 medium	90	3300
Pumpkin, canned, 1 cup	245	15,700
Sausage, liverwurst, 1 oz	30	1800
Squash, winter, cooked, 1/2 cup	120	4300
Sweet potatoes, cooked, 1 potato 5″ × 2″	145	9200
Tomato, raw, 1 medium	135	1100
Tomato juice, canned, 3/4 cup	180	1500
Turnip greens, cooked, 1/2 cup	70	4600
Watercress, raw, 10 sprigs	35	1700

Hypervitaminosis:

5. Vitamin deficiencies are caused by:
   A.

   B.

   C.

6. Hypervitaminosis is most often due to:

7. Define precursors.

8. Define antivitamins.

9. One of the fat-soluble vitamins is vitamin A. Its functions include:
   A.

   B.

   C.

   D.

E.

F.

G.

10. Vitamin A is stored in ________________ and ________________.

11. Deficiency of vitamin A causes ____________________________, ____________________________, ____________________________, ____________________, and ____________________.

12. Excessive intake of vitamin A results in:

13. The best sources of vitamin A are:

14. Vitamin A is easily destroyed by heat and light. Fats left in heat and light become ________________. Therefore, old fat would be lacking in ________________.

15. ____________________ and ____________________ cause poor absorption of vitamin A.

Vitamin D (Calciferol)

Vitamin D is known as the "sunshine" vitamin. There are several forms of vitamin D, and one form is made in the body following the action of certain sun rays on the skin. Vitamin D is necessary for absorption and utilization of calcium and phosphorus used for growth and bone structure. It promotes a normal level of calcium in the blood and is necessary for normal tooth eruption and formation.

The best sources of vitamin D are sunshine, cod liver oil, and other fish oils. Vitamin D is synthesized only when the skin is directly exposed to sunshine. But if the skin is covered with clothing or the sun's rays are obscured by clouds, fog or smog, or ordinary window glass, vitamin D is not produced. Heavy pigmentation of the skin also interferes with the synthesis of vitamin D. Small amounts of vitamin D are found in many foods including butter, cream, egg yolk, and liver. Because dietary sources do not provide enough vitamin D and because the amount produced in the skin varies widely with the amount of exposure to sunshine, the Council of Foods and Nutrition of the American Medical Association decided that milk should be fortified with 400 IU of vitamin D per quart. Vitamin D is stored in the liver, skin, brain, and bone.

The exact vitamin D requirement is still not known but 400 IU per day prevents symptoms of deficiency. A deficiency of vitamin D chiefly affects the bones and teeth, causing rickets in children and osteomalacia in adults.

Hypervitaminosis D is a toxic condition causing nausea, appetite loss, headache, and changes in bone structure. There is also a tendency to renal calculi formation.

Complete the following statements:

1. Since Middle Ages, cod liver oil has been used to treat rickets, although it was not known at that time that cod liver oil contained the substance we know as ________________ .

2. What are the functions of vitamin D?

3. Vitamin D is stored in ________________ , ________________ , ________________ , and ________________ .

4. Vitamin D deficiency results in ________________ in children and ________________ in adults because it is necessary for:

5. Too much vitamin D causes:

6. The best sources of vitamin D are:

7. Which foods are fortified with vitamin D?

8. What conditions prevent vitamin D synthesis in the skin?

Vitamin E (Tocopherol)

Vitamin E is an antioxidant, that is, it removes oxygen from a substance or prevents oxygen from combining with that substance. By reducing the amount of oxygen present, vitamin E prevents destruction of vitamin A, vitamin C, and fatty acids. It prevents the destruction of red blood cells by preventing the fatty acids in red blood cells from taking on too much oxygen. It stimulates the production of an enzyme necessary to cell respiration and protects the cell membrane. Some sources attribute the prevention of sterility to vitamin E; however, research has only shown this to be true in animals. It is doubtful that vitamin E is of much use in preventing sterility in humans.

Vitamin E is stored in fatty tissue throughout the body. The pituitary and adrenal glands store the most. It is the most easily obtained of all the vitamins and is found in abundance in seed germ oils, green vegetables, and egg yolk. No deficiency conditions in man have been proven for this vitamin. The RDA for vitamin E per day is: infants, 4 IU; children, 7 IU (depending upon age); men, 15 IU; women, 12 IU; and pregnant and lactating women, 15 IU.

Complete the following:

1. The best source of vitamin E is ______________________ .

2. Vitamin E is stored in ______________________ .

3. The functions of vitamin E are:

Vitamin K (Menadione)

Vitamin K is necessary for normal clotting of blood and for normal liver function. Vitamin K is also known as **menadione,** although this is actually the name of one of the three known K vitamins. One form of vitamin K is produced in the intestines by bacteria. Dietary sources of vitamin K are liver, milk, eggs, soybean oil, and green leafy vegetables. One of the K vitamins is found in fish meal.

Because it is found in so many foods, the usual cause of vitamin K deficiency is a condition interfering with the absorption process in the intestine. The cause of malabsorption is usually a liver disease because bile aids in absorption. The improper use of mineral oil and use of drugs such as antibiotics and salicylates also interfere with the absorption process and with the activity of the bacteria producing vitamin K in the intestine.

A deficiency of vitamin K results in slow blood clotting time and hemorrhages. Because newborn babies have no vitamin-K-producing bacteria in their intestines, they are subject to "hemorrhagic disease of the newborn" unless an injection of the vitamin is given shortly after birth.

It is not known how much vitamin K is needed, but doses of two milligrams daily will correct deficiencies.

Complete the following statements:

1. The sources of vitamin K are:

2. How often should leafy green vegetables be served?

3. The functions of vitamin K are:
   A.

   B.

4. A deficiency of vitamin K leads to ____________________.

5. The ingestion of mineral oil prior to mealtime is contraindicated because:

6. People with diseases of the liver and gallbladder have a tendency to hemorrhage because:

WATER-SOLUBLE VITAMINS

All the vitamins other than A, D, E, and K are water soluble. There is little storage of water-soluble vitamins and they must be ingested daily.

As a group, the more than 12 separate B vitamins are known as vitamin B complex. Although certain ones are studied separately, the deficiency of one of the B vitamins usually means that there is a deficiency of all B vitamins.

Thiamin (Vitamin B_1)

Vitamin B_1, also known as **thiamin,** is necessary for normal growth, normal carbohydrate metabolism, and normal functioning of the heart, nerves, and muscles.

Thiamin deficiency results in retarded growth, loss of appetite, and nerve disorders. The individual is easily fatigued and has digestive problems. A severe deficiency of thiamin causes **beriberi,** in which there is all of the above signs in addition to muscular pain and weakness, edema, and finally cardiac failure.

Although thiamin is very easily absorbed, there is almost no storage, so food containing thiamin must be eaten daily. The best sources of vitamin B_1, are pork, fish, poultry, eggs, soybeans, peanuts, and whole grain cereals and breads (Table 9).

During milling, the part of the grain containing thiamin is removed. To prevent deficiencies, most states require that bread and flour be thiamin enriched.

The average adult needs 1.5 milligrams of thiamin a day. Because few of the best sources of thiamin have more than 0.5 milligram in a serving, several servings of the good sources of thiamin should be on the daily menu.

TABLE 9. FOODS HIGH IN THIAMIN

	Grams	*Thiamin (mg)*
Asparagus, fresh, green cooked, 1/2 cup, cut	100	0.2
Bacon, broiled, drained, 2 strips	25	0.1
Bamboo shoots, 3/4 cup	100	0.15
Cashews, roasted, 1 oz	30	0.1
Cauliflower, raw, 1/2 cup, whole flower buds	50	0.1
Collards, cooked, 1/2 cup	70	0.1
Cowpeas or black-eyed peas, immature, 1/2 cup	80	0.2
Cowpeas or black-eyed peas, mature, dried, cooked, 1/2 cup	125	0.2
Crab meat, 1/2 cup, packed	100	0.2
Ham, baked, 3 oz	85	0.4
Kidney, braised, 3 1/2 oz	100	0.5
Lamb:		
Chop, 1 average	95	0.1
Leg, roasted, lean only, 3 oz	85	0.1
Shoulder, roasted, 3 oz	85	0.1
Liver:		
Beef, 3 oz	85	0.2
Calf, 3 oz	85	0.2
Chicken, 1/2 cup, chopped	70	0.1
Lobster, Northern, cooked, 2/3 cup	95	0.1
Melon, watermelon, 1/16 melon, 2 pounds with rind	425	0.1
Milk:		
2% low fat, 1 cup	245	0.1
Chocolate, low fat, 1 cup	250	0.1
Evaporated, 1 cup	250	0.1
Okra, cooked, 10 pods	105	0.1
Orange, raw, 1 medium	140	0.14
Orange juice, fresh or frozen, 3/4 cup	185	0.2
Oysters, raw, Eastern, 6	120	0.2
Peas, green, frozen, cooked, 1/2 cup	80	0.2
Peas, split, dry, cooked, 1/2 cup	100	0.2
Pecans, 1 oz, 20 halves	30	0.2
Pineapple, diced or crushed, raw, 1 cup	155	0.1
Pineapple juice, 3/4 cup	190	0.1

TABLE 9. *Continued*

	Grams	*Thiamin (mg)*
Pinenuts, piñon, 1 oz, 4 T	30	0.4
Plantain, 1 banana, 11″ × 2″	265	0.2
Pork sausage, 3 links	40	0.3
Potatoes:		
Baked, 1 large	200	0.2
Boiled, pared before cooking, 1 medium	135	0.1
Rice, cooked, white, enriched, 2/3 cup	135	0.2
Sprouts, Mung bean, raw, 1 cup	100	0.1
Sprouts, soybean, raw, 1 cup	100	0.2
Sunflower seeds, hulled, 1/4 cup	35	0.7
Sweet potato, baked in skin, 1, 5″ × 2″	145	0.1
Turnip greens, cooked, 1/2 cup	70	0.1
Walnuts, English, 1 cup halves	100	0.3
Wheat germ, raw, 1 oz	30	0.6
Yeast:		
Dry, active, 1 T	5	0.2
Brewer's, 1 T	5	1.2
Yoghurt, low fat, plain, 8 oz	230	0.1

Note: Many cereal products have been enriched with thiamin and are good sources of this vitamin.

Complete the following statements:

1. The water-soluble vitamins include:

2. Another name for vitamin B_1 is ____________ .

3. The functions of thiamin are:
   A.

B.

C.

4. The very best source of thiamin is ________________ . Other good sources are ______________________ , ______________________ , ________________ , and ________________ .

5. How many servings of whole grain cereals or breads per day are recommended by the National Nutrition Council?

How many servings have you had today?

6. What does a deficiency of thiamin cause?

7. What is the name of the severest form of thiamin deficiency?

What are its symptoms?

8. Where is thiamin stored?

Riboflavin (Vitamin B_2)

Riboflavin, another name for vitamin B_2, is also not stored in the body and must be ingested daily.

Riboflavin is necessary for:

1. Normal growth and vigor.
2. Health of skin and mucosa.
3. Carbohydrate metabolism.
4. Normal function of the eyes.

Riboflavin is found in milk and milk products, heart, kidney, and liver. Other sources are green leafy vegetables and eggs. When grain products are enriched, they contribute a considerable amount of riboflavin to the diet (Table 10). Adults require 1.7 milligrams of riboflavin daily.

A deficiency of this vitamin leads to lesions (cracks) in the corners of the mouth, retarded growth, glossitis, dry scaly skin, and cataract-like symptoms in the eyes. Riboflavin, thiamin, and niacin deficiencies usually occur together.

Complete the following exercise:

1. Riboflavin is another name for ________________ .

TABLE 10. FOODS HIGH IN RIBOFLAVIN

	Grams	*Riboflavin (mg)*
Kidney, braised, 3½ oz	100	4.8
Lamb, leg, roasted, 3 oz	85	0.3
Liver:		
Beef, fried, 3 oz	85	3.6
Calf, fried, 3 oz	85	3.5
Milk:		
Whole, 1 cup	245	0.4
2% low fat, 1 cup	245	0.5
Skim, nonfat, or buttermilk, 1 cup	245	0.4
Chocolate, low fat, 1 cup	250	0.4
Dried, instant, whole, ¼ cup	30	0.4
Dried, instant, nonfat, ¼ cup	35	0.5
Evaporated, 1 cup	250	0.8
Pork, spare ribs, braised, yield from ½ pound raw weight	90	0.4
Sausage, liverwurst, 1 oz	30	0.4
Wheat germ, raw, 1 oz	30	0.2
Yeast:		
Dry, active, 1 T	5	0.4
Brewer's, 1 T	5	0.3
Yoghurt, low fat, plain, 8 oz	230	0.5

2. The best sources of riboflavin are ________________ and ________________, ________________, ________________, and ________________. Other good sources are ________________ and ________________.

3. If grains are ________________, they are a good source of vitamin B_2.

4. Riboflavin deficiency is manifested by ________________ in the corners of the mouth, ________________ growth, ________________ ________________ in the eyes, ________________, and ________________ skin.

Niacin

Niacin is another B vitamin and is also known as nicotinic acid and nicotinamide in the form used as a drug. The amino acid tryptophan is a precursor of niacin. Niacin is necessary for normal growth and health of the skin; normal functioning of the stomach and intestines, nervous system, and circulatory system; and for carbohydrate, fat, and protein metabolism. Niacin is not stored and must be included in the diet each day.

The best sources of niacin are meat, liver, poultry, and peanuts. Other good sources are fish, beans, and whole grain cereals and breads (Table 11).

The recommended daily amount of niacin is 20 milligrams for adults. The greatest need for niacin is apparently during periods of growth.

Large doses of niacin given therapeutically cause flushing of the skin and a throbbing sensation in the head due to the vasodilating effect of the vitamin; however, it is not toxic.

Niacin deficiency is associated with a condition called **pellagra,** in which there are lesions at the corners of the mouth, diarrhea, muscle weakness, and soreness of the tongue. Skin lesions appear, and those on the forearms and backs of the hands are sensitive to light.

Complete the following exercise:

1. The B vitamin niacin is called ________________ or ________________ when it is given as a drug.

2. Functions of niacin include:
   A.

TABLE 11. FOODS HIGH IN NIACIN

	Grams	Niacin (mg)
Chicken:		
Canned, flesh only, 1/2 cup	100	4.5
Creamed, 1/2 cup	120	4.0
Fried breast, 1/2	95	11.5
Roasted, light meat, without skin, 3 1/2 oz	100	11.5
Fish:		
Mackerel, sauteed, 3 average	105	8.0
Salmon steak, broiled, 1 average 6″ × 2″	145	12.5
Salmon, canned, pink, 1/2 cup	110	9.0
Salmon, canned, red, 1/2 cup	110	8.0
Sardines, canned in oil, 3 oz, drained	85	4.5
Swordfish, broiled, 3 oz	100	10.5
Tuna, raw, 1/2 cup	100	6.6
Tuna, canned in oil, 1/2 cup	100	12.0
Tuna, canned in water, 1/2 cup	100	13.0
Kidney, braised, 3 1/2 oz	100	10.5
Lamb chops, loin, broiled, lean and fat, 1 average	95	5.0
Liver:		
Beef, cooked, 3 oz	85	14.0
Calf, cooked, 3 oz	85	14.0
Chicken, simmered, 1/2 cup, chopped	70	8.0
Peanuts, roasted, 1 oz or 30 nuts	30	4.9
Peanut butter, 1 T	15	2.4
Pork:		
Chops, broiled, lean and fat, 1 medium	80	4.5
Loin, roasted, lean and fat, 2 1/2″ × 2 1/2″ × 3/4″	85	4.8
Spare ribs, braised, yield from 1/2 pound raw weight	90	6.1
Tongue, beef, 3 1/2 oz	100	3.5
Turkey:		
Roasted, light meat, 2 slices, 4″ × 2″ × 1/4″	85	9.5
Roasted, dark meat, 4 slices, 2 1/2″ × 1 1/2″ × 1/4″	85	3.5
Veal cutlet, 3 oz	85	4.5

B.

C.

3. Niacin is not stored and must be ______________________.

4. The best sources of niacin are:

5. How many servings of meat should be in the daily diet?

6. How many servings of whole grain cereals or breads should be in the daily diet?

7. The deficiency condition found when niacin is lacking is __________ ____________________.

8. What effect does niacin have upon the blood vessels?

Pyridoxine (Vitamin B_6)

Pyridoxine, vitamin B_6, is necessary for fat, carbohydrate, and protein metabolism and is used in the treatment of nausea and vomiting in pregnancy and in deep x-ray treatment. Recent studies show that it is necessary for the production of antibodies.

The best sources of pyridoxine are liver, yeast, wheat germ, pork, milk, potatoes, and legumes. Pyridoxine deficiency is rare but can occur when a pyridoxine antivitamin, such as isoniazid (INH), is given. A pyridoxine deficiency results in dermatitis, anemia, and weakness.

The need for vitamin B_6 increases during pregnancy and periods of stress such as exposure to radiation and certain drug therapies. After large doses of vitamin B_6 the patient may complain of sleepiness. Otherwise, there is no toxic reaction.

Two milligrams of pyridoxine a day are recommended for adults.

Complete the following exercise:

1. Another name for vitamin B_6 is ______________________.

2. Vitamin B_6 is necessary for:

3. There should be no deficiency of pyridoxine because it is found in so many foods. The best sources are:

4. During pregnancy, pyridoxine is given to alleviate ______________ ______________________ and ______________________. It is also given for the same condition to patients who have had ____________ ______________________.

5. A side effect of therapeutic doses of vitamin B_6 is ______________ ______________________.

6. How many servings of potato should you have per day?

Vitamin B_{12} (Cyanocobalamin)

Combined with the protein of normal body tissue is a vitamin called cyanocobalamin, vitamin B_{12}. This vitamin is believed by some nutritionists to be the extrinsic factor necessary for the prevention of pernicious anemia. It is necessary for the health of nervous tissue and assists in the metabolism of iron and in the maturing of red blood cells. Often vitamin B_{12} is given to persons with nutritional anemia to hasten recovery from the condition.

Vitamin B_{12} is stored in the body, with the greatest amount found in the liver. A diet containing 6 micrograms per day will prevent symptoms of deficiency. Apparently, there is no toxic reaction to large therapeutic doses. Absorption of vitamin B_{12} is poor when the intrinsic factor or hydrochloric acid are lacking in the stomach.

The best sources of this vitamin are liver and kidney. Other good sources are milk, eggs, fish, cheese, and lean meat (Table 12).

Complete the following exercise:

1. Cobalamin is vitamin ________________ . It is necessary for:

2. Vitamin B_{12} is stored in the body, with the ________________ having the highest percentage.

3. The best sources of vitamin B_{12} are ________________________ and ________________ .

4. How often should liver be served?

TABLE 12. FOODS HIGH IN VITAMIN B_{12}

	Grams	*Vitamin B_{12} (mcg)*
Clams, canned with liquid, 3½ oz or ½ cup	100	20.0
Fish:		
Mackerel, sauteed, 3 average	105	9.4
Salmon, steak, broiled, 1 average, 6″ × 2″	145	5.8
Salmon, canned, pink, ½ cup	110	7.6
Salmon, canned, red, ½ cup	110	7.6
Sardines, canned in oil, 3 oz drained	85	8.5
Kidney, braised, 3½ oz	100	30.0
Liver:		
Beef, fried, 3 oz	85	68.0
Calf, fried, 3 oz	85	51.0
Chicken, simmered, ½ cup, chopped	70	17.5

5. Eggs, cheese, and lean meat belong to which group of nutrients?

Pantothenic Acid (Vitamin B_3)

Pantothenic acid, or vitamin B_3 as it was first known, is necessary for fat, carbohydrate, and protein metabolism. It is required for the production of cholesterol, adrenal steroids, and part of the hemoglobin. It is *not* a cure for gray hair in humans, as some advertisers claim.

Only 10 milligrams per day are required. Deficiencies occur only when pantothenic antivitamins are given while the individual's diet is deficient in this vitamin. The symptoms are fatigue, muscle cramps, burning feet, prickling hands, and susceptibility to upper respiratory infections.

Almost all foods contain pantothenic acid but the richest sources are egg yolk, liver, kidneys, yeast, whole grain cereals, and potatoes.

Biotin

Biotin is necessary for carbohydrate and protein metabolism. It aids in the synthesis of fatty acids and is involved in the synthesis of niacin and the digestive enzyme, pancreatic amylase, and other enzymes.

Although the daily requirements are not known, the RDA is 0.3 milligram per day.

Because the average diet provides biotin daily and biotin is also produced by intestinal bacteria, deficiencies occur only if absorption of the vitamin is interfered with. Drugs such as sulfonamide and tetracycline destroy the biotin-producing bacteria. Raw egg white contains an antivitamin that destroys biotin, but only if raw egg white is eaten in enormous amounts. The best sources of biotin are liver, kidney, egg yolk, milk, and yeast.

Folacin (Folic Acid)

Folacin is necessary for protein metabolism and helps convert some amino acids to other kinds of amino acids. Folacin is required for growth and is essential in the production of blood cells.

Adults require 0.4 milligram of folacin daily. The need for folacin is increased by anemia, leukemia, cancer, and alcoholism.

Some drugs used in treating leukemia are folacin antivitamins. Folacin is stored in the liver.

By law, vitamin preparations may not contain more than 0.1 milligram of folacin per dose because the vitamin changes the blood picture in pernicious anemia, a very serious condition, but does not cure the disease. Large amounts of folacin might prevent prompt diagnosis.

Good sources of folacin are liver, kidney, nuts, legumes, green leafy vegetables, and whole grain cereals.

Complete the following:

1. The functions of pantothenic acid are:

2. The symptoms of pantothenic deficiency are:

3. The richest sources of pantothenic acid are ________________, ________________, ________________, ________________, ________________, and ________________.

4. The functions of biotin are:

5. The best sources of biotin are ________________, ________________, ________________, ________________, and ________________.

6. The functions of folacin are:

7. Conditions that increase the need for folacin include ________________ ________________, ________________, ________________, and ________________.

8. Folacin is stored in the ________________.

9. Good sources of folacin are:

Vitamin C (Ascorbic Acid)

Vitamin C, or **ascorbic acid,** is a water-soluble vitamin that is easily destroyed by heat and exposure to air. The addition of alkaline substances to foods containing ascorbic acid also destroys it.

Vitamin C is easily absorbed, but must be consumed each day as the body cannot store it. The best sources are citrus fruits, tomatoes, and raw cabbage. Other good sources are raw leafy green vegetables, berries, and melons (Table 13).

Vitamin C is necessary for normal growth and cell activity. It maintains the strength of blood vessels so that the capillaries do not rupture so easily, helps the body resist upper respiratory infections, and is necessary for normal development of teeth and gums. It aids in the absorption of iron and the metabolism of protein. Wounds and burns require vitamin C for healing.

A deficiency of ascorbic acid causes the individual to bruise easily. Fractures fail to heal properly. There is a tendency to bleed during early stages of pregnancy. A severe deficiency of vitamin C leads to *scurvy,* a condition manifested by sore gums, loose teeth, and bleeding in the mouth.

The RDA for ascorbic acid is 60 milligrams per day. An average serving of citrus fruit juice yields 50 milligrams of ascorbic acid. Vitamin C is destroyed by heat, exposure to air, or alkalis such as baking soda.

Complete the following exercise:

1. Another name for vitamin C is ______________ .

2. Vitamin C deficiency causes:

3. The functions of ascorbic acid are:
   A.

   B.

TABLE 13. FOODS HIGH IN ASCORBIC ACID

	Grams	*Ascorbic Acid (mg)*
Broccoli, fresh or frozen, cooked, 1/2 cup	85	70
Brussels sprouts, fresh or frozen, cooked, 4 large	85	70
Cabbage, raw, 1 cup	70	35
Cauliflower, raw, 1/2 cup, whole flower buds	50	75
Grapefruit:		
raw, 1/2 medium	100	35
canned, unsweetened, 3/4 cup	180	65
canned, sweetened, 3/4 cup	180	60
Kale, cooked, without stems, 1/2 cup	55	50
Kohlrabi, cooked, 1/2 cup, diced	80	35
Lemon juice, 1 T	15	7
Lettuce, loose leaf, romaine, 1 cup, chopped	55	10
Lychee nuts, raw, 10	150	40
Mangos, raw, 1 cup, diced	165	60
Melons:		
Cantaloupe, 1/2	160	59
Honeydew, 1/8	170	40
Watermelon, 1/16, 2 pounds with rind	425	30
Mustard greens, cooked, 1/2 cup	70	35
Orange, raw, 1 medium	140	85
Orange juice, fresh or frozen, 3/4 cup	185	95
Papaya, raw, 1/2 papaya or 1 cup, cubed	225	85
Peppers, sweet:		
Green, raw, 1/2 cup, chopped	75	95
Red, raw, 1 medium	90	150
Pineapple, diced or crushed, raw, 1 cup	155	25
Plantain, 1 banana, 11″ × 2″	265	35
Potato, baked, 1 large	200	30
Tomato, raw, 1 medium	135	30
Tomatoes, canned, 1/2 cup	120	20
Tomato juice, canned, 3/4 cup	180	30
Turnip greens, cooked, 1/2 cup	70	50
Watercress, raw, 10 sprigs	35	30

C.

D.

E.

F.

G.

4. The best sources of vitamin C are:

5. Name the citrus fruits.

6. How often should citrus fruits be served?

7. What are the best substitutes for citrus fruits in the diet?

8. What food have you had today that is high in vitamin C?

9. What happens to a leafy green vegetable that "wilts"?

OPTIONAL ACTIVITIES TO ENHANCE LEARNING

ACTIVITY 1

Obtain labels, or the information from the labels, of vitamin compounds that can be purchased without a prescription. Be sure to include compounds most advertised in the local community. Compare the RDA with the amount of vitamins in the compound. Discuss in class the implication of your findings—possible overdoses, cost, and so forth. Discuss ways to include extra vitamins in the diet without taking vitamin compounds.

ACTIVITY 2

Water-soluble vitamins, particularly ascorbic acid, are lost when produce is exposed to heat and light. Visit the grocery store, the produce market, and any other sources of fresh vegetable in the community. Compare the quality of the produce and discuss in class the implications of your findings.

ACTIVITY 3

Select a group of foods such as cereals. Obtain labels and make a list of the vitamins that have been added. Compare the amounts added to the foods with the RDA. Discuss in class the implications of your findings.

BIBLIOGRAPHY

ANDERSON, TW: *Vitamin C and the common cold.* Contemporary Nutrition 3(10), October, 1978.

BRIGGS, GM AND CALLOWAY, DH: *Bogert's Nutrition and Physical Fitness,* ed 10. WB Saunders, Philadelphia, 1979. Chapter 6, *Vitamins—General information.* Chapter 7, *Fat-soluble vitamins.* Chapter 8, *Vitamin B complex.* Chapter 9, *Vitamin C (ascorbic acid).*

CHANEY, MS, ROSS, ML, AND WITSCHI, JC: *Nutrition,* ed 9. Houghton Mifflin, Boston, 1979. Chapter 11, *The fat soluble vitamins.* Chapter 12, *The water soluble vitamins.*

DELUCA, HF: *Modern views on vitamin D.* Contemporary Nutrition 6(2), February, 1981.

DOWLING, JA: *Human Nutrition: Readings from Scientific American.* WH Freeman & Company, San Francisco, 1978, pp 205–211, *Night blindness.*

HALPERN, SL ET AL: *Quick Reference to Clinical Nutrition: A Guide for Physicians.* JB Lippincott, Philadelphia, 1979. *Rational use of vitamins in practice.*

HERBERT, VD: *Megavitamin therapy.* Contemporary Nutrition 2(10), October, 1977.

KRAUSE, MV AND MAHAN, LK: *Food, Nutrition and Diet Therapy,* ed 6. WB Saunders, Philadelphia, 1979. Chapter 8, *Vitamins.*

LYNCH, SR: *Ascorbic acid and iron nutrition.* Contemporary Nutrition 5(9), September, 1980.

ROBINSON, CH: *Basic Nutrition and Diet Therapy,* ed 4. Macmillan, New York, 1980. Chapter 11, *Vitamins: Introduction and fat-soluble vitamins.* Chapter 12, *water-soluble vitamins.*

Vitamin E. Contemporary Nutrition 2(11), November, 1977.

Vitamin E—Miracle or Myth? FDA Consumer Memo, July/August, 1973.

WILLIAMS, SR: *Mowry's Basic Nutrition and Diet Therapy,* ed 6. CV Mosby, St Louis, 1980. Chapter 7, *Vitamins.*

WORTHINGTON-ROBERTS, BS: *Contemporary Developments in Nutrition.* CV Mosby, St Louis, 1981. Chapter 5, *Vitamin E and the accessory lipid antioxidants.* Chapter 6, *The fat-soluble vitamins A and D.* Chapter 7, *The water-soluble vitamins.*

10

WATER

OBJECTIVES

Upon completion of this chapter the student should be able to:

- Describe the location of water in the body and the results of water deficiency.
- Give the functions and sources of water.
- List the ways the body loses water, differentiating between the normal and abnormal.
- List some fluids that have "empty" calories.

Almost three fourths of total body weight is water. Next to oxygen, it is the most important factor for maintenance of life. A person can live several weeks without food but only a few days without water. Loss of 10 percent of the water in the body causes severe disorders; a loss of 20 percent causes death (Fig. 3). Water is found within and between the tissue cells and is an important component of all body fluids.

About half of the water in the body is found inside the cells, 15 percent is found in the fluid around the cells, and 5 percent in the blood. The remainder

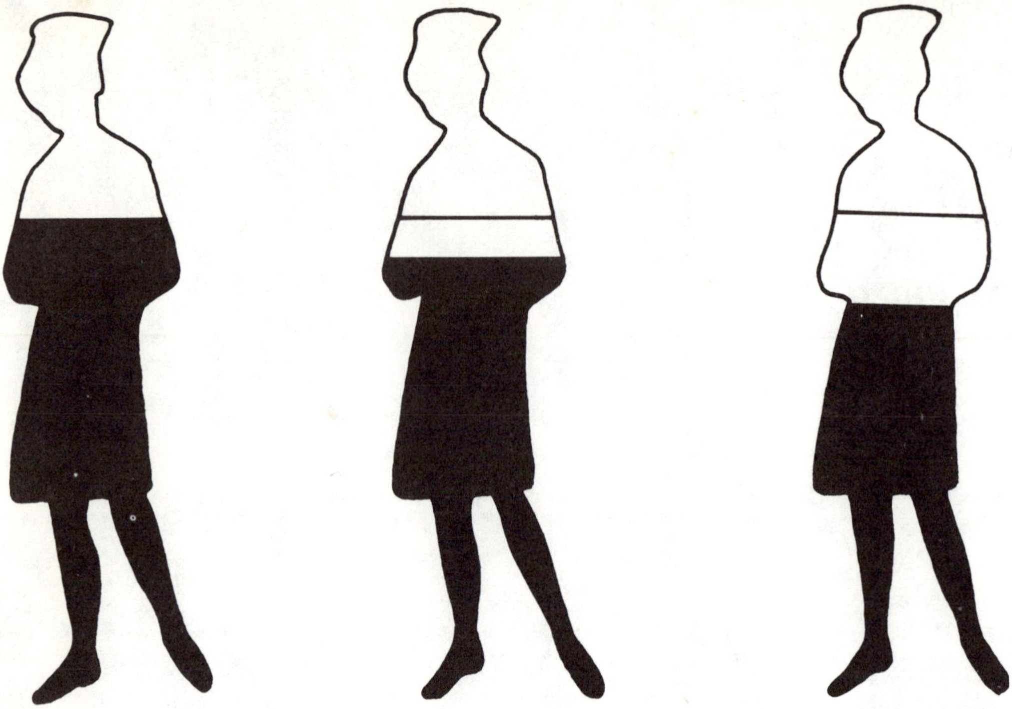

FIGURE 3. *Left,* Almost three fourths of the body is water. *Center,* A 10 percent loss results in severe disorders. *Right,* A 20 percent loss results in death.

is in the other bodily fluids (Fig. 4). Water does not stay in one compartment but moves as conditions change.

The body expresses the need for water as **thirst**. Thirst is controlled by a center in the hypothalamus that reacts to osmotic pressure changes in the blood and fluids. The first signs of water deficiency are dry lips, dry mucous membranes, and dry tongue.

Water in the body fills the following roles:

SOLVENT. Most of the chemicals in the body are in solution. Water aids digestion by softening and liquifying food.

REGULATOR OF BODY TEMPERATURE. As water moves in and out of the cells, it equalizes temperature throughout the body. Water lost through the skin in perspiration and from the urinary tract acts to cool the body.

TRANSPORTATION. Nutrients and body secretions are moved throughout the body as the water moves in and out of the cells.

EXCRETORY AGENT. Waste products are removed from the body dissolved in urine, perspiration, and feces. Water adds bulk in the intestinal tract.

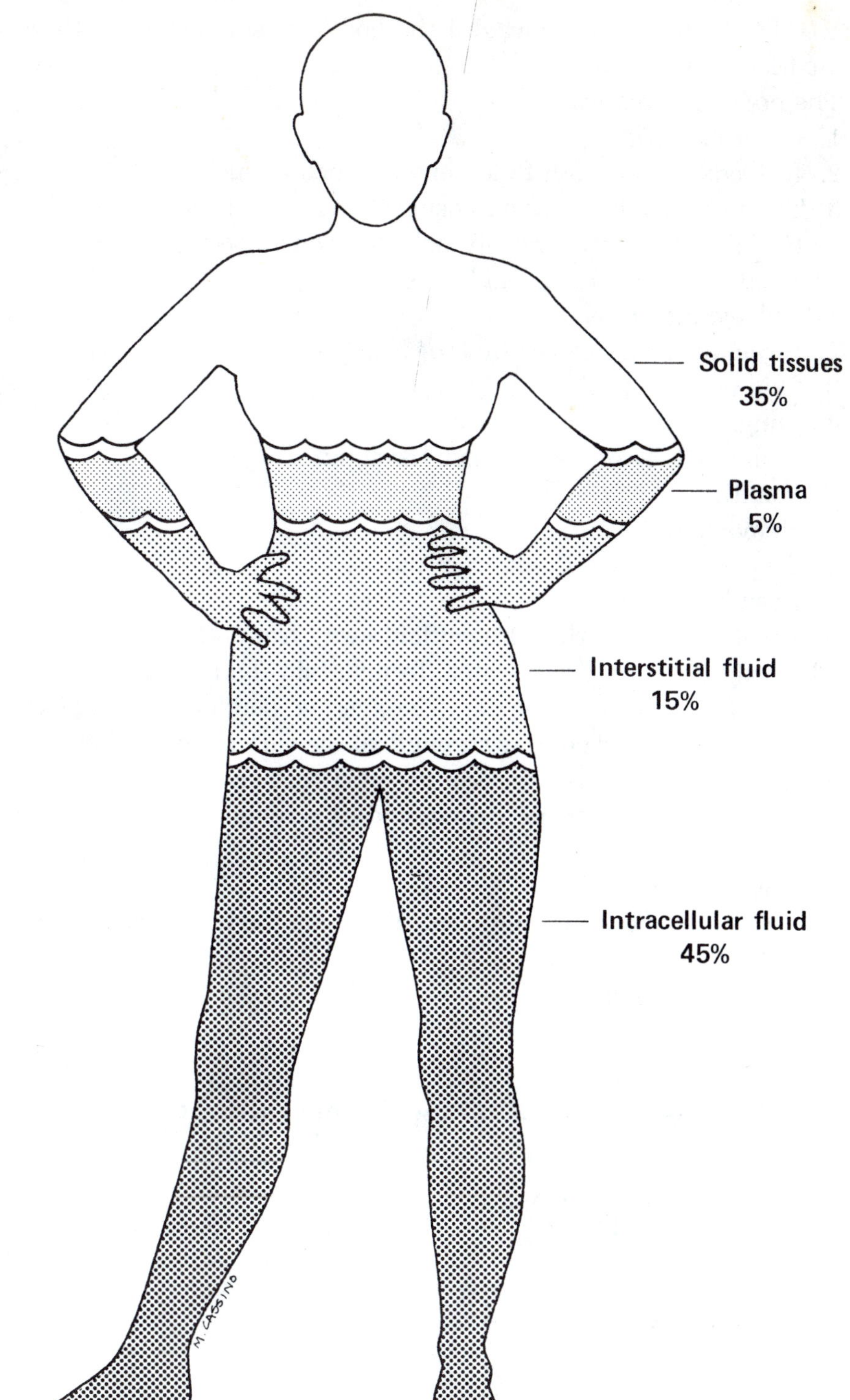

FIGURE 4. Fluid content of the body.

LUBRICANT. The moving parts of the body are surrounded with water to prevent friction and wear.

The body receives water:

1. By drinking it.
2. In foods with a high fluid content, such as melon.
3. Through metabolism and chemical changes of food.
4. By injection (intravenously, subcutaneously, rectally).

The body loses water through the:

1. Kidneys as urine.
2. Bowel as a part of the bulk of feces.
3. Skin as perspiration.
4. Lungs as moisture in the air.

Abnormal losses of water occur through:

1. Vomiting.
2. Hemorrhaging.
3. Seepage of tissue fluids from burns.
4. Draining wounds.
5. Localized edema that draws fluid away from other parts of the body.

The body does not store water. To maintain fluid balance, water intake must equal water output each day. The average person loses approximately 3,000 milliliters of water per day through all the outlets listed above and must take in the same amount. It is recommended that six to eight cups (1,500 to 2,000 milliliters) of water be drunk and the remainder come from other sources.

Complete the following:

1. Water is an essential nutrient. What are the functions of water in the body?

   A. Solvent

   B. Regulation of body temperature

   C. transportation

   D. excretory Agent

   E. Lubricant

2. How does the body receive water?

Drinking, Foods, metabolism & chemical Changes of Food.

3. How much water can the body lose before becoming seriously ill?

10%

4. How much water loss results in death?

20%

5. How does the body lose water?

Urine, Feces, sweat

6. What are the signs of dehydration?

Dry lips, Tongue & mucous membrane

7. What nutrients that we have already studied help the body to retain water?

Sodium

8. Name some fruits and vegetables that have an obvious abundance of water.

Water melon

9. When planning the menu, what dishes can be planned to increase the fluid intake?

Anything that become liquid AT Room Temperature, soup

10. Why are salty broths good for dehydrated patients?

Many fluids we drink have value other than water content. For example, orange juice has water, carbohydrates, and is also an excellent source of vitamin C. A cup of milk yields 170 calories and is a complete protein food.

Some fluids have little value except for carbohydrate content, which adds calories, and water. As sufficient calories are usually ingested in solid foods each day, fluids that contain essential nutrients such as minerals and vitamins should be chosen. Fluids containing nothing but water and calories are called "empty" calorie drinks. For example, a coke, has 68 calories but almost no other valuable factor.

Complete the following exercises:

1. Keep a record of your water and other fluid intake for a 24-hour period. Use the same method as you did in recording your food intake.

Fluid	*Amount*	*Essential Nutrients in Fluid Other than Carbohydrate*

Total:

2. Did your fluid intake for the 24-hour period equal the amount recommended?

3. How many milliliters of the fluids contain "empty" calories?

4. What foods did you eat during the 24-hour period that were high in water content?

OPTIONAL ACTIVITIES TO ENHANCE LEARNING

ACTIVITY 1

Some foods contain approximately 90 percent water. Select samples of celery, melon, lettuce, green beans, and orange. Weigh each sample on a scale that is calibrated in milligrams. Take each sample and crush or press as much water from it as possible. Weigh the sample again and compute the amount of water that was in the food.

ACTIVITY 2

The oxidation of food in the body produces water as an end product. It is obvious that this end product leaves the body through urine, perspiration, and feces, but it is not so obvious that water also leaves the body during respiration. Obtain a large test tube and breathe into it. Observe what happens. Then jog in place for five minutes. Again breathe into the test tube. Compare the findings.

BIBLIOGRAPHY

BRIGGS, GM AND CALLOWAY, DH: *Bogert's Nutrition and Physical Fitness,* ed 10. WB Saunders, Philadelphia, 1979. Chapter 10, *Water and minerals: The electrolytes (sodium, potassium, and chlorine).*

CHANEY, MS, ROSS, ML, AND WITSCHI, JC: *Nutrition,* ed 9. Houghton Mifflin, Boston, 1979. Chapter 13, *Water and electrolyte balance.*

ROBINSON, CH: *Basic Nutrition and Diet Therapy,* ed 4. Macmillan, New York, 1980. Chapter 10, *Fluid and electrolyte balance.*

SUITOR, CW AND HUNTER, MF: *Nutrition: Principles and Application in Health Promotion.* JB Lippincott, Philadelphia, 1980. Chapter 28, *Alteration in fluid and electrolyte balance.*

11

NUTRITION IN PREGNANCY, INFANCY, ADOLESCENCE, AND OLD AGE

OBJECTIVES

Upon completion of this chapter the student should be able to:

- Adjust the daily diet of a woman to meet the nutritional requirements for pregnancy and lactation.
- List the advantages of breast feeding, comparing human milk and cow's milk.
- Describe formulas, their preparation, and sterilization.
- Given a child's age, plan the daily diet of the child and discuss some points to remember about feeding a child.
- Plan the daily diet of an adolescent, and discuss some of the points to remember about feeding an adolescent.
- Discuss snacks and convenience foods as sources of nutrients.
- Plan the daily diet of an elderly person, and discuss some principles involved.

PREGNANCY

Nutrition for pregnancy does not start with conception; it starts many years before. Both mother and baby will fare better if the mother enters a pregnancy well nourished and in the habit of eating a well-balanced diet. Frequent pregnancies can deplete a woman's nutritional reserves.

The pregnant woman should have an adequate diet based upon the recommendations in Chapter 2 (The Daily Diet) and should increase her milk intake to one quart per day. She is not "eating for two" and excessive food intake should be avoided, at the same time neither should she be on a starvation diet. Her caloric intake should remain at the nonpregnant level until the last three months of pregnancy, at which time a 300 calorie increase may be allowed. A nutritionally adequate diet helps prevent toxemia, premature birth, and infant death.

Normal weight gain is about 24 pounds, with most of this gain occurring in the last trimester. By six months postpartum, the woman should be at her normal weight.

The menu of the pregnant woman should include foods that increase her daily intake of the following substances for the reasons given:

PROTEIN. To provide for the tissue growth of the fetus and for tissue maintenance in the mother's body, she should choose complete proteins. She will receive sufficient essential amino acids if at least two thirds of the proteins are from meat, eggs, cheese, and fish. An extra 30 grams of protein per day is recommended. (One ounce of meat and one pint of milk will add needed protein, calcium, phosphorus, zinc, chromium, and iron.)

CALCIUM. To provide for skeletal growth in the fetus, the mother needs 1.2 grams per day. One quart of milk per day is recommended. When caloric intake is a problem, skim milk can be used. If the mother does not like the taste of milk, she can use dried skim milk in her cooking. (Five tablespoons of dried milk equals one pint of whole milk in calcium content.)

PHOSPHORUS. To provide for skeletal and muscle growth in the fetus, the mother should have adequate phosphorus. (Refer to Chapter 8 for sources of dietary phosphorus.)

IRON. A diet high in iron is necessary to counteract tendencies toward anemia in the mother and to build an iron reserve for the fetus. The RDA is 18 milligrams. Supplementary iron is needed if the woman enters pregnancy in a poor nutritional state.

IODINE. This mineral is needed to provide the thyroxine necessary for growth and development of the fetus. The mother will also need more thyroxine because of her increased metabolism. The RDA for iodine during pregnancy is 125 micrograms. Iodized salt will supply this.

VITAMIN A. The RDA for vitamin A is 8,000 IU. This is necessary for cell integrity and tooth formation in the fetus. Excessive intake should be avoided as it can cause malformations in the fetus.

VITAMIN B COMPLEX. Although these vitamins should be increased, the need will be met as food intake increases. The RDA for the B vitamins are: thiamin, 1.7 milligrams; riboflavin, 2 milligrams; niacin, 20 milligrams; pyridoxine, 2.5 milligrams; folacin, 0.8 milligram; B_{12}, 8 micrograms; biotin, 0.3 milligram; and pantothenic acid, 10 milligrams.

VITAMIN C. The RDA is 60 milligrams. This vitamin aids in iron absorption in the mother and is so essential to tissue development in the fetus that the vitamin C content in the fetus' blood is two to four times as much as the mother's blood.

VITAMIN D. This vitamin is necessary to aid in absorption of calcium and phosphorus. One quart of vitamin-D-fortified milk supplies the required 400 IU. Excessive vitamin D should be avoided because it can cause abnormalities in the fetus.

VITAMIN E. Although this vitamin is necessary for normal development of the fetus, a well-balanced diet supplies all that is needed.

VITAMIN K. There is no recommended allowance but a well-balanced diet provides an adequate amount. Vitamin K is important, especially during the last three months of pregnancy, to protect the fetus from prothrombin deficiency, which leads to hemorrhagic disease of the newborn. To prevent this, some physicians give the infant vitamin K immediately after birth.

The pregnant woman should be encouraged to eat whole grain cereals and breads, green leafy and yellow vegetables, and fresh fruits for their cellulose content as well as for their vitamin and mineral content. Iron can be provided by eating liver once a week and one egg each day. Having several small meals during the day helps prevent nausea, controls the appetite, and prevents discomfort from pressure within a crowded abdomen.

Because before birth, waste products from the fetus must be excreted by the mother, an adequate amount of water each day is important. Six to eight glasses are recommended.

Complete the following exercises:

1. The pregnant woman requires ________________ of milk daily.

2. How many calories per day should the pregnant woman have during the first six months of pregnancy?

3. Why is milk so important in the diet of the pregnant woman?

4. Including milk, how much fluid should the pregnant woman have per day?

5. The pregnant woman has a tendency toward constipation, which is alleviated by a diet high in roughage, or cellulose. What foods can she eat to obtain needed cellulose?

6. Why should the pregnant woman be sure to include liver and egg in her diet?

Pregnancy during adolescence must be treated individually. The diet must be planned to meet the needs of the mother's growing and maturing body as well as the needs of the fetus. The energy output of teenagers may be greater than that of a woman. All too often, the young mother-to-be already has poor dietary habits and enters the pregnancy with a deficient nutritional status. More infants born of teenagers die than those born to mature women.

Nutrition During Labor

During labor, the woman's body concentrates upon the activities leading to the child's birth. Those systems not directly involved temporarily suspend or slow their activity. Activity of the digestive system is slowed and food ingested during labor is usually retained in the stomach for 12 to 48 hours. The woman in active labor should not have foods or fluids as she may regurgitate stomach contents into the lungs, particularly if she receives an anesthetic. If she becomes dehydrated, fluids can be given intravenously.

Lactating Women

The lactating mother produces approximately 850 milliliters of breast milk per day. She must receive adequate nourishment to produce this. Her caloric intake should be increased (over the nonpregnant needs) by 500 calories per day and five cups of milk and about one quart of other fluids should be taken each 24 hours. Because breast milk is a protein food, her protein intake should increase (over the nonpregnant needs) by 20 grams per day. She needs an increased amount of calcium, phosphorus, and iron, as well as vitamins A, riboflavin, thiamin, and ascorbic acid. The calcium intake should be 400 milligrams more (over the nonpregnant needs).

The caloric increase is needed to replace the energy expended in caring for a small baby and in producing the breast milk. The greater amount of protein increases the yield of breast milk. Iron is needed to replace iron lost in the postpartum menstrual flow. Little iron is transferred to breast milk.

The only dietary restriction for lactating women is to avoid gas-forming, spicy, or otherwise irritating foods.

Complete the following exercises:

1. The lactating woman requires ________________ of milk daily.

2. In addition to milk, she should also have about ________________ of other fluids.

3. The lactating woman will want to continue eating liver and egg because:

4. Why should the lactating woman be careful to include proteins in her diet?

5. The lactating woman continues to need an increased amount of calcium and phosphorus. What food should she include in her diet to obtain these?

INFANCY

Breast Feeding

The advantages of breast feeding are:
1. Breast milk is the correct formula for the baby.
2. Breast milk is of the right temperature.
3. Immune bodies are present in breast milk.
4. The milk is bacteria free when the baby gets it.
5. It is convenient, as the milk does not have to be prepared or stored.
6. Breast milk is more economical.
7. Infants on breast milk develop fewer allergies.

A comparison of human milk and cow's milk reveals that:
1. The caloric value is about the same.
2. Cow's milk is more constipating because it contains less sugar (lactose) than human milk.
3. Cow's milk has more protein and calcium.
4. Cow's milk forms large hard curds in the stomach; breast milk forms small soft curds.
5. Human milk contains antibodies to prevent disease in the baby, which cow's milk does not.
6. Human milk has slightly more iron and vitamins A and C than cow's milk.

Feeding of Formulas

Formulas are made of milk, sugar, and water.

Milk provides the protein in the formula, and the type of milk used varies with the need of the infant. It can be homogenized, evaporated, dried, specially prepared (such as acidified milk, which forms smaller curds), cow's milk, or milk from other animals.

Corn syrup or cane sugar are the easiest forms of sugar to use, although the doctor may prescribe special preparations of lactose or maltose. The caloric content of the formula is easily varied by adjusting the amount of sugar.

The amount of water added to the formula will be determined by the amount of milk used and the total volume of formula needed for the day's feedings. The baby requires about two ounces of water per pound of body weight per day.

If the infant is allergic to animal proteins, a soybean formula may be given. If the baby has difficulty digesting milk proteins, lactic acid may be added to the formula to make smaller curds, which are easier to digest.

There are two methods of preparing formulas. In the older method, all equipment and the water are sterilized, and the formula is prepared under aseptic conditions. In the *terminal sterilization method*, the equipment and the water are clean but not sterile. After preparation of the formula, the bottles are filled; then, the bottles of formula are sterilized. The terminal sterilization method is easier, and there is less danger of contaminating the formula. This method can be used on all types of formula except those containing lactic acid.

Disposable containers can be purchased today and are usually used with a holder. The collapsible portion is filled with sterilized formula in such a manner that no air is left in the container. As the infant nurses, the container collapses like a balloon and the infant has less chance of sucking air. The empty container is thrown away.

Schedule of Feeding

The newborn baby may require as many as 12 feedings per day. At about six weeks of age, the 2:00 AM feeding is usually discontinued. By the sixth month, the baby will no longer need the 10:00 PM feeding and will sleep all night.

A baby from 2 to 7 months old requires 117 calories per kilogram of body weight. From the sixth through the twelfth month, the baby needs 108 calories per kilogram. A baby's stomach has a capacity of about 2 tablespoons at birth. As the baby grows, the size of the feedings should be increased. Most pediatricians add cereals, pureed foods, and mashed egg yolk to the diet. Because milk is deficient in iron, vitamin D, and vitamin C, pureed liver, and mashed egg yolk are given to furnish iron. (Egg whites are not usually given until the baby is a year old as they sometimes cause allergic reactions.) Vitamin compounds high in vitamins A and D, or cod liver oil, are usually ordered daily. Diluted orange juice may be given to increase the vitamin C intake. Between feedings, the baby should be offered water, which has been boiled, particularly during hot weather.

When starting solid foods, one new food should be introduced at a time. Mild flavored foods are most readily accepted, although it is the feel of the food, not the taste, that the baby may object to. At the age of 1 year, chopped vegetables are substituted for strained ones.

Between the ninth and the twelfth months, the mother will begin to wean the baby. The number of feedings and the amount fed should be gradually decreased. By this time, the child should be accepting solid foods well. It is wise to start teaching the baby to drink milk from a cup a few months before starting to wean.

When teething, the baby enjoys chewing on zwieback or oven-dried bread.

As baby develops:

1. Use a feeding schedule but be flexible.
2. Remember that each baby is an individual.
3. Allow the child to self-feed as soon as the child wishes to.
4. Help the child when the child tires.
5. Remember that manners can be taught after the child masters the fundamental skills of eating.
6. Remember the size and strength of baby hands when purchasing utensils or sizing the baby's food.
7. At birth, the stomach holds 2 tablespoons; at 1 year, it holds 1 cup; as an adult it will hold 2 quarts. Plan meals accordingly.
8. Remember that overfeeding the infant can lead to a lifelong habit of overeating. Satisfy the child's hunger; do not force feed.

Complete the following exercises:

1. The advantages of breast feeding are:

   A.

   B.

   C.

   D.

   E.

   F.

   G.

2. What are the differences between breast milk and cow's milk?

   A.

   B.

C.

D.

E.

F.

3. What is the primary function of milk in a formula?

4. Why is sugar added to the formula?

5. What is the usual age for weaning an infant? How is this best accomplished?

6. Milk is deficient in iron, vitamin C, and vitamin D. What foods are added to the baby's diet to make up for this deficiency?

7. Describe the terminal method of sterilization of formula.

8. Which feeding is usually discontinued first?

9. As the baby gets older, the rate of growth is less in proportion to the baby's size. How does this affect the child's caloric need?

10. Common sense should govern the mother's attitude toward her baby's feeding as the baby develops. What are some of the common-sense rules she should remember that will help to make mealtime more pleasant for her and the baby?

CHILDHOOD

A well-balanced diet is as important for a child as for an adult. Because children grow rapidly, they need approximately 2 grams of protein for each kilogram of body weight. Children need food high in calcium, iron, and vitamin D. They should get at least one pint of milk each day. Additives to milk, such as chocolate, should be avoided. Stimulants such as coffee or tea should be restricted. Four to six glasses of water are needed daily.

The child's attitude toward eating will change several times during childhood. Patient, consistent parental discipline will help prevent formation of bad habits. A healthy attitude toward eating will be encouraged if:

1. Mealtimes are happy times.
2. Foods are simply prepared and easily handled by a child.
3. A short "settling down" time is provided before meals so that the child will not come to the table excited and boisterous.
4. It is recognized that a child's appetite varies at each stage of growth. As long as weight and growth are maintained, parents should not worry.
5. Meals are served at fairly regular times.
6. Simple, nutritional snacks are provided between meals as long as they do not interfere with the appetite at mealtimes.
7. Small servings are provided, as they are more appetizing.
8. Children are allowed to help to plan and prepare their meals. This may help them to accept a wider variety of foods.
9. A variety of foods are presented at an early age to prevent the formation of food dislikes.

10. The child is not allowed to use not eating as an attention getter.
11. Eating with the family is used to teach manners. (It is an excellent method, but the adult members of the family must remember that the child observes *all* things, bad as well as good.)

Complete the following exercises:

1. The young child is going through a period of rapid growth and development. Which nutrient is especially needed?

2. Which nutrients are needed for skeletal growth?

3. What foods supply the nutrients needed for bones?

4. A child's nervous system is sensitive to even mild stimulants. Therefore, stimulating foods should be avoided. Name some stimulating foods.

5. Which would be the better way to prepare carrots for a young child?

   ________ Buttered carrots ________ Carrots timbale

6. Which of the following would be a good mid-afternoon snack for a child?

   ________ Peanut butter sandwich ________ Jelly sandwich
   ________ Orange ________ Popsicle
   ________ Chocolate kisses ________ Carrot and celery sticks

7. What size should a child's serving be?

8. One of your neighbors has a 3-year-old child whose appetite has declined. The neighbor tells you that the child has maintained weight and has even grown a little taller. After suggesting that the neighbor consult the child's doctor if the loss of appetite is really alarming, you can explain that a child's appetite ______________________________ ____.

ADOLESCENCE

The adolescent period is also one of growth, although it may occur in spurts. The following should be borne in mind when planning the teenager's diet:

1. There is still a great need for protein, from 1½ to 2 grams per kilogram of body weight.
2. Milk is still important although ingenuity may be necessary to get the adolescent to take it.
3. A well-balanced diet high in calcium, iron, and vitamin D is important, especially for girls past the menarche.
4. Teenagers should be made to understand the importance of eating raw fruits and vegetables for their vitamin content.
5. They should drink four to six glasses of water a day to help in eliminating waste products from the body, which in turn will help to keep the skin clear.
6. Stimulants such as coffee and tea should be restricted.

Because adolescence is a time of emotional as well as physical development, parents may find it difficult to control dietary habits as the youngsters try to assert their maturity. At this age, children want to be like, eat like, and act like their peers. As a group, they try to emulate their hero or heroine. Parents can use this desire to encourage good diet habits. For the boys, the nutritional program of a favorite athlete can be a good example. Girls may desire to have the figure or skin of a well-known actress. A discussion of the necessary dietary regimen may help.

Many teenagers, particularly girls, skip breakfast. The omission of breakfast seriously depletes energy—many active adolescents still need to take between meal nourishment to prevent fatigue. Without breakfast, the body never gets a chance to prepare for the day. There is no reason that breakfast has to be the traditional eggs and bacon. A peanut-butter sandwich is better than no breakfast at all; our ancestors enjoyed steak or fish as their first meal of the day.

Provide answers to the following questions:

1. The adolescent needs $1\frac{1}{2}$ to 2 grams of protein per kilogram of body weight each day. Why?

2. What are some ways for the teenager who is "too big to drink milk" to get the milk needed?

3. How much water should a teenager have each day?

4. Charles is 15 years old. When he gets hungry at school, he can purchase a coke, a candy bar, or ice cream in the snack bar. Which would be the best choice?

   Why?

5. Mary is "going through a phase." She refuses to eat the same breakfast as the rest of the family and has asked for one of the following menus. Place a check before any you would allow her to prepare for herself.

   _____ Hamburger and glass of milk.
   _____ Peanut butter and mashed banana sandwich with a glass of pineapple juice.
   _____ Vanilla malt and cream puff.
   _____ Tuna fish salad.

ATHLETES

The athlete should have a well-balanced diet with an increase in calories, sodium, and water. The amount of physical activity and its duration determines the number of calories required by the athlete, male or female. Sodium, potassium, and other electrolytes lost in perspiration can be replaced by the addition of salt to season foods and by eating a variety of fruits, such as oranges, and vegetables. Water loss, as evidenced by weight loss and concentrated urine, should be replaced at frequent intervals.

If the activity takes place in a very hot atmosphere, potassium loss as well as sodium and water loss is increased. Drinks advertised almost always have too much sodium and potassium and should be used sparingly. Salt tablets should be taken only on a physician's advice; an overdose of sodium can occur and severe dehydration result.

Protein, carbohydrates, minerals, and vitamins are readily supplied in sufficient quantity by a well-balanced diet. No supplement is needed although many athletes attempt to better their performance by "dosing" themselves.

Prior to an activity, the athlete will probably want to eat a meal that is easily and quickly digested, usually with limited fat. There should be sufficient calories to sustain the athlete throughout the activity.

Complete the following:

1. What nutrients are increased in the athlete's diet?

2. What foods are high in sodium?

3. What foods are high in potassium?

4. How much water should an individual drink per day?

5. Name three signs that someone should drink more water.

6. What is the effect of fat on digestion time?

7. An excessive intake of salt tablets can lead to ______________________ ______________________.

OLD AGE

Changes in metabolism, lessened functioning of the digestive tract, and reduced activity reduce the need of the elderly for some nutrients and increase the need for others.

The senses of taste and smell change, causing food to apparently change flavor. For many, the only taste buds that retain acute function are those that record sweet tastes.

Reduced salivary gland activity leads to a dry mouth, making it difficult to chew and swallow with ease. Loss of teeth is common, causing problems with biting and chewing.

Digestive problems include weakness of intestinal movement and decreased secretion of digestive enzymes. Weakened intestinal movement predisposes the elderly to constipation. Intestinal gas is increased when food is improperly digested and remains in the intestines longer than usual.

CALORIES. Caloric content of the diet depends largely upon the level of physical activity maintained and the physical condition of the individual. Aging is not a calendar affair; people age at their own rates. However, all should reduce caloric content in the diet as the metabolism slows. A diet of fewer than 1800 calories does not provide all needed nutrients.

CARBOHYDRATES. Because starches contain many essential vitamins and minerals, calories should be reduced by restricting sugars. Whole grain cereals and breads, potatoes, and dried legumes supply vitamins, minerals, and fibers.

FATS. Fat consumption by the elderly should be reduced. Fats often cause indigestion in the elderly due to reduction in flow of gastric, liver, and pancreatic juices necessary for the assimilation of fats and their consumption can contribute to problems with blood cholesterol and arteriosclerosis. Their "concentrated energy" is not necessary with the reduced caloric requirement in old age.

PROTEIN. Protein needs increase to 1 gram per day because there is less digestion and absorption of protein. Protein is necessary to prevent the wasting away of muscle tissue.

MINERALS. Calcium and iron are important in the diet of the elderly as absorption and utilization of minerals are not as efficient as in younger persons. Most elderly persons neglect to select foods high in minerals.

VITAMINS. A sufficient intake of vitamins is important. Niacin and vitamin A are of primary importance in preventing senility.

WATER. Water is needed to ease the burden of the "tired" kidney and to help with the problem of constipation. Because of lessened activity, the elderly seldom drink enough fluids.

CELLULOSE. The diet of the elderly is usually deficient in bulk due to denture problems. Bulkage is necessary to prevent constipation and can be supplied by preparing foods high in cellulose in ways in which they are chopped finely or ground.

In planning a diet for the elderly, the following principles should be observed:

1. Avoid foods that might cause digestive disturbances, such as cabbage, fried foods, rich dressings, gravies, and sauces.
2. When chewing is difficult, meat may be chopped or ground, and vegetables may be chopped or pureed.
3. Plan to serve a hot dish at each meal.
4. Clear soups and relishes help stimulate the appetite.
5. If the main meal is served in the middle of the day and the lighter, more easily digested meal in the evening, there are fewer digestive upsets and sleep is less likely to be disturbed. However, if the evening meal is served early, it is best for it to be the main one as the patient is less likely to complain of hunger during the night, and the early hour allows sufficient time for digestion before sleep.
6. It may be desirable to divide the food for the day into five light meals instead of three large ones. This will aid in digestion and avoid distress.
7. Foods should be simply prepared. Combination dishes are not well accepted or desired.
8. A cup of warm milk at bedtime will often help to induce sleep.
9. Older persons tend to take an inadequate amount of fluids. They will take warm fluids more readily than cold; warm tea and broth taken either between meals or at mealtime will help increase their fluid intake.

10. Meals should be attractive in color, texture, and flavor in order to appeal to the appetite.
11. Serve smaller helpings to whet the appetite.
12. The diet should include all essential nutrients. (Often older people will neglect protein, vitamin C, and calcium intake.)
13. Milk is important and, if the elderly person objects to drinking milk, whole or skim milk can be added to recipes. Dried milk is excellent used in cooking.
14. The general attitude of the older person should be evaluated; indifference to life will be reflected in indifference to food.

Complete the following exercises:

1. In planning the diet of the elderly, certain nutrients should be increased and others decreased. Write "increased" or "decreased" in the spaces below:

   Carbohydrates ________________ Minerals ________________
   Fats ________________ Vitamins ________________
   Protein ________________ Water ________________

2. Why should cabbage, dried beans, and fried foods be avoided in the diet of the elderly?

3. If the elderly person has no appetite, what foods could you give to stimulate it?

4. Name some ways to increase the daily intake of milk by the elderly.

5. How should the food for the elderly be prepared?

Plan a day's menus including snacks, following the basic four groups and including all the essential nutrients, for the following persons:

DAY'S MENU

	5-Year-Old Boy	*14-Year-Old Girl*	*75-Year-Old Man with Dentures*
Breakfast:			
Lunch:			
Dinner:			

OPTIONAL ACTIVITIES TO ENHANCE LEARNING

ACTIVITY 1

Case Study

Marcia J., 24 years old, is in her second month of pregnancy. She is five feet four inches tall and weighs 106 pounds. This is her first pregnancy. Her appetite has been good up until three weeks ago, at which time she developed some nausea early in the morning. She complains of some frequency of urination but has no burning or discomfort on voiding. She works as a program analyst with a computer service. She usually has toast and coffee for breakfast and again during morning break. Her lunch often consists of yoghurt and a cookie. The evening meal is the largest, usually composed of a meat, vegetable, and green salad. She is allergic to oranges and seldom eats tomatoes. Beverages at dinner consist of iced tea and wine. Her obstetrician wants her to have a balanced diet with additional calcium intake.

Prepare a nutritional care plan. (See Appendix for example.)

OPTIONAL ACTIVITIES—*Continued*

ACTIVITY 2

Obtain a list of infant formulas sold in the local area. Identify the main ingredient of each, its cost, and the method of preparing for use.

ACTIVITY 3

Visit a kindergarden during mealtime. Observe the size of portions given the children, the children's behavior, the atmosphere of the dining area, and the variety of foods offered. Ask whether or not the children helped plan the menu. List the foods the children ate and those that they did not want to eat. Note whether or not adults ate with the children. Discuss the findings in class and their implications in developing healthy attitudes toward eating.

BIBLIOGRAPHY

AFTERGOOD, L AND ALFIN-SLATER, RB: *Women and nutrition.* Contemporary Nutrition 5(3), March 1980.

BUSSE, EW: *Eating in late life: Physiologic and psychologic factors.* Contemporary Nutrition 4(11), November, 1979.

CARRUTH, BR: *Adolescent pregnancy and nutrition.* Contemporary Nutrition 5(10), October, 1980.

CHANEY, MS, ROSS, ML, AND WITSCHI, JC: *Nutrition,* ed 9. Houghton Mifflin, Boston, 1979. Chapter 14, *Nutrition during the reproductive period.*

CHOI, MW: *Breast milk for infants who can't breast-feed.* American Journal of Nursing 78(5), May, 1978.

CHOW, BF: *The imprint of maternal dietary protein on the metabolic development of the offspring.* Food and Nutrition News, June, 1968.

COMBS, KL: *Staying well while growing old: Preventive care in the elderly.* American Journal of Nursing 78(8), August, 1978.

FORD, B: *Apple pie for breakfast? Mmm. . . .* RN, August, 1970.

HALPERN, SL ET AL: *Quick Reference to Clinical Nutrition: A Guide for Physicians.* JB Lippincott, Philadelphia, 1979. Chapter 3, *Nutrition in pregnancy.* Chapter 5, *Nutrition in the adolescent.* Chapter 6, *Geriatric Nutrition.*

HENTHORN, FY: *Better breakfasts.* American Journal of Nursing 63(8), August, 1963.

HODGES, RE: *Nutrition in Medical Practice.* WB Saunders, Philadelphia, 1980. Chapter 2, *Nutrition in pregnancy and lactation.*

HOFMANN, L: *The Great American Nutrition Hassle.* Mayfield, Palo Alto, California, 1978. Chapter 12, *The elderly.*

Infant Care. DHHS Publication No (OHDS) 80-30015, US Government Printing Office, Washington, DC, 1980.

KRAUSE, MV AND MAHAN, LK: *Food, Nutrition and Diet Therapy,* ed 6. WB Saunders, Philadelphia, 1979. Chapter 13, *Nutrition for pregnancy and lactation.* Chapter 15, *Nutrition in childhood and adolescence.* Chapter 16, *Nutrition in adulthood and later years.*

LAMY, PP: *Nutrition and the elderly.* Journal of Practical Nursing Vol 30, August, 1980.

LEVINE, AS: *The relationship of diet to intestinal gas.* Contemporary Nutrition 4(7), July, 1979.

LINKSWILER, HM AND ZEMEL, MB: *Calcium to phosphorus ratios.* Contemporary Nutrition 4(5), May, 1979.

LOCKHART, JD: *Breast milk.* Contemporary Nutrition 4(1), January, 1979.

LUKE, B: *A lesson in eating for two.* RN 38(11), November, 1975.

MAYER, J: *Nutrition: The secret ingredient in graceful aging?* Family Health Vol 11, November/December, 1979.

MAYER, J: *Eating well after 50.* Family Health, Vol 12, June, 1980.

SELECT COMMITTEE ON NUTRITION AND HUMAN NEEDS, US SENATE: *Medical Evaluation of the Special Supplemental Food Program for Women, Infants and Children.* US Government Printing Office, Washington, DC, August, 1976.

MCWILLIAMS, M: *Nutrition for the Growing Years,* ed 3. John Wiley & Sons, New York, 1980. Chapter 4, *Pregnancy and lactation.*

Nutrition Education for Young Children. DHEW Publication No (OHDS) 76-31035, US Government Printing Office, Washington, DC, 1976.

PHILLIPS, MG: *Food for the Teenager During Pregnancy.* DHEW Publication No (HSA) 77-5106, US Government Printing Office, Washington, DC, 1977.

SERFASS, RC: *Nutrition for the athlete.* Contemporary Nutrition 2(5), May, 1977.

NUTRITION DEPARTMENT: *Special Nutrition Needs for Women.* General Mills, Inc, Minneapolis, 1980.

SUITOR, CW AND HUNTER, MF: *Nutrition: Principles and Application in Health Promotion.* JB Lippincott, Philadelphia, 1980. Chapter 7, *Promoting sound eating habits in pregnancy and lactation.* Chapter 9, *Promoting sound eating habits during childhood and adulthood.*

WILLS, B: *Food becomes fun for children.* American Journal of Nursing 78(12), December, 1978.

WINICK, M: *Nutrition and aging.* Contemporary Nutrition 2(6), June, 1977.

WOODRUFF, CW: *Supplementary foods for infants.* Contemporary Nutrition 6(1), January, 1981.

WORTHINGTON-ROBERTS, BS: *Contemporary Developments in Nutrition.* CV Mosby, St Louis, 1981. Chapter 16, *Nutritional issues related to pregnancy.* Chapter 20, *Diet and athletic performance.*

12

CHOOSING, STORING, AND PREPARING FOODS

OBJECTIVES

Upon completion of this chapter the student should be able to:

- Make the best choice as to purchase of milk, meat, fish, cheese, eggs, legumes, nuts, fruits, and vegetables.
- Select the best method of storing and preparing these foods.
- Differentiate among the various kinds of milk: homogenized, pasteurized, fortified, evaporated, condensed, skim, fermented, and buttermilk.
- Discuss processed foods and give the reasons for their use, their deficiencies and excesses in nutrients, and some advantages in use.
- Suggest snack foods that are nutritious.

Space is too limited in this text for a complete discussion of the choosing, storing, and preparing of food. However, this chapter covers pertinent points on the most common purchases.

MILK

A complete protein food, milk contains all the essential amino acids, is the most important source of calcium, and is one of the best sources of riboflavin. When cow's milk cannot be obtained, milk from other sources can be used.

The number of bacteria present in milk determines the grade. Grade A has the fewest bacteria; grade C has the most. Grades B and C can be used in cooking; only grade A should be served as a drink.

Milk is sold as:

FORTIFIED MILK. Milk that has vitamin D added.

PASTEURIZED MILK. Milk that has been heated to 140°F for 30 minutes to inhibit the bacterial growth.

HOMOGENIZED MILK. Pasteurized milk in which the fat particles have been broken into smaller particles and distributed evenly throughout the milk.

EVAPORATED MILK. Milk from which 50 percent of the water has been removed.

CONDENSED MILK. Evaporated milk with sugar added.

SKIM MILK. Milk from which most of the butter fat has been removed.

DRIED MILK. Milk from which all water has been removed. This can be either whole milk or skim milk.

FERMENTED MILK. Milk that has had bacteria added to cause changes.

BUTTERMILK. Commercially, milk that has had bacteria added.

Milk and all milk products must be stored in the coolest part of the refrigerator as milk is an excellent media for bacterial growth. Containers should be meticulously cleaned before milk is put into them and preferably kept covered.

There are many ways to include milk on the menu other than as a drink. Cream soups are nutritious and delicious. Milk can be served as a dessert in ice cream, puddings, and custards. Either dried whole milk or dried skim milk can be added to dishes such as mashed potato. With a little imagination, the necessary daily requirement of milk for everyone in the family can be met. Milk and milk products should be cooked at low temperatures.

MEAT

Meat forms the "backbone" of a meal. It provides taste and satiety and furnishes protein, iron, phosphorus, and vitamin B complex. Meat can be beef, veal, mutton, lamb, pork, or poultry. Meat is almost entirely digested but the fat content and cooking method determine how fast it is digested. Meat such as beef is usually "aged" to allow enzymes time to tenderize tough connective tissue.

BEEF AND VEAL. Beef is from cattle and veal is from very young calves—the nutritive value is essentially the same. Beef is graded by the amount of fat marbling, the firmness, the redness, and the juiciness of the lean meat. High-quality beef is red and liberally marbled with white fat. Available grades are prime, choice, good, standard, and commercial. The shopper should purchase good to prime beef, depending upon the amount of money budgeted for this item. If in doubt about the grade of beef you are purchasing, look for the small purple United States Department of Agriculture stamp on the meat, which gives the grade.

LAMB AND MUTTON. Lamb is from young sheep and mutton is from mature sheep. Mutton is graded as choice, medium, and cull. Lamb or yearling mutton (from sheep one to two years old) is the best buy for home consumption. In high-quality mutton, the lean meat is deep pink and the fat covering is creamy white and well distributed on the outside. Most people in the United States prefer lamb to mutton. However, removing the fat covering or rubbing mutton with lemon before cooking removes part of the strong flavor some find objectionable.

PORK. Most pork is from mature pigs and is graded choice, medium, and cull. Roasting pigs, commonly called "suckling pigs," are immature and are usually available at holiday time. Fresh, good quality pork has firm, fine-grained lean meat of bright, light red color and firm, white fat evenly distributed over the meat. Pork should always be cooked to the well-done stage.

POULTRY. Chicken, turkey, duck, and goose are all classified as poultry. The best poultry has firm tissue, smooth, blemish-free skin, and well-distributed fat. Poultry of all ages is used in various ways. Chickens may be purchased as fryers, broilers, roasters, or stewing chickens. Turkeys are marketed as fryers and roasters. The shopper who desires a young bird should look for one with a flexible breastbone. The fat content is high in duck and goose and higher in a younger chicken than an older one. Turkey contains approximately the same amount of fat as a stewing chicken. Although poultry is very digestable, white meat is often preferred in special diets as it has less connective tissue and fat than dark meat and is easier to digest. The white and dark meat are equal in nutritive value.

Purchase and Preparation of Meat

Meat can be purchased fresh, frozen, dried, cured, or smoked. Fresh meat should be stored uncovered or loosely covered in the coldest part of the refrigerator.

Pork, veal, and poultry must be cooked until well done to prevent transmission of diseases. The temperature for cooking meat is determined by the method, but a low to moderate temperature generally will yield a tastier, more tender dish. The methods and temperatures used are as follows:

roasting	low temperature
broiling	high temperature
pan-broiling	high temperature
braising	moderate to low temperature
frying	moderate temperature

Boiling meat is not advised except in preparing a base for soup or sauces because the flavor and nutrients are removed.

FISH

Fish has almost the same nutritive value as beef, except that saltwater fish contains more iodine, fluorine, and other minerals. Shellfish, such as oysters and scallops, are especially rich in calcium and iodine. Fresh fish, saltwater or freshwater, should be chosen for firm tissue, clear bulging eyes, and tight scales. Fish, except for shellfish, is usually less expensive than meats. It is sold fresh, frozen, canned, dried, or salted. Shellfish should be fresh and kept thoroughly chilled until used. All fish spoils easily and must be kept in cold storage or frozen. It should be stored in a covered container to prevent transmission of odor to other foods. Fish is cooked only until tender and flaky.

CHEESE

Cheese is made from milk solids. An excellent protein food, about 1/2 pound of cheese provides the same amount of protein as 1 pound of meat. Although it has lost a few nutrients found in the liquid portion of the milk, it is a good source of calcium. Most Cheddar cheese is high in fat and vitamin A. Cottage cheese is a low-fat cheese.

Cheese is classified as hard, semihard, or soft. Processed cheese is made by blending and pasteurizing several varieties. Processed cheeses keep the best; all cheeses should be wrapped thoroughly and kept refrigerated. Domestic cheeses are the least expensive.

Cheese is easily digested. It should be cooked slowly at a low temperature, as a high temperature causes it to become tough and rubbery. Avoid overcooking cheese dishes. The many different flavors of cheese and the many ways it can be used add infinite variety to the diet. Combined with a cereal product, such as macaroni, it can be the main dish at a meal. Cheese sauces can be used on vegetables, and it makes a good protein base for a salad. In many countries, fresh fruit and cheese is a popular dessert.

EGGS

Eggs are a good source of complete protein, vitamin A, phosphorus, sulfur, and iron. The yolk contains most of the minerals and vitamins found in an egg. The fats in an egg yolk are unsaturated. Easily digested, eggs are almost completely assimilated by the body and are a good meat substitute.

The color of the shell or the egg yolk has nothing to do with the nutritive value of the egg. Most eggs used in this country are from chickens, although eggs from other sources are edible and nutritious. Egg shells should be scrupulously clean as they are porous and admit microorganisms.

The larger the egg the more it will cost, but size does not appreciably affect nutritive value. The finest egg is grade AA, which is recommended for poaching and frying. Grade A eggs are more economical and are suitable for most uses. Other grades are used for baking and cooking. Eggs can be purchased fresh, frozen, or dehydrated.

A fresh egg has a thick white and a firm yolk that stands above the white. As the egg ages, the white becomes thinner and spreads out and the yolk becomes flat. Eggs can be kept for long periods in cold storage.

A low temperature is best for cooking eggs or egg dishes. Overcooking toughens the protein and makes it difficult to digest. Too high a temperature curdles egg dishes or causes discoloration.

The recommended number of eggs are easily included in the diet, as they are used to leaven baked goods, to bind ingredients of dishes together, and to thicken liquids. They can be served fried, poached, boiled, scrambled, baked, or in an omelet. Hard-boiled, they are used as a garnish or mixed in a salad. In fact, it is hard to plan a day's menu that does not include egg.

CEREALS

Cereals include all the foods made from grains such as wheat, rice, oats, barley, and rye. They furnish carbohydrates, vitamin B complex, bulkage, and some amino acids. When milk is added to breakfast cereals or used in preparing breads, pancakes, and so forth, the dish becomes a complete protein food.

Refined cereals have had the bran layer removed. There is no bulkage, and little residue is left after digestion. Low-residue cereals include white rice, white flour, corn flakes, and farina. High-residue foods include oatmeal, whole corn, bran cereals, and whole wheat.

During the milling of cereal grains, many vitamins and minerals are lost. Many cereal products are treated to make up for this loss. *Enriched* products have had minerals and vitamins added. *Restored* products have had minerals and vitamins added to the level present before processing. Enriched or restored cereal products should always be chosen.

Cereals should be kept in tightly closed containers. Flour products, such as bread, keep best stored in cool, well-ventilated areas. Many cereal foods can be frozen after being cooked.

An economical source of energy, cereals can be used as breakfast foods; in breads, cakes, and pastry; as side dishes such as steamed rice; as part of a main dish as in macaroni casseroles; or as filler in soups as noodles or dumplings.

The most inexpensive cereals are those that have to be cooked. To soften the cellulose walls and release the starch granules, cereals are cooked with moderate heat, usually with a liquid.

LEGUMES

Legumes are good sources of protein, iron, thiamin, and riboflavin and are one of the most inexpensive meat substitutes. For economy, they can be used as the main dish several times a week.

Legumes include kidney beans, pinto beans, split peas, lentils, black-eyed peas, field peas, chick peas, and lima beans. Only those legumes that are free from defects and have a bright, uniform color should be purchased. They should be stored in a covered container in a dry, cool place.

Dried legumes are usually soaked in water before cooking over low heat. The water in which they were soaked should be used in cooking. They are usually eaten boiled or baked. Pinto beans may be boiled, mashed, and then fried. Bean curds are used in some countries. While legumes are easily digested, some individuals have a tendency to have flatulence after eating.

Soybeans are the only plant source of complete protein; however, they must be processed before they can be eaten by humans. Because they contain a substance that inactivates trypsin, soybeans must be heated before they are dried and made into a flour. Soybean products that simulate the taste of meat are used both as meat substitutes and to extend various meat products such as hot dogs. In protein-deprived communities in Africa and South America, teams of experts sent by the United Nations are teaching the people to grow, process, and utilize soybeans as a flour for breadmaking in an effort to increase protein intake.

NUTS

Nuts, except chestnuts, are high in proteins, B vitamins, manganese, phosphorus, and fat. They are used as snack foods and as meat substitutes and extenders. Peanut butter is an excellent substitute for meat in sandwiches. Nuts can be used to stuff meats, poultry, and peppers. They can be added to vegetable fritters and to desserts.

FRUITS AND VEGETABLES

Fruits and vegetables furnish carbohydrates, vitamins, minerals, and cellulose and add variety and flavor to the menu. They are often classified according to the amount of carbohydrate they contain. If the fruit or the vegetable contains 3 grams of carbohydrate in each 100 grams of the fruit or the vegetable, it is classified as a 3 percent fruit or vegetable. If there are 20 grams of carbohydrate in each 100 grams, it is said to be a 20 percent fruit or vegetable. The higher the percentage of carbohydrate in the fruit or vegetable, the more calories it contains. Therefore, 3 percent fruits and vegetables are lower in caloric content than 20 percent fruits and vegetables.

Three percent fruits and vegetables include:

Asparagus	Mustard greens
Beans, young green	Radishes
Broccoli	Rhubarb
Cabbage	Sauerkraut
Cauliflower	Spinach
Celery	Squash, summer
Cucumbers	Tomatoes
Lettuce	Turnip greens

Six percent fruits and vegetables include:

Beans, mature, green	Peppers, green
Cantaloupe	Pumpkin
Dandelion greens	Squash, winter
Eggplant	Strawberries

Honeydew melon	Turnips
Okra	Watermelon

Nine percent fruits and vegetables include:

Artichokes	Lemons and lemon juice
Beets	Limes and lime juice
Blackberries	Onions
Brussels sprouts	Papayas
Carrots	Rutabagas
Cranberries	

Twelve percent fruits and vegetables include:

Apricots	Pineapples and pineapple juice
Oranges and orange juice	Plums
Peaches	Raspberries

Fifteen percent fruits and vegetables include:

Apples	Nectarines
Blueberries	Parsnips
Grapes	Pears
Loganberries	Peas

Eighteen percent fruits and vegetables include:

Beans, kidney	Figs
Cherries, sweet	Potatoes, white

Twenty percent fruits and vegetables include:

Bananas	Corn
Beans, lima	Prunes

Thirty percent fruits and vegetables include:

Sweet potatoes

Fresh vegetables should be crisp and firm when purchased. Fruit should be firm and unblemished but fully ripe. The sugars in fruit develop as it ripens and are at their most digestible when the fruit is fully ripe. Wilted fruits and vegetables have lost much of their vitamin content. Foods that are in season are most economical, but when unavailable, frozen or canned ones can be very nutritious.

Fresh fruits and vegetables should be used as soon as possible or stored in the vegetable bin of the refrigerator. Root vegetables such as potatoes should be stored in cool, dark, well-ventilated bins. Dried vegetables should be stored in tightly closed containers to prevent insect damage.

Properly cooked vegetables are firm but tender. As much of the vegetable or fruit as possible should be served, as minerals and vitamins are lost with the peelings. The following principles of cookery should be followed for best results:

1. Cook fruits and vegetables as soon as possible after preparation.
2. Use the smallest amount of water possible.

3. Cook for as short a time as possible. Food should be done but not overcooked.
4. In preparing canned or frozen foods, heat the liquid to boiling before adding the fruit or vegetable.
5. Cover the pot with a tight lid to minimize water loss during cooking.
6. Use moderate heat.
7. Serve the fruit or the vegetable as soon as possible after cooking.

Complete the following exercise:

1. Define the following terms:

   Pasteurized milk:

   Homogenized milk:

   Evaporated milk:

   Dried milk:

   Condensed milk:

2. Milk is an excellent source of ________________, ______________, and ________________.

3. What grade of milk should be purchased for children to drink?

4. What determines the grade of milk?

5. How should milk be stored?

6. Everyone in the family requires milk in the daily diet. Name some of the ways it can be included.

7. At what temperature should milk be cooked?

8. Cheese is a good substitute for meat in the diet because it is a ________________ food.

9. Which cheese has the lowest fat content?

10. Cheese is an excellent source of which mineral?

11. How can you prevent cheese used in cooking from becoming tough and rubbery?

12. How should cheese be stored?

13. Name some ways cheese can be used in the daily menu.

14. Eggs are good sources of ________________, ________________, ________________, ________________, and ________________.

15. After breaking an egg in a dish, how can you tell if it is fresh or not?

16. Which are the most nutritious, white or brown eggs?

17. When purchasing chicken eggs, you should choose those with clean, unstained shells because:

18. The most economical grade of egg for frying is:

19. Why should a low temperature be used in cooking eggs or egg dishes?

A.

B.

20. What have you eaten today that was made with egg?

21. What is a cereal?

22. Cereals furnish ____________________, ____________________ ________________, and ________________.

23. What is the difference between refined and unrefined cereals?

24. Define the following terms:
    Enriched cereals:

    Restored cereals:

    Low-residue cereals:

    High-residue cereals:

25. Name four low-residue cereals:

26. Name four high-residue cereals:

27. Why is water added in cooking cereals?

28. At what temperature should cereals be cooked?

29. How are cereals used in the diet?

30. Meat furnished the nutrients, ______________________________, ______________________, ______________________, and ______________________.

31. What are the characteristics to watch for in choosing beef?

32. What are the characteristics to watch for in choosing mutton?

33. What are the characteristics to watch for in choosing poultry?

34. Which is the most nutritious, dark or white meat?

35. Which is easier to digest, dark or white meat?

Why?

36. If the patient were on a low-fat diet, which poultry would be the best?

37. How do you check the age of dressed chicken?

38. Fish has almost the same nutritive value as beef but in addition it is a good source of ________________, ________________, and ________________.

39. Shellfish also are good sources of ________________ and ________________.

40. Fish that is fresh has ________________, ________________, and ________________.

41. Pork, veal, and poultry should be cooked until well done to ________________________.

42. Fish is cooked until ____________________________________.

43. The temperature for cooking meat is determined by the method chosen, but in general a ________________________ temperature will yield a tastier, more tender dish.

44. What are the methods used in cooking meats?

45. Why is boiling of meat not advised as a method of cookery?

46. How should beef, veal, mutton, and poultry be stored?

47. Why is it advisable to cover fish tightly when storing it in the refrigerator?

48. Fruits and vegetables furnish ____________________________, ________________, ________________, and ________________.

49. If there are 15 grams of carbohydrate in 100 grams of apple, it is a ____________ percent fruit.

50. If there are 6 grams of carbohydrate in eggplant, it is a ____________ percent vegetable.

51. If 18 grams of carbohydrate were desired in the diet, this could be supplied by:

________	grams cherries	________	grams carrots
________	grams eggplant	________	grams asparagus
________	grams sweet potato	________	grams apples

52. How many grams of carbohydrate in:
100 grams of Brussels sprouts? ________
200 grams of lettuce? ________
400 grams of watermelon? ________
75 grams of orange juice? ________
50 grams of sweet potatoes? ________

53. List the principles of cooking fruits and vegetables.

A.

B.

C.

D.

E.

F.

G.

54. Many markets sell wilted fruits and vegetables at cheaper prices. Why isn't purchasing these a good practice?

55. What nutrient is lost when a vegetable wilts?

56. Why should fruit be purchased when fully ripe?

57. Where should potatoes be stored?

58. Meat is one of the more expensive food items. What foods mentioned in this chapter are good substitutes for meat?

59. Legumes are inexpensive meat substitutes that are good sources of ________________, ________________, ________________, and ____________.

60. Legumes should be stored:

61. Legumes should be cooked at a ____________ temperature.

62. ________________ are the only plant source of complete proteins.

63. Soybeans must be heated before processing because:

64. Soybeans are used as ______________________________,
______________________________, and ______________________________.

65. Nuts provide ______________________, ______________________,
______________________, ______________________, and
__________________ in the diet.

66. An excellent meat substitute sandwich, which children usually accept eagerly, is __________________ .

67. Name some ways in which nuts can be used in the diet.

PROCESSED FOODS

Today, people purchase more processed foods than ever before. With the majority of the population of the United States living in cities and their suburbs, food must be brought long distances from the areas in which it is grown. There is increased availability of a variety of foods due to modern processing, transporting, and marketing methods. Kiwi fruit from New Zealand can be found in most grocery chain stores. Advertisements lead people to try foods they have not been accustomed to in their diets. Fried, puffed pork skins is an example of a regional snack that can now be purchased in any part of the United States. Shrimp Creole is enjoyed in Kansas where it can be purchased from the frozen food section; formerly this dish could be obtained only in coastal areas.

The changing life style of the American people has an effect on eating patterns. The shorter work week gives people time for leisure, which means more time to eat out either in a restaurant or in a fast-food place. Before family units became as small as they are today, it was too expensive to eat out often. In addition, more women work outside the home than ever before. There is less time to prepare meals from "scratch." In households where the women work, or where there is no woman, men are responsible for meals and usually choose easily prepared foods because they have had little or no training in food preparation. It is extremely important that everyone, men and women, understand the principles of nutrition and the impact processed foods have on nutritional status.

Processed foods are those that have been altered before being placed on the market. This includes all except the fresh fruits, vegetables, and meats. Processed foods include those that have been canned, frozen, dehydrated, sterilized, or altered as to content. Vitamin C and thiamin are the nutrients in which processed foods are most often deficient. TV dinners and many other processed foods are low in folic acid and pyridoxine.

So much sodium is used in processing and flavoring foods that most Americans receive an excessive amount of sodium each day. Fat is used in numerous foods in preparation and to extend shelf life. Most of this fat is saturated. Another excess in the American diet is sugar, used to preserve and add flavor.

Many of the ingredients in processed foods are substitutes for the "real" food. Among the most common are substitutes for milk and cream in ice cream and substitutes for natural flavors, such as maple.

Processed foods can be nutritious if chosen and used carefully. They do save time and effort. Someone who finds it difficult to see the measurement markings on a cup finds it much easier to prepare biscuits from a mix. The person with arthritis of the hands finds it easier to use precut frozen vegetables. A greater variety of foods are available throughout the year; the canned food section of the grocery has a tremendous selection with something for everyone.

Fabricated foods, sometimes called *food analogs,* are those that are produced with technology and are not found in nature. Among the most common are the "meats" from soybean and cereal bases, nondairy creamers, and imitation bacon. The Federal Food and Drug Administration requires that fabricated foods that resemble real food be labeled "Imitation." If the fabricated food contains as much protein, vitamins, and minerals as the real food, the company can give it a descriptive name instead.

Formulated foods have been prepared to meet specific needs. Food supplements and infant formulas come under this category.

Dietetic foods are modified as to the amount of one or more of the nutrients—sodium, sugar, cholesterol, saturated fats, or other nutrients. Dietetic foods should be used only on the advice of the physician.

Americans are addicted to *snack foods*; quite often these are obtained from vending machines and are substitutes for full meals. Vitamin A and calcium are the nutrients in which snack foods are most deficient. Vitamins C, E, and folic acid and trace minerals are also lacking. Snack foods contain excessive calories, sugars, saturated fats, and sodium. Because snack foods are usually highly refined, bulkage is missing.

In a few places, an effort is being made to replace traditional snack foods in vending machines with a more nutritious selection. Milk, fruit juices, and cheese cubes have been placed in vending machines. Fresh fruits, such as apples and oranges, are being offered in cafeterias. Packages of nonsalted roasted peanuts are available.

Healthful snack foods are easily available to persons interested in preserving nutritional balance. Among the most nutritious and easily prepared are:

Raw vegetables — carrot and celery sticks, green pepper slices, tomatoes, sliced cucumbers, and zucchini squash.

Fruits — apples, peaches, pears, oranges, grapes, cherries, pineapples, tangerines, grapefruits.

Melons — watermelon, cantaloupe, Persian melon.

Milk, fruit juices, vegetable juices.

Broth and bouillon (especially good on cold days).

Peanuts, walnuts, pecans, and popcorn (without butter).

Various cheeses and yoghurt.

Complete the following:

1. Some of the reasons that Americans eat so many processed foods are:

   A.

   B.

   C.

   D.

   E.

   F.

2. Processed foods are those that:

3. Which processed foods have you had today?

4. Which nutrients are usually lacking in processed foods?

5. Which nutrients are usually in excess in processed foods?

6. Which nutrients were probably in excess in the processed foods you have had today?

7. Which foods could you add to your diet to overcome the deficiencies in the processed foods you had today?

8. Which food have you had this week that had a substitute in it? (You may need to consult the nutrition labeling.)

9. What are some of the advantages of processed foods?

10. Define:
    Fabricated food:

Formulated food:

Dietetic food:

11. Which nutrients are lacking in snack foods?

12. What is found in excess in snack foods?

13. Which snack foods do you most often eat?

14. How often do you substitute snack foods for a meal?

15. Take a typical day when you have substituted snacks for a meal and list all foods taken that day.

Check this against the basic four food groups. Was your diet adequate? ________ Did your snack supply anything your other foods did not? ________

OPTIONAL ACTIVITIES TO ENHANCE LEARNING

ACTIVITY 1

Many foods are labeled with a date indicating when the food should no longer be sold. Visit the grocery store and find which foods contain this labeling. Note whether or not the grocery store has removed those foods that are out-of-date and how the dated foods are placed on the shelf. Discuss the implications of your findings to someone responsible for the food budget.

ACTIVITY 2

Ask several persons to bring eggs to school. Attempt to include eggs from fowl other than chickens. Make a note when and where the eggs were purchased. Observe for differences in the shells of the various varieties and in eggs bought at different times. Crack each egg and empty into a saucer. Was the egg easy to crack? Observe the yolk and white to determine its freshness. Discuss your findings in class, indicating their implications to someone responsible for the food budget.

ACTIVITY 3

Select three meats (beef, lamb, pork, poultry). Divide each portion into two. Season the meats as desired. Fry one piece of each meat using a low to moderate heat. Then fry the other piece of each meat using a high temperature. Taste each piece of the first meat. Repeat with the other meats. Discuss the taste, the tenderness, and the probable food value of each meat as it was prepared over moderate heat and over high heat.

BIBLIOGRAPHY

BRIGGS, GM AND CALLOWAY, DH: *Bogert's Nutrition and Physical Fitness, ed 10.* WB Saunders, Philadelphia, 1979. Chapter 17, *Food: From the producer to the consumer.*

US DEPARTMENT OF AGRICULTURE: *Home Freezing of Fruits and Vegetables.* Home and Garden Bulletin No 10, US Government Printing Office, Washington, DC, November, 1971.

US Department of Commerce: *How to Eye and Buy Seafood.* US Government Printing Office, Washington, DC, 1976.

US Department of Agriculture: *USDA Public Hearings on Sale of "Competitive Foods" in Schools.* Nutrition Policy Issues, No 4, US Government Printing Office, Washington, DC, February, 1979.

Consumer and Food Economics Institute: *Keeping Food Safe to Eat—A Guide for Homemakers.* US Government Printing Office, Washington, DC, October, 1978.

Krause, MV and Mahan, LK: *Food, Nutrition and Diet Therapy,* ed 6. WB Saunders, Philadelphia, 1979. Chapter 18, *Food and nutrition in the community.* Chapter 40, *Choosing food for nutrition and health.*

Martin, AA: *Diet Against Disease—A New Plan for Safe and Healthy Eating.* Houghton Mifflin, Boston, 1980. Part II, *Selecting, storing, and preparing foods: Making the goals a reality.* Part III, *Recipes and cooking procedures.*

McNutt, KW: *How contemporary is our nutrition education?* Contemporary Nutrition 6(6), June, 1981.

Some Questions and Answers About Canned Foods. FDA Consumer Memo, US Government Printing Office, Washington, DC, 1974.

Suitor, CW and Hunter, MF: *Nutrition: Principles and Application in Health Promotion.* JB Lippincott, Philadelphia, 1980. Chapter 11, *Menu planning and the purchase of food.* Chapter 12, *Food preparation and the safe handling of food.*

Williams, SR: *Mowry's Basic Nutrition and Diet Therapy,* ed 6. CV Mosby, St Louis, 1980. Chapter 11, *Basic principles of cooking.*

Worthington-Roberts, BS: *Contemporary Developments in Nutrition.* CV Mosby, St Louis, 1981. Chapter 11, *The American food supply.*

REVIEW QUESTIONS FOR SECTION 1

Circle the letter of the phrase that best completes each statement in the exercise below:

1. Nutrition is:
   A. Food that nourishes the body cells.
   B. The state of complete physical, mental, and social well-being and not merely the absence of disease or infirmity.
   C. The combination of processes by which the body receives and uses food for growth, development, and maintenance.

2. The functions of food in the body are to:
   A. Alleviate hunger and thirst.
   B. Give energy, aid in growth and repair, and regulate life processes.
   C. Prevent disease and deformities.

3. The daily diet is adequate when:
   A. It supplies the essential nutrients to perform all the functions of food.
   B. The caloric intake does not exceed caloric output.
   C. The body gains weight and height.

4. The daily diet will be balanced if the:
   A. Basic four food plan is followed.
   B. Allowance of protein exceeds 1 gram per person.
   C. Foods chosen are fresh.

5. A calorie is defined as the:
   A. Amount of heat required to raise the temperature of 1 kilogram of water 1° centigrade.
   B. Amount of heat required to raise the temperature of 1 kilogram of water 10° centigrade.
   C. Amount of heat required to raise the temperature of 10 kilograms of water 1° centigrade.

6. Which of the following is most likely to be found in improperly handled and refrigerated milk and egg dishes such as custards and cream puffs?
   A. Botulism B. Tularemia C. Staphylococii

7. The major sources of food for all people in the world are those which are predominantly:
   A. Fat B. Carbohydrate C. Protein

8. The quickest source of energy is:
   A. Sucrose B. Galactose C. Glucose

9. Fats are important in the diet because they:
   A. Carry fat-soluble vitamins.
   B. Are less expensive than protein.
   C. Provide satiety.

10. The best sources of protein in the diet are:
    A. Lean meat and eggs.
    B. Fruits and cereals.
    C. Gelatins and dried beans.

11. The individual who needs the most protein intake in relation to body weight is:
    A. Father B. Baby John C. Grandpa

12. The mineral most often found to be deficient in the diet is:
    A. Calcium B. Iron C. Phosphorus

13. The best source of iron is:
    A. Milk B. Bread C. Liver

14. The most common source of iodine for most people in the United States is:
    A. Milk B. Table salt C. Codfish

15. Potassium deficiency occurs after:
    A. Surgery, diabetic coma, and vomiting.
    B. A salt-free diet.
    C. Radiation therapy and starvation.

16. The best sources of vitamin A are:
    A. Liver, egg yolk, butter, and yellow vegetables.
    B. Lean meat, milk, and egg white.
    C. Citrus fruits, cabbage, and tomatoes.

17. The best sources of vitamin D are:
    A. Fruits and cereal grains.
    B. Sunshine and fish oils.
    C. Green vegetables and shellfish.

18. The functions of vitamin K include:
    A. Production of heat and energy.
    B. Assistance in normal red-cell production.
    C. Assistance in blood-clotting mechanism.

19. In general, the water-soluble vitamins are:
    A. Stored in the liver.
    B. Stored in fatty tissue.
    C. Not stored at all by the human body.

20. The best sources of ascorbic acid are:
    A. Citrus fruits, tomatoes, and cabbage.
    B. Liver, kidney, and brains.
    C. Milk, eggs, and lean meat.

21. In addition to other sources of fluid, it is recommended that an individual drink:
    A. 250 to 500 ml water per day.
    B. 1500 to 2000 ml water per day.
    C. 3000 to 4000 ml water per day.

22. Ruth has just found out that she is two months pregnant. Her physician has given her instructions about her diet. Her physician's instructions would include all the following statements except:
    A. "As you are not overweight and have been eating a well-balanced diet, it will not be necessary for you to increase your caloric intake until the last three months of your pregnancy."
    B. "If you do not like milk, use Sanka instead."
    C. "Increase the amount of fresh fruits and vegetables in your diet, and don't neglect to drink plenty of water each day."

23. Ruth had a baby boy. She and her husband wanted the baby to be breast fed because:
    A. All of these. B. All but (1) and (3). C. All but (2).
    (1) The baby would get the correct formula at all times.
    (2) Breast milk contains some immune bodies needed by the newborn.
    (3) The baby would be less likely to be constipated than on cow's milk formula.
    (4) It would be convenient and economical.

24. George is 5 years old. His mother has consulted her pediatrician because George has not been eating well. The pediatrician would be most likely to tell George's mother:
   A. "If he won't eat enough at one meal, double his portions at the next one to make up for it."
   B. "The child's appetite will vary at each stage of growth—as long as his weight and growth are maintained, there is nothing to worry about."
   C. "If he decides not to drink milk, use chocolate or cocoa to flavor it."

25. Because her teenagers are often hungry between meals, Mrs. J. tries to keep her refrigerator stocked with foods for snacks. Which of the following would be the best selection?
   A. Ice cream, soda, cheese crackers, and pickles.
   B. Peanut butter, apples, and hamburger patties.
   C. Chocolate milk, lemon pie, and cheese.

26. Mrs. J.'s father lives with her. For his meals, Mrs. J. should:
   A. Remember to include extra protein.
   B. Give him what he wants even if it is starchy.
   C. Serve her father the same number of calories as her son receives.

27. Mrs. J. chooses pasteurized milk for her family because:
   A. The fat particles have been evenly distributed throughout the milk.
   B. The milk has been heated to inhibit the growth of bacteria.
   C. She can add water to increase the amount.

28. Little Mary J. is learning to cook. She was very disappointed that the eggs she cooked were tough and unappetizing. She probably used:
   A. Old, dark-shelled eggs.
   B. Grade B eggs.
   C. A high temperature to cook them.

29. When Mrs. J. purchases cereals, she should be sure the refined cereals have had minerals and vitamins added because:
    A. During the milling process, many minerals and vitamins are lost.
    B. Her teenagers need extra minerals and vitamins.
    C. Minerals and vitamins are costly in the pill form.

30. As soon as she brings her vegetables and fruits home, Mrs. J. stores them in the vegetable bin of her refrigerator because she knows that:
    A. They might sprout if left in the heat.
    B. Her family prefers cold produce.
    C. When vegetables and fruits wilt, they lose vitamin C.

Complete the following statements:

31. When the body does not receive the necessary amount of nutrients, it suffers from ____________________ .

32. The normal adult requires ____________ of milk per day.

33. There should be ________ or more servings per day from the meat, poultry, fish, and egg group.

34. When nutrients are added that were not in the food before processing, the food is said to be ____________________ .

35. ____________________ includes the processes by which the body uses food for growth, maintenance, and repair and the processes in which the tissues are broken down into wastes.

36. Sugar is stored in the muscles and liver as ________________ .

37. Table sugar is a double sugar known as ________________ .

38. There are ________ calories in 1 gram of carbohydrate.

39. There are ________ calories in 10 grams of fat.

40. Butter, lard, and hydrogenated shortenings are classified as ________________ fats.

41. The only vegetable that supplies a complete protein is ________________ .

42. There are ________ calories in 1 gram of protein.

43. One reason milk is so important in the diet is that it is the best source of the mineral ________________ .

44. A deficiency of ________________ results in dehydration even when the patient is taking enough water.

45. Vitamin ________ is important for maintaining good night vision and resisting infection.

46. The fat-soluble vitamins are ________________________ .

47. A deficiency of vitamin D and calcium causes ________________ in children.

48. A deficiency of vitamin ________ leads to a disturbance in the blood clotting mechanism and to hemorrhage.

49. A severe deficiency of ________________ results in a condition called beri-beri.

50. The deficiency of one of the B vitamins usually means that there is a deficiency of ________________ .

51. A deficiency of niacin is associated with a condition called ______________________.

52. Another name for vitamin C is ______________________.

53. Scurvy is caused by a deficiency of vitamin ________.

54. A ________ percent loss of water from the body is critical and a ________ percent loss results in death.

55. The body loses water through the ____________, ____________, ____________, and ____________.

56. ________________ furnishes bulk in the diet.

57. The framework of fruits and vegetables is formed by ____________.

58. The pregnant woman requires ________________ of milk in some form each day.

59. The woman who is nursing her baby will need ________________ of milk each day.

60. During lactation, the diet should be increased by ____________ calories.

61. During lactation, the protein allowance in the diet should be ________________.

62. In comparing cow's milk and human milk, ________________ milk is apt to be more constipating for an infant.

63. The baby's formula is usually made from _______________, _______________, and _______________.

64. In the terminal sterilization method of preparing formulas, the bottles are filled _______________ sterilization.

65. Milk that has had part of the water content removed and sugar added is _______________ milk. .

66. Cheese can be used on the menu as a substitute for _______________.

67. _______________ is a low-fat cheese and is an excellent choice for a low-calorie diet.

68. Eggs can be used on the menu as a substitute for _______________ _______________.

69. Whole grain cereals are excellent sources of the _______ vitamins.

70. To soften the cellulose walls and make the starch available, cereals must be _______________.

71. When cooking meats, a ___________ temperature will yield a tastier, more tender dish.

72. Which would be higher in calories, a 12 percent fruit or a 20 percent vegetable? _______________

73. The sugar content of a fruit is highest when it is _______________ _______________.

74. Dried beans, peas, and lentils can be used on the menu as a ____________ substitute.

75. When cooking fruits or vegetables, how much water should be used? ____________

76. The foods usually consumed by a particular individual include fried chicken, hominy grits, kale, okra, and cornbread. This person is probably from:
   A. Topeka, Kansas.
   B. Mobile, Alabama.
   C. Hartford, Rhode Island.

77. The patient's religion is Jewish. For this patient's breakfast you would order:
   A. Cheese omelet and coffee.
   B. Ham and eggs with milk.
   C. Pork sausage and pancakes.

78. The label on a dessert reads: Ingredients: Sugar, gelatin, adipic acid, disodium phosphate, artificial flavor, artificial color. Which ingredient is in the greatest abundance in the dessert?

79. Which two ingredients on the label described above are fabricated foods?

80. Checking the nutrition labels on two vegetables you are considering for lunch, you find this.

	Peas	*Tomatoes*
Serving size	1 cup	1 cup
Calories	120	50
Protein	6 gm	2 gm
Carbohydrate	20 gm	11 gm
Fat	1 gm	0

	Peas	*Tomatoes*
Percentage RDA:		
Protein	10%	2%
Vitamin A	15%	30%
Vitamin C	30%	60%
Thiamin	8%	8%
Riboflavin	4%	2%
Niacin	6%	10%
Calcium	2%	8%
Iron	10%	4%

A. Which vegetable would you choose if you were limiting calories?

B. Which gives you the most vitamins?

C. Which would you choose for its protein and iron content?

D. Which would you choose for a diet free of fat?

81. Polyols, such as sorbitol, are used in a diabetic diet because they:
    A. Are sweeteners.
    B. Are alcohols.
    C. Require less insulin to metabolize.

82. The athlete should:
    A. Eat a well-balanced diet providing enough calories for the physical activity involved.
    B. Increase vitamin and mineral intake with supplements.
    C. Double protein and vitamin intake.

83. Processed foods are frequently deficient in:
    A. Folic acid
    B. Protein
    C. Sodium

84. Dietetic foods are foods that are:
   A. Altered as to content to meet special needs.
   B. Better for you.
   C. Grown in organic gardens.

85. Snack foods usually contain too much:
   A. Saturated fat and sodium.
   B. Fiber and Vitamin A
   C. Folic acid and tryptophan.

SECTION 2

DIET THERAPY

Diet is an integral part of the prevention and treatment of disease. In this section, the student applies the basic principles of nutrition learned in Section 1. To understand Diet Therapy fully, the student must be able to correlate the facts learned in Body Structure and Function and in Medical and Surgical Nursing with Nutrition.

13

MODIFICATIONS OF THE NORMAL DIET

OBJECTIVES

Upon completion of this chapter the student should be able to:

- List the responsibilities of the nurse in diet therapy for the patient and give some examples of how these responsibilities are met.
- Plan a day's menu for a patient on one of the standard hospital diets: general, light, soft, full liquid, clear liquid.
- Given the name of a special diet, give the characteristics of that diet and select foods that are allowed on that diet.

Diet therapy is the treatment of a disease or condition by modification of the diet. In some instances, diet therapy is the only treatment for a condition; in others, it is part of the treatment.

Although the dietitian plans the patient's diet, the nurse has the following definite responsibilities:

1. The nurse must know what the diet prescription consists of. For example, the nurse must know which foods are included in a bland diet and how they should be prepared. The nurse should know how bland foods are served (the temperature and so forth).

2. The nurse should understand what is to be accomplished with the diet. For example, it must be understood that a low-fat diet will relieve the liver of the need to produce a large amount of bile and the gallbladder will not be stimulated to empty itself, thereby resting these organs and giving them a chance to heal.
3. The nurse should understand the problem in the functioning of the body created by the condition being treated. For example, know that following a subtotal gastrectomy, the patient needs extra iron and vitamin B_{12} as the loss of stomach mucosa results in decreased production of the intrinsic factor necessary to stimulate production of erythrocytes by the red bone marrow.
4. The nurse must be aware of the patient's reactions to the diet to be able to explain the diet to the patient and obtain the patient's cooperation. For instance, diabetic patients should be taught the relationship between their insulin and the amount of food consumed. If they understand the problems and are shown that they can continue to eat most of their favorite foods, they will be more likely to remain on the diet.
5. The nurse must be aware of the patient's home situation and the problems the diet will cause in order to help plan for the patient's continued care. Most patients are hospitalized only during the acute and early convalescent phases of their illness so that a special diet may be necessary for some time at home. Chronic conditions, such as peptic ulcers, require permanent dietary alteration. The patients and their families will have to adjust family meal planning to meet the patients' needs. The nurse can help the family plan for this.

There are certain standard modifications of the normal diet. Although these modifications may vary somewhat in different hospitals, the general principles remain the same. Table 14 outlines the diets, their characteristics, foods allowed, foods to be avoided, and a list of typical conditions in which a particular diet may be ordered. Because of their complexity, the sodium-restricted diet and the diabetic diet will be discussed in the chapters relating to the conditions in which they are used.

Occasionally, a patient's condition, or conditions, may require a combination of two or more modifications of the normal diet. For example, a patient with cirrhosis of the liver would have difficulty digesting fats and the doctor would probably order a diet low in fat. Also, the liver would have difficulty metabolizing carbohydrates, making increased carbohydrate intake necessary. The diet needed would be a high-carbohydrate, low-fat diet. Sometimes cirrhosis is accompanied by edema and ascites. In which case, the dietary prescription would be for a high-carbohydrate, low-fat, low-sodium diet.

Many hospitalized patients do not require a diet in which the ratio of the nutrients is altered. For such patients "hospital diets" or "house diets" are provided, which consist of a normal diet modified only as to consistency and ease of digestion.

TABLE 14. DIET THERAPY

Diet	*Characteristics*	*Food Allowed*	*Food Not Allowed*	*Conditions in Which Prescribed*
High-calorie	1. Calories increased to 3000 to 5000 per day 2. Food intake gradually increased 3. Treatment may be individualized: a. men prefer extra portions of usual food at meal times b. women, concentrated foods c. children, between-meal snacks	Extra portions of sugars, butter, cream, sauces	Large amounts of low-calorie foods such as lettuce; too many fats, as they affect appetite	Hyperthyroidism, tuberculosis, pneumonia, typhoid fever
High-protein	1. Normal diet with increased amount of protein 2. Fat reduced	Extra portions of milk, eggs, lean meat, cheese	High fat foods such as cream, gravy, avocado; incomplete plant proteins	Nephrosis, tuberculosis, fevers, burns, before and after surgery
High-carbohydrate	Balanced diet with added carbohydrates	Extra portions of fruits, vegetables, sugars, starches	Fatty foods, spicy foods that may cause digestive upsets	Toxemia of pregnancy, liver and gallbladder conditions
High-iron	Balanced diet choosing foods high in iron and vitamin B_{12}	Meats (especially glandular meats such as liver), oysters, leafy green vegetables, egg yolk, peas, beans (dried), fruit, whole grain cereals		Iron-deficiency anemia, pernicious anemia
High-fiber (High-residue)	Normal diet with increased fiber content	Raw fruits and vegetables (use skins when possible), whole-grain cereals, leafy green vegetables	Excessive seasoning, refined cereal, concentrated foods	Atonic constipation

TABLE 14. *Continued*

Diet	*Characteristics*	*Food Allowed*	*Food Not Allowed*	*Conditions in Which Prescribed*
Low-fiber (Low-residue)	1. Foods must be completely absorbed 2. Should be used for a limited time only 3. Diet rests the gastrointestinal tract but lacks minerals and vitamins	Tender meats, clear fat-free soup, eggs, refined cereals, fruit juice, gelatins, milk-free beverages	Whole-grain cereals, milk, cheese, fruits, vegetables, excessive seasoning	Severe diarrhea, ulcerative colitis, before and after surgery of intestinal tract
Low-protein	Protein is kept at low normal level	Limited amount of complete protein foods such as milk, cheese, eggs, meat; bland, easily digested fruits and vegetables	Incomplete proteins, excessive seasoning	Nephritis, cardiac conditions
Low-fat	1. Only most easily digested fats are used 2. Lacks vitamin A that must be given as a supplement	Lean meat, egg white, cottage cheese, skim milk, fruits, and vegetables low in fat	Egg yolk, fat meats, sauces, gravies	Obesity, liver and gallbladder conditions, digestive disturbances
Bland	1. Prevents peristalsis and flow of gastric juices 2. Normal diet modified as to consistency and choice of foods 3. Small frequent feedings that keep food in stomach but avoid overloading	Tender meat, milk, eggs, puréed fruits and vegetables, refined cereals, white potatoes, macaroni, rice, custards, gelatins	Strong flavors, spicy seasoning, high-residue foods, raw fruits and vegetables	Peptic ulcers, gastritis, diarrhea, fevers
Low-calorie	1. Normal diet with reduced caloric intake	Bulky low-calorie fruits and vegetables, adequate fluids, lean meats, egg, skim milk	Fats, pastries, creams, sauces, and gravies	Obesity

TABLE 14. *Continued*

Diet	*Characteristics*	*Food Allowed*	*Food Not Allowed*	*Conditions in Which Prescribed*
	2. If less than 1000 calories, it is deficient in minerals and vitamins 3. Calories reduced by eliminating some carbohydrates and fats 4. Protein intake remains normal			

GENERAL DIET

This is an adequate, normal diet of 2000 to 2500 calories containing all the protective foods (meat, eggs, milk, citrus fruits, vegetables, whole-grain or enriched bread, and butter). Foods causing digestive disturbances are avoided. The general diet may also be called regular, full, or house diet.

LIGHT DIET

Similar to the general diet, the light diet is adequate but monotonous. Fatty foods and highly spiced dishes are avoided. Preferred meats are lamb and chicken, or fish. Bran, celery, melon, apple, and other coarse foods are omitted.

SOFT DIET

If the hospital serves a light diet, the soft diet is usually omitted. Adequate diet low in cellulose, the soft diet is planned for mechanical ease in eating and digesting. Some hospitals omit all meats and serve all vegetables pureed. Others allow broiled, roasted, or boiled ground meats and fish, as well as cooked low residue vegetables. There are usually 1800 to 2000 calories in the soft diet, slightly fewer than in the general.

LIQUID DIET

FULL LIQUID DIET. Usually the bridge between the clear liquid diet and the soft diet, this diet is adequate for maintenance only and should be used for a limited time. The diet produces 1300 to 1500 calories and usually consists of all foods that are liquid at room and body temperature. Foods allowed include milk beverages, strained soups, tea, coffee, fruit juices, ice cream, gelatins, and carbonated drinks.

CLEAR LIQUID DIET. Sometimes known as a surgical liquid diet, the clear liquid diet is mostly water and carbohydrates, furnishes about 500 calories, and is very inadequate. Its purpose is to relieve thirst and dehydration and to start peristalsis in recent postoperative patients. It consists of clear liquids such as tea, coffee, and fat-free broth served at frequent intervals. Carbonated drinks are allowed in selected cases.

Complete the following exercises:

1. Define "diet therapy."

2. What is the nurse's responsibility in the treatment of a patient by modification of the diet:

   A.

   B.

   C.

   D.

   E.

3. If food intake is suddenly increased greatly, the patient may become nauseated or have a loss of appetite. So, when the patient is placed on a high-calorie diet, the caloric allowance should be ______________ .

4. If you wanted a man to increase his caloric intake, how could you best accomplish this?

5. What foods would you add to change a normal diet to a high-calorie diet?

6. ________________, ________________, and ________________ are added to a normal diet to make it a high-protein diet.

7. With the high-carbohydrate diet, it is important to avoid ____________ and ____________ that may cause digestive upsets.

8. How is a normal diet modified to become a high-carbohydrate diet?

9. Liver is important in the diet for anemias because it is high in ____________ content.

10. Which part of the egg contains the most iron?

11. The high-fiber diet is the same as a ________________ diet. What foods are added to the high-fiber diet?

12. What foods are avoided on the high-residue diet?

13. The low-fiber diet is the same as a _______________ diet.

14. What foods are allowed on the low-fiber diet?

15. What foods are avoided on the low-residue diet?

16. On the low-protein diet, the protein content is kept at what level?

17. Complete proteins are chosen on the low-protein diet. Complete proteins contain the _______________ amino acids. Legumes, nuts, lentils, and corn are restricted on the low-protein diet because they are _______________ protein foods.

18. The low-fat is deficient in _______________ .

19. What foods are allowed on the low-fat diet?

20. What foods are avoided on the bland diet?

21. Why is the bland diet given in small frequent feedings?

22. What is the objective in giving the patient a bland diet?

23. In the low-calorie diet, the protein intake is ________________ .

24. What foods are avoided on the low-calorie diet?

25. Low-calorie diets of fewer than ________ calories are deficient in vitamins and minerals.

26. How could you modify a breakfast menu of orange juice, toast, poached egg, and black coffee to change it to a high-caloric diet?

27. Is the following a high-protein luncheon? Grilled pork chop, baked beans, buttered spinach, egg custard, and milk.

28. Cross out the one of the following dishes that should not be on this high-carbohydrate menu.
Macaroni and cheese with chili sauce, English peas, candied carrots, mixed fruit salad, vanilla ice cream, and tea with sugar and lemon.

29. Mrs. H. has to prepare her daughter a diet high in iron. Is the following diet high in iron?
Braised liver, black-eyed peas, stewed tomatoes, tossed green salad, stewed apricots, and whole-wheat bread.

30. Name several salads that could be used on a high-residue diet.

31. Plan a luncheon for someone on a low-residue diet.

32. Cross out dishes on the following menu to change the menu to a low-protein diet.
Roast beef, gravy, baked beans, corn, fresh pear, and milk.

33. Place a check before those of the following foods that would be allowed on a low-fat diet.

________	Bacon	________	Cottage cheese and onion salad
________	Apple	________	Deviled eggs
________	Peanuts	________	French dressing

34. What is the difference between a normal diet and a general or regular diet in the hospital?

35. The soft diet is an adequate diet low in ________ .

36. How many calories are usually found in the soft diet?

37. The two types of liquid diet are:

38. The full liquid diet usually consists of foods that are ____________ ________________ at room temperature.

39. Check those of the following foods that would be allowed on a full liquid diet.

________ Iced tea	________ Ice cream
________ Coffee	________ Consomme
________ Jello	________ Strained cereal gruel
________ Orange juice	

40. What is another name for the clear liquid diet?

41. What is the purpose of the clear liquid diet since it is so inadequate?

OPTIONAL ACTIVITIES TO ENHANCE LEARNING

ACTIVITY 1

Visit a clinic and obtain copies of the materials used in teaching patients about special diets. Select one special diet and prepare a lesson plan to use in teaching an adult about the diet. If permitted, teach a patient at the clinic.

ACTIVITY 2

Visit a clinic and ask the nurse to introduce you to a patient who has been on a special diet. Interview the patient, asking what problems the patient has encountered in trying to adhere to the diet.

ACTIVITY 3

Divide into 15 groups. Each group selects one of the special or hospital diets. Prepare a lunch menu for that diet. Then prepare the foods. (This can be done at home and the meal brought to school.) Observe the amount of food allowed, its attractiveness, and its smell. Then eat the meal. Discuss in class how you would like to be on the chosen diet and the problems you might have in remaining on the diet.

BIBLIOGRAPHY

HALPERN, SL ET AL: *Quick Reference to Clinical Nutrition: A Guide for Physicians.* JB Lippincott, Philadelphia, 1979. Chapter 7, *Principles of therapeutic nutrition.*

KRAUSE, MV AND MAHAN, LK: *Food, Nutrition and Diet Therapy,* ed 6. WB Saunders, Philadelphia, 1979. Chapter 20, *The nutritional care process.*

NEWTON, M AND FOLTA, J: *Hospital food can help or hinder care.* American Journal of Nursing 67(1), January, 1967.

ROBINSON, CH: *Basic Nutrition and Diet Therapy,* ed 4. Macmillan, New York, 1980. Chapter 20, *Modification of the normal diet for texture.*

SALMOND, SW: *How to assess the nutritional status of acutely ill patients.* American Journal of Nursing 80(5), May, 1980.

WILLIAMS, SR: *Mowry's Basic Nutrition and Diet Therapy,* ed 6. CV Mosby, St Louis, 1980. Chapter 14, *Routine hospital diets.* Chapter 15, *Modifications in individual constituents.*

WILL, B: *Food becomes fun for children.* American Journal of Nursing 78(12), December, 1978.

14

DIET IN DISEASES OF THE GASTROINTESTINAL TRACT

OBJECTIVES

Upon completion of this chapter the student should be able to:

- List the factors that predispose a patient to gastric, duodenal, and stress ulcers and give the signs and symptoms.
- Discuss the objectives of ulcer therapy and outline the dietary prescriptions that may be ordered.
- Compare the diet therapy of hyperchlorhydria and hypochlorhydria.
- Discuss the diet therapy for acute gastroenteritis, chronic gastritis, indigestion, and hiatal hernia and give the dietary care for each.
- Select the diet for each type of constipation and give the reasons for the selection.
- Discuss the diet therapy for diverticuli, hemorrhoids, diarrhea, and colitis and give the dietary care for each.

GASTRIC AND DUODENAL ULCERS

An eroded lesion in the gastrointestinal mucosa is termed an ulcer. Gastric ulcers are found in the stomach; duodenal ulcers are located in the duodenum; and both may be called *peptic ulcers.* The exact cause of peptic ulcers is not known. Some of the factors involved may be:

1. Emotional tension and stress
2. Bad dietary habits.
3. Excessive smoking.
4. Overindulgence in alcohol.
5. Impaired circulation.
6. Infected teeth and tonsils.
7. Heredity, possibly.

The signs and symptoms of peptic ulcers include:

1. Burning pain when the stomach is empty.
2. **Melena** (tarry stools due to blood content).
3. Gastric hyperacidity.
4. Vomiting.
5. Feeling of weakness.

Medical treatment of the patient with peptic ulcers attempts to:

1. Control the hyperacidity of the stomach by giving the patient antacids.
2. Control tension and aid the patient to relax by giving the patient drugs.
3. Keep the stomach and intestines quiet by serving small frequent meals of nonirritating and nonstimulating foods.

When medical treatment does not achieve the desired result, surgical treatment may be instituted. Surgery is usually a last resort after a hemorrhage or perforation and may be the resection of the affected part or total removal of the stomach. Surgery is sometimes necessitated by the patient's failure to cooperate with the medical routine.

Sippy Diet

At one time, the Sippy diet was the most commonly used in treatment of ulcers. One of the first ulcer diets, it is a progressive diet, divided into five or more stages. Although very severe ulcer cases usually start with the first stage, the physician may decide that the patient may start at one of the later stages. Or the physician may keep the patient at one of the stages where the patient is doing well, and not allow progress to the last stage of the diet.

The foods on the Sippy diet are of soft consistency with little fiber content. Serving size is small, and servings are given as frequently as the patient requires. The patient should be encouraged to make mealtimes as unhurried and pleasant as possible.

FIRST STAGE. A serving of not more than 3 ounces of milk and cream (half and half) is given every hour. The nurse should see that the milk and cream mixture is always served at a temperature only slightly cooler than room temperature. It may be necessary to awaken the patient at night.

SECOND STAGE. Small amounts of milk toast, poached egg, strained cereals, custard, and gelatin are given in three to four servings a day. The patient still takes milk and cream between meals.

THIRD STAGE. Strained cream soups, toasted bread with butter, and vanilla ice cream are added to the diet. The nurse should caution the patient to eat slowly and chew the food well.

FOURTH STAGE. The patient receives six feedings a day with milk and cream between meals. Ground tender beef, liver, fish, cottage cheese, macaroni, noodles, rice, white potatoes, pureed bland fruits and vegetables, and bland dilute fruit juices are added to the diet.

FIFTH STAGE. The fifth stage is a *bland convalescent ulcer diet* and is simply a bland diet served at frequent intervals. Although this is a rather monotonous diet, it is adequate, and the patient can subsist on it indefinitely.

Today, physicians tend to be more liberal in prescribing diets for ulcer patients as trying to stay on a strict diet is in itself tension-causing. Also, the strict ulcer diet is high in saturated fats, which can lead to atherosclerosis, and in calcium, which can lead to renal calculi formation.

Bland Convalescent Ulcer Diet

The *bland convalescent ulcer diet* is the one most frquently used today. The patient and physician work out a dietary regimen that the patient is able to follow. This usually means that the patient must make some changes in life style and eating habits. The diet is individualized as much as possible to make it acceptable to the patient.

Foods that cause gastric irritation or increase acid secretion in the stomach are avoided. These foods include alcoholic drinks, beverages with caffeine in them (some colas), coffee, tea, and spices. Aspirin and other salicylate drugs should not be taken, particularly on an empty stomach. The patient should never eat just before going to bed as there is then a tendency toward acid production during the night. Foods listed in the bland diet in Chapter 13 are included in this diet.

Meulengracht Diet

The Meulengracht diet is frequently ordered for patients with gastric hemorrhage. As the hemorrhage is controlled, a clot is formed. Because blood is a protein, the clot will be digested if the stomach is not kept full. Thus, an abundant pureed diet consisting of milk, eggs, bread and butter, bland fruits and vegetables, pudding, and custard is given on the first day of the hemorrhage. Feedings are given every two hours. After the second day, ground or scraped meat is allowed.

Andresen Diet

Patients who are hemorrhaging or who have gastric surgery are given the Andresen diet, which consists of 6-ounce feedings of a milk-cream-gelatin mix every two hours. The nurse mixes the gelatin into the milk and cream at the patient's bedside after allowing the milk and cream to warm to room temperature. If mixed too early, the gelatin will cause the mixture to get too thick to drink. After a week of milk-cream-gelatin mixture, the patient may be allowed selected foods such as jello, custards, and puddings.

STRESS ULCERS

Stress ulcers differ from gastric and duodenal ulcers in that they occur after major physical stress and they commonly occur anywhere in the alimentary canal. Some of the conditions that may lead to stress ulcers are severe burns, brain injuries, and critical major surgery. Steroids given over a long period of time can also cause ulcers. The dietary prescription is a *bland pureed diet or milk-based formulas.*

HYPERCHLORHYDRIA

In hyperchlorhydria, the gastric juice secreted by the stomach contains an excess of hydrochloric acid, which can be irritating to the stomach lining. The cause is unknown. A *bland diet* is usually ordered for the same reason that a bland diet is given to a convalescent ulcer patient—to control the amount of free acid in the stomach.

Individuals with hyperchlorhydria usually benefit by changing their food habits; a regular, pleasant mealtime helps.

HYPOCHLORHYDRIA

In hypochlorhydria, the stomach does not produce enough hydrochloric acid. Lack of hydrochloric acid can cause diarrhea and improper digestion of proteins and fats. (An acid environment is necessary to trigger the emptying of bile from the gallbladder.) Hypochlorhydria can indicate pernicious anemia, cancer, and chronic gastritis. A *bland, low-fiber, low-fat diet* is usually given. Very hot or very cold foods are contraindicated. Because the lack of acid makes the digestive tract susceptible to bacteria, care must be used to prevent the introduction of pathogens with food.

ACUTE GASTROENTERITIS

Acute gastroenteritis is the common "upset stomach" in which there is nausea, vomiting, and intestinal cramping. It is caused by overeating, eating foods the individual cannot tolerate, "bolting" of food, fatigue, highly seasoned food, toxins, and infections.

The initial treatment is to allow the stomach to empty itself. No food is given for 24 to 48 hours. Cracked ice may be given to relieve thirst. Following the period of fasting, liquids such as hot tea, ginger ale, and tart carbonated drinks may be given at the discretion of the physician. Later, as the patient can tolerate them, small amounts of *bland foods* may be taken until the patient is on a *soft diet.*

CHRONIC GASTRITIS

Chronic gastritis often occurs when cancer or ulcers are present, but its exact cause is probably related to those of acute gastritis. The physician usually prescribes a *low-fiber diet* to eliminate very fibrous and highly seasoned foods from the diet. There is a tendency toward flatulence and meals should be served with little liquids as liquids will tend to cause gas. Very hot or very cold foods should not be served.

INDIGESTION

The term indigestion is used to describe any discomfort occurring from a digestive tract disorder. Symptoms vary with the individual and are usually vague. A therapeutic diet is seldom necessary. A well-balanced diet and *correct eating habits* are usually all that is necessary.

SLIDING HIATAL HERNIA

Herniation of the diaphram close to the esophagus is termed hiatal hernia. When pressure is exerted on the abdomen as happens when the patient bends or lifts heavy objects, a portion of the stomach slips up into the thoracic cavity. Occasionally, it happens when the patient lies down immediately after eating a heavy meal. The patient complains of pain and burning and occasionally bleeding occurs. The dietary treatment is a *low-fiber diet,* usually in small amounts at frequent intervals.

CONSTIPATION

Constipation is the retention of feces in the colon beyond the normal length of time. The normal length of time varies with the individual; some people have a bowel movement each day; others may have two a day; and still others may have one every other day. Good hygiene, regular eating and defecation habits, and stable emotional status help prevent constipation.

Atonic Constipation

Atonic constipation, the most common type, occurs because the muscles of the colon have lost their tone. It is commonly found in the elderly, in the obese, during pregnancy, and following surgery. The most frequent causes of atonic constipation are faulty diet and failure of the individual to establish a regular time for defecation. The dietary treatment is to include adequate bulk in the diet and to drink at least 8 to 10 glasses of fluids daily. The *high-residue diet* includes whole-grain cereals and breads, vegetables high in cellulose content, and fruits, especially raw fruits with peels.

Spastic Constipation

Overstimulation of peristaltic waves in the digestive tract causes spastic constipation characterized by frequent ineffectual movements, which cannot move the contents of the colon along. The causes are excessive use of cathartics, spices, and tobacco, excessive ingestion of very coarse foods, and drinking excessive amounts of tea, coffee, and alcohol. The dietary treatment is a *low-residue diet* including such foods as milk and milk products, refined cereals and breads, pureed and strained vegetables, pureed fruits, fruit juices, syrups, sugars, and jellies.

Obstructive Constipation

A partial or complete closure of the intestinal tract results in obstructive constipation. The cause may be adhesions, cancer, tumors, or impaction of feces. Dietary treatment tries to provide nourishment and to keep the amount of residue to a minimum. Intravenous fluids providing all the essential nutrients may be necessary if the obstruction is too great. Injection of fluids rapidly into the superior vena cava by pump is called *hyperalimentation,* which is discussed more fully in Chapter 24.

DIVERTICULITIS

Occasionally, small sacs or pockets, known as diverticuli, appear on the colon. Recent studies have suggested that the lack of sufficient fiber in the highly refined foods of the modern diet causes these. Some authorities recommend a *high-fiber diet,* both for prevention and treatment of diverticuli. Traditionally, physicians have ordered a *low-fiber* or *bland diet* when the diverticuli have become irritated and inflamed. Often food is withheld for 48 hours during an acute attack. Fluid intake should be normal.

HEMORRHOIDS

Hemorrhoids are varicose veins in the rectum. Although they are not treated by diet, a *low-residue diet* is more comfortable for the patient both before and after surgery. The patient should avoid constipation by ingesting an adequate amount of fluids.

DIARRHEA

In diarrhea, the stools are frequent and liquid. Although diarrhea is usually a symptom rather than a disease, it is serious in that nutrients and fluids are passed through the body before they can be absorbed. Diarrhea can be caused by improper digestion, overeating, allergic reaction, emotional reaction to a situation, spoiled food, or ingestion of pathogens.

During the acute phase, the physician may recommend that nothing be taken by mouth. In cases of severe loss of electrolytes and fluids, intravenous solution may be given. As soon as possible, oral fluids such as tea and fat-free broth are introduced. Dry toast is often tolerated at this stage. Gradually, a *low-fiber, high-calorie, high-protein diet* is added until the patient can tolerate a normal diet.

COLITIS

Colitis is an inflammation of the lining of the colon. There are three types: mucous, simple, and ulcerative.

Mucous Colitis

This form of colitis usually occurs in emotional individuals. The stools are frequent and full of mucus. To prevent further stimulation of the colon, a *low-residue, bland diet* is usually ordered.

Simple Colitis

This form of colitis may be called *spastic or irritable bowel* and is usually found in tense or overly fatigued persons. Again, the diet of choice is a *low-residue, bland diet.*

Ulcerative Colitis

Ulcerative colitis may be caused by infection, deficiencies, or allergy and the diet depends upon the cause. Often the physician will order a *low-residue diet with extra milk* to be given in frequent small feedings. If it is determined that the cause of the colitis is a food allergy, the offending food will be excluded from the diet.

Complete the following exercises.:

1. The three diets commonly used for peptic ulcer patients are:
   A.

   B.

   C.

2. The patient with a hemorrhaging peptic ulcer may have a ________________ or ________________ diet ordered.

3. After gastric surgery, the ________________ diet may be ordered.

4. In the Meulengracht diet, the patient receives an abundance of pureed foods to ________________________________ ________________.

5. How often is milk and cream given with the first stage of the Sippy diet?

6. The Sippy diet is known as a progressive diet because:

7. What are the characteristics of the foods served on the Sippy diet?

8. What are some of the instructions the nurse should give to the patient on an ulcer diet?

9. When is the gelatin mixed with milk and cream in the Andresen diet?

10. What diet is prescribed for hyperchlorhydria?

11. A bland, low-fiber, ________________ diet is usually ordered for the patient with hypochlorhydria because hydrochloric acid is necessary to trigger the excretion of bile by the gallbladder.

12. In acute gastroenteritis, the initial treatment is to have the patient ________________ for 24 to 48 hours, followed by liquids such as ________________, ________________ and ________________. After that the patient may have ________________ as tolerated.

13. In chronic gastritis, the physician usually orders a low-fiber diet because:

14. What is the dietary treatment of indigestion?

15. The most common type of constipation is ________________, for which the dietary treatment is ________________________ and ________________.

16. Plan a high-residue diet for one day for a patient with atonic constipation.
Breakfast:

Lunch:

Dinner:

17. What is the difference between a high-fiber and a high-residue diet?

18. The dietary treatment for spastic constipation is ________________.
What foods would you include in the diet of this patient?

19. The dietary prescription for mucous colitis and spastic colitis is the same; it is ________________________.

20. For the patient with hemorrhoids, a ______________ diet usually causes the least discomfort.

OPTIONAL ACTIVITY TO ENHANCE LEARNING

ACTIVITY 1

Case Study

Mr. M., a 40-year-old football coach, was admitted to the hospital Friday night with severe pain in the epigastric region. He has had a history of pain and burning in the upper abdomen occurring, usually around 9:30 AM, 3:30 PM, and during the night. He regularly takes a common commercial antacid tablet for this. His hematocrit on admission was 42; all other blood work was within normal limits. Mr. M. chews gum constantly and is always on the telephone to his assistant at school. Stool studies for occult blood were 1+. An upper GI series has been ordered. Because the physician has never succeeded in getting Mr. M. to stay on a strict ulcer diet, the physician has ordered a convalescent bland ulcer diet. (Mr. M. prefers highly spiced foods "because they have more flavor.") Maalox has been ordered to be given between meals and at bedtime. Mr. M. has no known food allergies and no food preferences, "except he does not like 'baby food'."

Prepare a nutritional care plan. (See Appendix for example.)

BIBLIOGRAPHY

BRENEMAN, JC: *Food allergy.* Contemporary Nutrition 4(3), March, 1979.

THE INSTITUTE OF FOOD TECHNOLOGISTS EXPERT PANEL ON FOOD SAFETY AND NUTRITION AND THE COMMITTEE ON PUBLIC INFORMATION: *Dietary fiber.* Contemporary Nutrition 4(9), September, 1979.

HALPERN, SL ET AL: *Quick Reference to Clinical Nutrition: A Guide for Physicians.* JB Lippincott, Philadelphia, 1979. Chapter 12, *Nutrition and upper gastrointestinal disorders.* Chapter 13, *Nutrition and disorders of the colon.*

HODGES, RE: *Nutrition in Medical Practice.* WB Saunders, Philadelphia, 1980. Chapter 3, *Nutrition and the digestive system.*

KRAUSE, MV AND MAHAN, LK: *Food, Nutrition and Diet Therapy,* ed 6. WB Saunders, Philadelphia, 1979. Chapter 22, *Nutritional care for patients with esophageal and gastric diseases.* Chapter 23, *Nutritional care for patients with intestinal diseases.* Chapter 35, *The metabolic stress response and methods for providing nutritional care to stressed patients.*

LEVINE, AS: *The relationship of diet to intestinal gas.* Contemporary Nutrition 4(7), July, 1979.

ROBINSON, CH: *Basic Nutrition and Diet Therapy,* ed 4. Macmillan, New York, 1980. Chapter 28, *Diseases of the gastrointestinal tract.*

RYNBERGEN, HJ: *In gastrointestinal disease fewer diet restrictions.* American Journal of Nursing 63(1), January, 1963.

SHERMAN, WC: *Reflex or functional disorders of the stomach.* Food and Nutrition News December, 1968.

SUITOR, CW AND HUNTER, MF: *Nutrition: Principles and Application in Health Promotion.* JB Lippincott, Philadelphia, 1980. Chapter 33, *Alteration in digestion and/or absorption.*

WILLIAMS, SR: *Mowry's Basic Nutrition and Diet Therapy,* ed 6. CV Mosby, St Louis, 1980. Chapter 8, *Digestion.* Chapter 16, *Diseases of the gastrointestinal tract.*

WORTHINGTON-ROBERTS, BS: *Contemporary Developments in Nutrition.* CV Mosby, St Louis, 1981. Chapter 2, *Dietary fiber.*

15

DIET IN DISEASES OF THE LIVER AND GALLBLADDER

OBJECTIVES

Upon completion of this chapter the student should be able to:

- Give the etiology, signs and symptoms, and dietary prescription for cirrhosis, infectious hepatitis, hepatic coma, obstructive jaundice, cholecystitis, cholelithiasis, and pancreatitis.

CIRRHOSIS

Cirrhosis is the most serious or final stage of liver injury or degeneration. It is caused by dietary deficiencies, injury, toxic agents, or infections. Cirrhosis related to alcoholism is classified as due to dietary deficiency as the person with alcoholism often does not eat properly.

The dietary prescription is a *high-calorie, high-carbohydrate, high-protein diet with moderate fat and an abundance of vitamins.* The extra calories help to prevent loss of weight and strength often seen because of impaired digestion and disturbed metabolism in patients with liver disease. The extra proteins, which should be complete proteins, are needed for the repair of damaged tissue. Carbohydrates "spare the protein" and extra vitamins help protect the liver. Extra vitamin K may be necessary when prothrombin levels are low.

Highly seasoned foods and gas-forming foods should be omitted. As dietary treatment is very important in these patients, the food should be made as appealing and as attractive as possible. When *ascites* is present, sodium and fluids will have to be restricted.

INFECTIOUS HEPATITIS

Infectious hepatitis is inflammation of the liver caused by a virus. Symptoms are: loss of appetite, fatigue, drowsiness, weakness, nausea and vomiting, chills, fever, constipation, and tenderness over the liver. The fever may be as high as 104°F. Jaundice of the skin and eyes appears within two weeks.

Treatment consists of complete bed rest and the same diet as for cirrhosis of the liver. Every effort is made to spare the liver and alcoholic beverages are counterindicated. If the appetite is poor, the patient can be given small feedings at frequent intervals. Often hard candies are left at the bedside in an effort to increase the caloric intake.

Infectious hepatitis is usually contracted through contaminated water and food. Another more severe form of hepatitis, *serum hepatitis,* is transmitted through articles that have come into contact with contaminated blood or serum, such as hypodermic needles that have not been properly sterilized. The signs and symptoms are usually more acute. The dietary prescription is the same as for other types of hepatitis.

HEPATIC COMA

Severe liver damage from disease or impaired circulation in the area of the liver causes a toxic condition leading to coma. Interference with the liver's ability to metabolize protein substances causes the level of ammonia in the blood to increase, producing symptoms of coma.

Proteins cannot be completely withheld from the diet indefinitely, but during the most severe stage of intoxication, the patient may be given a *protein-free diet* that consists of salt-free fat and sugar usually served as chilled balls. Vitamin and mineral supplements are necessary. Ham, hamburger, chicken, salami, peanut butter, and gelatin increase the amount of ammonia in the blood and should be avoided.

As the patient improves, a *low-protein diet* may be tolerated. Complete proteins such as meat or milk should be used. To assure an adequate caloric intake, the remainder of the diet should consist of foods that contain no protein.

OBSTRUCTIVE JAUNDICE

In obstructive jaundice, an obstruction within the common bile duct keeps the gallbladder from emptying. Absorption of bile salts into the blood stream causes yellow appearance. Treatment is usually surgical.

A *high-calorie, high-carbohydrate, high-protein, and moderate-fat diet* is usually ordered. As bile is necessary for the absorption of vitamin K in the digestive tract, patients with obstructive jaundice have a tendency to bleed. Vitamin K may be given by injection to prevent this. As with liver disease patients, alcohol is forbidden.

CHOLECYSTITIS

In cholecystitis, the gallbladder is inflamed. Factors predisposing to this fairly common condition are infections of the tonsils, teeth, or sinus; overweight; pregnancy; constipation; improper diet; and digestive upsets. Symptoms are pain in the region of the gallbladder, nausea, flatulence, soreness in the upper right quadrant of the abdomen, and occasional jaundice.

The dietary treatment is a *low-fat, nonirritating diet* with avoidance of gas-forming foods. The following foods are considered to be gas-forming although reactions to foods differ with individuals and the dietary prescription must take this into account.

Apples, raw	Cauliflower	Peppers
Beans, dried	Corn	Radishes
Broccoli	Lentils	Rutabagas
Brussels sprouts	Onions	Sauerkraut
Cabbage	Peas, dried	Turnips

Foods should be prepared simply. Some patients also require a *low-residue diet.*

CHOLELITHIASIS

Gallstones are formed from the concentration of mineral salts in the bile. Cholelithiasis may result from a sluggish gallbladder or an infection. The stones can slip out of the gallbladder and pass through the bile ducts when small, but frequently they must be removed surgically. The patient complains of severe pain, particularly after eating a diet high in fat. The dietary prescription is the same as in cholecystitis.

PANCREATITIS

Infectious organisms in the common bile duct may lead to inflammation of the pancreas, or pancreatitis. Bile, which is irritating to the pancreatic duct, sometimes backs into the pancreatic duct when the common duct is obstructed. Jaundice may occur. The patient complains of pain in the epigastric region. In severe pancreatitis, the patient may go into shock. The dietary treatment is individualized; usually a *low-fat diet* is given in six small feedings between severe attacks. Alcoholic beverages and foods that increase pancreatic and gallbladder activity must be avoided. During severe attacks, all food is usually withheld.

Answer the following questions:

1. The diet ordered for cirrhosis of the liver is:

2. The prescribed diet for cirrhosis of the liver is also the dietary treatment for:

3. In cirrhosis of the liver:

   A. Why are extra calories ordered?

   B. Why is a high-protein diet needed?

   C. What is the role of the extra carbohydrates?

   D. What do the extra vitamins do?

   E. What foods should be avoided?

4. What restrictions are ordered when the patient has ascites?

5. What diet is ordered for obstructive jaundice?

6. What diet is ordered for cholecystitis and cholelithiasis?

7. How is pancreatitis treated by diet?

8. Why is fat difficult to digest when the pancreas does not function?

9. Plan a breakfast menu for a patient on a high-calorie, high-carbohydrate, high-protein, moderate-fat diet.

10. Plan a luncheon menu for a patient on a low-fat, nonirritating diet.

11. Plan a dinner menu for a patient on a low-fat, low-residue diet.

OPTIONAL ACTIVITY TO ENHANCE LEARNING

ACTIVITY 1

Case Study

Mrs. M. is 70 years old, five feet tall, and weighs 180 pounds. She is a good cook and regularly treats her friends and family to traditional Mexican foods, such as enchiladas and homemade tortillas with butter. She was admitted to the hospital because of recurring abdominal pain after eating. The pain was located in the right upper quadrant of the abdomen and was frequently accompanied by belching and nausea. There is no jaundice, diarrhea, or fever, and, upon examination, the conformation of the liver appeared normal. Her blood pressure was 170/100. A blood count revealed no leukocytosis or anemia. Examination of her heart revealed a slight arrhythmia and an electrocardiogram was ordered. A cystogram revealed evidence of chronic cholecystitis with many small stones in the gallbladder. Mrs. M. was placed on a 1500-calorie, low-fat, bland diet and is to be maintained medically because her age and heart condition make her a poor surgical candidate.

Prepare a nutritional care plan.

BIBLIOGRAPHY

HALPERN, SL ET AL: *Quick Reference to Clinical Nutrition: A Guide for Physicians.* JB Lippincott, Philadelphia, 1979. Chapter 12, *Nutrition and upper gastrointestinal disorders.* Chapter 21, *Nutrition and liver disease.*

HODGES, RE: *Nutrition in Medical Practice.* WB Saunders, Philadelphia, 1980. Chapter 3, *Nutrition and the digestive system.*

KRAUSE, MV AND MAHAN, LK: *Food, Nutrition and Diet Therapy,* ed 6. WB Saunders, Philadelphia, 1979. Chapter 24, *Nutritional care for patients with diseases of the liver, exocrine pancreas and biliary system.*

LIEBER, CS: *Alcohol-nutrition interaction.* Contemporary Nutrition 3(9), September, 1978.

ROBINSON, CH: *Basic Nutrition and Diet Therapy,* ed 4. Macmillan, New York, 1980. Chapter 30, *Diseases of liver, gallbladder, and pancreas.*

SUITOR, CW AND HUNTER, MF: *Nutrition: Principles and Application in Health Promotion.* JB Lippincott, Philadelphia, 1980. Chapter 33, *Alteration in digestion and/or absorption.*

WILLIAMS, SR: *Mowry's Basic Nutrition and Diet Therapy,* ed 6. CV Mosby, St Louis, 1980. Chapter 8, *Digestion.* Chapter 17, *Diseases of the liver and gallbladder.*

16

DIET IN DISEASES OF THE CARDIOVASCULAR SYSTEM

OBJECTIVES

Upon completion of this chapter the student should be able to:

- List the objectives of dietary management of cardiac patients and the rules to follow.
- Give four reasons why the cardiac patient should not be obese.
- Discuss the dietary regimen of the cardiac patient and give the limitations and the reasons for these.
- Select foods for the mildly, moderately, and strictly restricted sodium diets.
- Select foods for the Karell and Kempner diets, and give the conditions in which these diets are used.
- Discuss the etiology, signs and symptoms, and dietary prescriptions for hyperlipidemia, arteriosclerosis, and hypertension.

More people die of heart disease in the United States than from any other cause. It has been estimated that 1 in every 15 persons has some type of heart or circulatory disease. Ninety percent of those persons with heart and circulatory diseases have either rheumatic heart disease, hypertensive heart disease, or a coronary condition. Interestingly, even where there is no actual heart disease, malnutrition affects the heart to such an extent that the patient may exhibit signs and symptoms of heart disease. These include dyspnea, palpitation, enlargement of the heart, and systolic murmurs.

The major objective in care of the cardiac patient is *rest.* The objectives of dietary management for cardiac patients are:

1. Maximum rest for the heart.
2. Prevention or elimination of edema.
3. Maintenance of good nutrition.
4. Acceptance of the nutrition program by the patient.

There are four reasons why the cardiac patient should not be obese:

1. The heart must work harder as the body pushes and pulls the extra weight around.
2. Fat deposits in the myocardium decrease efficiency of these muscles.
3. Abdominal fat interferes with movement of the diaphragm and thus with free action of the heart. Breathing is more difficult.
4. Arteriosclerosis often follows obesity. It is more difficult for the heart to push blood through vessels narrowed by arteriosclerosis.

In general, diet therapy for all types of cardiovascular conditions follows these four simple rules:

1. Give the patient only the amount of food actually needed. The patient must not overeat and may be placed on a low-calorie diet.
2. Plan the menu around those foods that are easier to digest.
3. Restrict stimulants such as tea, coffee, cocoa.
4. Limit sodium. If edema is present, the sodium intake may be severely restricted.

The cardiac patient may have to learn to accept new foods and to avoid foods normally eaten. Bulky foods that distend the stomach or gas-forming foods that distend the colon should be omitted as should foods that require a lot of effort to eat. If the patient has known food idiosyncrasies or allergies, this should be noted. In many cases, several small meals a day are better than three large ones. Mealtimes should be pleasant and unhurried. The nurse must remember this when feeding the cardiac patient. When the condition is severe, the patient will not be allowed to make the effort necessary to eat without assistance.

Cardiac conditions may be acute or chronic. *Acute cardiac diseases* may be due to an inflammation of the lining of the heart (endocarditis) or to loss of function of the muscles because of lack of stimulation (cardiac failure). *Chronic heart conditions* usually involve the muscles or the valves.

Because proteins take more energy to digest and metabolize, they are kept at a low-normal level in the cardiac diet. Also, the end product of protein metabolism is excreted through the kidneys, and frequently the kidneys do not function as well as usual in the presence of heart disease. Carbohydrates are easily digested, so many of the dietary calories are carbohydrates. Fats in the cardiac diet should be in an easily digested form. Both fat and carbohydrates are reduced when it is necessary to limit the total number of calories in the diet.

Low-Sodium Diet

Often cardiac patients have edema or retention of fluids because sodium cannot be handled normally by the body. In such cases, the physician will order a low-sodium diet. The amount of sodium restriction necessary will depend upon the amount of edema.

Foods naturally high in sodium are:

Milk	Poultry	Kale
Cheese	Fish	Carrots
Eggs	Beets and beet greens	Turnips
Meat	Celery	Spinach

A *mildly restricted sodium diet* limits dietary sodium to 1 to 2 grams per day. (The ordinary daily diet contains 3 to 6 grams of sodium.) Salty foods such as those listed below are avoided, and salt is not added to food during cooking or at the table.

Baking soda	Biscuit and pancake mixes
Baking powder	Hominy
Graham crackers	Pretzels and potato chips
Crackers	Cheese
Pudding mixes	Bacon and bacon fat
Ice cream mixes	Mayonnaise and salad dressings
Nuts, salted	Brined meats
Peanut butter	Prepared meats such as bologna
Canned soups	Shellfish
Celery and garlic salt	Jellies preserved with sodium benzoate
Worcestershire sauce	Sauerkraut
Chili	Bouillon
Pickles and relishes	Meat tenderizers
Prepared mustard	Butter, unless prepared without salt

A *moderately restricted sodium diet* limits sodium to 1 gram per day. The patient must have all food prepared without salt and will need to take salt-free bread. A *strictly restricted sodium diet* limits the patient to ½ gram sodium per day.

On occasion, the patient's condition requires that sodium be restricted to less than ½ gram per day. Low-sodium milk and distilled water must be substituted for regular milk and water. The sodium content of the drugs the patient is taking must be noted; even the patient's dentifrice should be examined for sodium content. Fruits and vegetables low in sodium content should be chosen. In general, foods that have been processed contain more sodium but it is possible to purchase specially processed, low-sodium canned food. The patient on 1/2 gram or less of sodium is usually hospitalized.

The low-sodium diet is tasteless, and it is very difficult to get the patient to accept it. Salt substitutes should be given only on the doctor's order as many are potassium salts and ammonium salts, which could be harmful to patients with kidney or liver disease. The patient should be urged to use herb seasonings, except for celery and parsley flakes. Allspice, mace, lemon juice, or thyme can be added to food to improve its flavor. Lemon juice can be sprinkled on vegetables after cooking. If the caloric content of the diet is not significant, sugar added to cooking vegetables improves the flavor. Any seasoning that does not contain sodium and is not contraindicated by the patient's diagnosis may be used to flavor food during the cooking process.

Karell Diet

On occasion, the patient with cardiac failure is placed on the *Karell diet.* This diet consists of 800 ml of milk per day in four equal servings. The diet provides only 600 calories and 1 gram of salt per day. It is a very deficient diet and can be prescribed for only four to seven days at a time. Milk is given because it is easily digested and is a complete protein.

HYPERLIPIDEMIA

Hyperlipidemia is a condition in which there are excessive lipids (fats) in the blood. There are many forms in which fats are found in the blood. Some are in the blood serum as *triglycerides;* some are combined with proteins as *lipoproteins.* When the lipid content of the blood exceeds the normal amount, the risk of cardiovascular problems is increased. Blood cholesterol levels are elevated and *plaque* is deposited on blood vessel walls.

Hyperlipidemia occurs when a high-fat diet is ingested (particularly one high in saturated fats), when an individual habitually takes in excessive alcohol, or when the individual does not exercise sufficiently. The tendency toward hyperlipidemia is hereditary and can occur as the result of liver disease, diabetes, nephrosis, or hypothyroidism.

Dietary prescription depends upon the type and severity of the hyperlipidemia. In general, the caloric intake is restricted to prevent obesity or to cause weight loss. Saturated fats and high-cholesterol foods are avoided. Carbohydrates should consist of the more complex kinds, such as starches; sugars should be avoided. Foods high in residue apparently help to lower the serum cholesterol level. Alcohol should be avoided as it increases the level of serum triglycerides.

ARTERIOSCLEROSIS

Arteriosclerosis (also known as *atherosclerosis*) and hypertension are usually found together, although hypertension can be due to other causes.

Arteriosclerosis is characterized by a narrowing of the lumen of the blood vessels and by loss of elasticity of the walls of the blood vessels. Inside the blood vessels, small particles of cholesterol and fat are deposited on the lining. The heart must work harder to push the blood through; thus the blood pressure becomes elevated.

Although the exact cause of arteriosclerosis is not known, the following factors seem to predispose to the condition:

1. Heredity.
2. A diet high in fat, especially saturated fats.
3. High blood cholesterol level.
4. Sex hormones. (Studies indicate that female hormones offer protection from arteriosclerosis.)
5. Excessive smoking.
6. Obesity.
7. Certain diseases, such as diabetes.

Because a high level of fat is found in the blood in many patients with arteriosclerosis and because consumption of saturated fats tends to increase the cholesterol level, some authorities recommend reducing the amount of saturated fats in the diet and substituting polyunsaturated fats in an attempt to reduce the blood cholesterol level. Many physicians order a *low-cholesterol diet* for their patients to decrease the chance of developing arteriosclerosis. Foods to avoid on a low-cholesterol diet are brains, kidneys, liver, heart, egg yolk, butter, milk, and milk products.

The low-cholesterol diet has become very popular with self-diagnosing laymen. However, a physician should *always* be consulted before a dietary plan is followed.

HYPERTENSION

Recent surveys show that many more Americans have hypertension than expected. Hypertension is usually treated medically with drugs and diet. Many patients with hypertension are overweight and may be placed on a *low-calorie diet.* In general, the physician will limit stimulants and excessive amounts of proteins, sodium, and fat. Stimulants such as tea and coffee cause the heart to accelerate. Sodium causes fluid retention and thus elevates the blood pressure. The product of protein metabolism, urea, must be excreted by the kidneys, which are often affected by arteriosclerosis. Fats are concentrated sources of calories and are therefore limited.

In addition to antihypertensive drugs, the physician may prescribe diuretic agents to reduce blood volume and thus the blood pressure. Potassium deficiency can occur and the patient should be encouraged to include high-potassium foods in the daily diet. These include melons, bananas, orange juice, and avocados.

Kempner Diet

In cases of severe hypertension that do not respond to ordinary diet therapy, the Kempner diet is ordered. It consists of rice, fruit, and sugar. The Kempner diet is cholesterol-free, contains only 5 grams of fat, and is high in carbohydrate and low in sodium. It is an inadequate diet, and the patient is kept on it only for a few days until the blood pressure begins to drop.

Complete the following exercises:

1. The main objective in the care of a cardiac patient is ____________ .

2. The four objectives of dietary management of cardiac patients are:
   A.

   B.

   C.

   D.

3. The four reasons the cardiac patient should not be obese are:
   A.

   B.

C.

D.

4. Describe the typical cardiac diet.

5. Why are proteins kept at a low-normal level in the cardiac diet?

6. Why are most of the calories in the cardiac diet in the form of carbohydrates?

7. The salt-free diet is misnamed. Actually, it is only the ___________ part of the salt that is restricted.

8. The sodium-restricted diet is very tasteless, and most patients resent it. Some physicians allow salt substitutes. Can you think of other ways to add flavor to the patient's food without adding sodium?

9. Plan a menu for a patient on a low-sodium diet. Indicate when the food must be prepared without salt.
Breakfast:

Lunch:

Dinner:

10. What modifications of the above menu would be necessary to reduce the sodium content to less than 1/2 gram?

11. The Karell diet consists of ____________ given in ____________ equal servings. It provides ____________ calories and ____________ sodium every day.

12. The ____________ diet is used in cases of severe hypertension, which does not respond to ordinary means. This diet is composed of ____________, ____________, and ____________. It contains ____________ cholesterol and ____________.

13. Foods to avoid on the low-cholesterol diet are:

14. Foods high in potassium include:

15. Hyperlipidemia occurs when:

A.

B.

C.

D.

E.

16. In hyperlipidemia, the following elements of the diet must be adjusted. How?
    Calories:

    Carbohydrates:

    Fats:

    High-residue foods:

    Alcohol:

OPTIONAL ACTIVITY TO ENHANCE LEARNING

ACTIVITY 1

Case Study

One week ago Mr. P. was admitted to the Coronary Care Unit with a myocardial infarction. He is the president of an oil drilling company, 35 years old, married, and a self-made man. Mr. P. regularly has "martini" business lunches. He is 30 pounds overweight; he belongs to a golf club but seldom has time to play. He drinks about 10 cups of coffee each day. On admission his blood pressure was 166/100, and on transfer to this unit it was 140/88. Upon transfer to this unit, the cardiologist changed his diet to low cholesterol, low fat, low calorie, to be given in six equal portions during the day as Mr. P. develops angina-like pain after eating. Blood lipids, cholesterol, and triglycerides are elevated. Mr. P. has known of his tendency toward hypertension but "forgot" to take his medications, even though he knew his headaches indicated that his blood pressure was elevated. Prior to hospitalization, Mr. P. treated himself frequently for indigestion. He prefers casserole and creamed dishes. He does not like vegetables and says that milk makes his stomach hurt.

Prepare a nutritional care plan.

BIBLIOGRAPHY

CALIENDO, MA: *Nutrition and Preventitive Health Care.* Macmillan, New York, 1981. Chapter 7, *Diet, nutrition and heart disease.*

DARBY, WJ: *Why Salt? How Much?* Contemporary Nutrition 5(6), June, 1980.

FLYNN, MA: *The cholesterol controversy.* Contemporary Nutrition 3(3), March, 1978. 1978.

HALPERN, SL ET AL: *Quick Reference to Clinical Nutrition: A Guide for Physicians.* JB Lippincott, Philadelphia, 1979. Chapter 9, *Nutrition and cardiovascular disease.*

HILL, M: *Helping the hypertensive patient control sodium intake.* American Journal of Nursing 79(5), May, 1979.

HODGES, RE: *Nutrition in Medical Practice.* WB Saunders, Philadelphia, 1980. Chapter 4, *Diet, cholesterol and coronary heart disease.*

THE INSTITUTE OF FOOD TECHNOLOGISTS EXPERT PANEL ON FOOD SAFETY AND NUTRITION AND THE COMMITTEE ON PUBLIC INFORMATION: *Dietary fiber:* Contemporary Nutrition 4(9), September, 1979.

KRAUSE, MV AND MAHAN, LK: *Food, Nutrition and Diet Therapy,* ed 6. WB Saunders, Philadelphia, 1979. Chapter 28, *Nutritional care for patients with cardiovascular diseases.*

KRITCHEVSKY, D AND CZARNECKI, SK: *Lipoproteins.* Contemporary Nutrition 5(5), May, 1980.

MALLISON, M: *Updating the cholesterol controversy: Verdict—Diet does count.* American Journal of Nursing 78(10), October, 1978.

MARSH, AC, KLIPPSTEIN, RN, AND KAPLAN, SD: *The Sodium Content of Your Food.* Home and Garden Bulletin No. 233, US Government Printing Office, August, 1980.

MAYER, J: *Don't salt it: Season it.* Family Health, December, 1971.

ROBINSON, CH: *Basic Nutrition and Diet Therapy,* ed 4. Macmillan, New York, 1980. Chapter 25, *Hyperlipidemia and atherosclerosis.* Chapter 26, *Diseases of the heart.*

ROCKWELL, SM: *Low-cholesterol meats for cardiologists—And for you.* RN, May, 1972.

ROSEN, E: *Hypertension: Nutrition guidelines in the treatment and control of hypertension.* Journal of Practical Nursing Vol 27, December, 1977.

SEARIGHT, MW: *A low-sodium potluck luncheon.* Nursing Outlook, August, 1968.

SPAIN, DM: *Human Nutrition: Readings from Scientific American.* WH Freeman & Company, San Francisco, 1978, *Atherosclerosis,* p 221.

WILLIAMS, SR: *Mowry's Basic Nutrition and Diet Therapy,* ed 6. CV Mosby, St Louis, 1980. Chapter 20, *Diseases of the cardiovascular system.*

17

DIET IN DISEASES OF THE GENITOURINARY SYSTEM

OBJECTIVES

Upon completion of this chapter the student should be able to:

- Discuss the diet therapy and the rationale for its selection for: glomerulonephritis, nephrosis, nephrosclerosis, uremia, and urinary calculi.
- Select a diet that would alter the alkaline or the acid condition of urine.
- Discuss diet therapy for a patient on renal or peritoneal dialysis.

NEPHRITIS

Nephritis, or Bright's disease, includes three types of kidney conditions: glomerulonephritis, nephrosis, and nephrosclerosis.

Glomerulonephritis

An inflammation within the nephron of the kidney where the fluids are filtered from the blood results in glomerulonephritis. The dietary objective is to rest the kidney. The protein intake may be reduced as the end product of protein metabolism is urea, which must be excreted by the kidneys. The proteins selected must be complete proteins in order to give the patient the essential amino acids needed. Vegetable proteins are restricted. To prevent use of protein for energy, the diet must include sufficient carbohydrate and fat. Sodium is restricted when edema is present.

Nephrosis

Nephrosis, also known as *degenerative Bright's disease,* causes a severe loss of body proteins. Therefore, the required diet is *high in protein.* Frequently, it is also a *low-sodium diet* as the patient may be quite edematous.

Nephrosclerosis

This condition, also called *malignant hypertension,* is usually found in the young or in adults past age 35. The blood supply to the kidneys is poor, and the waste products cannot be filtered out of the blood into the nephron. It is a progressively fatal condition. A *200 milligram sodium diet* is given if edema is severe and has offered some success in reducing blood pressure. Obesity should be avoided to reduce the work load of the cardiovascular system. The protein allowance is adjusted as the severity of the condition indicates.

UREMIA

Uremia is a toxic condition caused by retention of urinary substances in the blood. Its cause is severe kidney diseases. As the kidneys cannot eliminate urea, it stays in the blood and the patient progresses to convulsions, coma, and death. A few patients can be saved if the toxic substances can be removed by use of the artificial kidney or if enough of the kidney function is left to rid the body of the toxin gradually. Exceptionally good nursing care is required. The diet is usually *low-protein, high-carbohydrate. Fluids are given only in amounts equal to output. Sodium and potassium intakes* are carefully monitored in severe cases.

Butter balls, made of sugar, flour, unsalted butter, water, and flavoring, are given to those patients who require a *protein-free, potassium-free diet.* Patients who do not tolerate butter balls can be given substitutes such as glucose candy or protein-free formulas.

URINARY CALCULI

Urinary calculi are composed of mineral salts that have precipitated from urine. They are found in the kidneys, ureters, bladder, or urethra and vary in size and shape. Alkaline stones are found in alkaline urine; acid stones are found in acid urine. The condition cannot be cured by diet alone, but by adjusting the diet, an acid or alkaline urine can result. This may make medication more effective and help prevent the formation of more stones.

A patient with *alkaline calculi* would receive acid medication and a diet that would result in acid ashes after metabolism. Such a diet is known as an *acid-ash diet.* Foods that yield acid ash upon metabolism are meat, eggs, fish, poultry, bread, and cereal. As these foods are high in sodium, salt is omitted in preparation.

A patient with *acid calculi* would receive alkaline medication and a diet that would result in alkaline ashes after metabolism, the *alkaline-ash diet.* This would tend to neutralize the urine or make it alkaline. Foods that yield alkaline ash upon metabolism are fruits (except cranberries and plums) and vegetables.

The mineral in 90 percent of all calculi is calcium. The physician may suggest that the patient avoid milk and oxalates such as tea, spinach, beets, and rhubarb.

Complete the following exercises:

1. In glomerulonephritis, the diet is usually ____________ in protein. In order that the patient receive all the essential amino acids, ____________ proteins should be chosen.

2. Because the patient with nephrosis is suffering from a loss of body protein, the dietary prescription would be ____________________ .

3. The uremic patient must be strictly regulated as to intake and output of fluid because:

4. If the renal calculi are acid, the diet must be an ________________ diet and may include:

5. If the renal calculi are alkaline, the diet must be an ________________ diet, and may include:

6. Plan a day's menu for a patient on a low-protein diet.
Breakfast:

Lunch:

Dinner:

7. How would you modify the low-protein diet, you have planned to make it a low-protein, low-sodium diet?

8. Plan a high-protein diet for one day.
Breakfast:

Lunch:

Dinner:

9. Which foods would you have to delete from your high-protein diet above if you also had to restrict the calcium intake?

PATIENTS ON DIALYSIS

Patients are placed on dialysis when the kidneys can no longer remove waste products in sufficient quantity to maintain a healthy state. The usual reason for placing a patient on dialysis is renal failure. Because these treatments are not selective regarding which elements are removed from the blood, excess water and electrolytes are removed during the process of removing urea and other nitrogen waste products.

The objectives of diet therapy for patients on dialysis are to:

1. Balance the protein intake with urea removal.
2. Preserve fluid and electrolyte balance.
3. Prevent bone diseases due to low calcium stores.
4. Provide a diet adequate for energy, growth, and maintenance.
5. Obtain the cooperation of the patient in maintaining the dietary regimen.

Dialysis patients may have loss of appetite or nausea due to taste change brought on by the disease. The *hemodialysis* patient can usually have a tray during treatment but the patient on *peritoneal dialysis* should have only small amounts of non-gas-forming and nonirritating foods as food is poorly tolerated during the treatment.

The dietary prescription must be highly individualized. Protein intake is usually slightly restricted and composed of complete proteins. Although hyperlipidemia is almost always present, the diet is not altered from the normal diet as to the percentage of fats. Carbohydrates are utilized to increase the calories in the diet and to prevent the use of protein as energy. By giving appropriate medications, calcium intake is increased and phosphorus intake is decreased to prevent the loss of bone. Potassium is usually restricted. Sodium intake depends upon the amount lost. Some patients go through a phase in which much sodium is lost; others retain sodium and become edematous. Liver and other foods high in iron are recommended. Water-soluble vitamins are lost during dialysis and a supplement may be ordered.

Complete the following:

1. The objectives of diet therapy for dialysis patients are:

   A.

   B.

   C.

D.

E.

2. What are some of the problems the nurse may encounter in getting the dialysis patient to eat?

3. What are the recommendations for each of the following for the dialysis patient?
   Calories:

   Protein:

   Fats:

   Carbohydrates:

   Calcium:

   Phosphorus:

   Sodium:

   Potassium:

   Iron:

   Water-soluble vitamins:

OPTIONAL ACTIVITY TO ENHANCE LEARNING

ACTIVITY 1

Case Study

After a severe streptococcal infection of the throat, which she neglected several days before seeking medical attention, Mrs. A. was admitted to the hospital. The 24-year-old mother was complaining of weakness, headaches, shortness of breath, and loss of appetite. Her throat had apparently healed before admission. Upon examination her blood pressure was 156/98; other vital signs were within normal limits. Mrs. A. stated that she did not seem to be urinating as much as usual. A stat urinalysis revealed that the specific gravity was elevated and that there were large amounts of proteins and blood in the urine. She exhibited pitting edema of both lower extremities. Mrs. A. has always eaten a well-balanced diet with a variety of fruits and vegetables. She states she usually has meat at each meal. She is fond of cola drinks and tea, and drinks copious amounts of these during the day. She is allergic to chocolate. The evening meal is the largest as she likes to serve her husband a balanced diet when he comes from work. Mrs. A. was placed on complete bed rest, with recording of intake, output, and daily weight. Her blood pressure is to be taken twice a day. Pencillin was re-instituted and she was ordered a low-sodium diet.

Prepare a nutritional care plan.

BIBLIOGRAPHY

DARBY, WJ: *Why Salt? How Much?* Contemporary Nutrition 5(6), June, 1980.

HALPERN, SL ET AL: *Quick Reference to Clinical Nutrition: A Guide for Physicians.* JB Lippincott, Philadelphia, 1979. Chapter 15, *Diet therapy of renal failure.*

HEDTRICK, A, GILMAN, CM, AND FRAUMAN, AC: *Nutrition in renal failure: When the patient is a child.* American Journal of Nursing 79(12), December, 1979.

HODGES, RE: *Nutrition in Medical Practice.* WB Saunders, Philadelphia, 1980. Chapter 10, *Nutrition and the kidney.*

KRAUSE, MV AND MAHAN, LK: *Food, Nutrition and Diet Therapy,* ed 6. WB Saunders, Philadelphia, 1979. Chapter 30, *Nutritional care for patients with diseases of the kidney.* Chapter 35, *The metabolic stress response and methods for providing nutritional care to stressed patients.*

LUKE, B: *Nutrition in renal disease: The adult on dialysis.* American Journal of Nursing 79(12), December, 1979.

MARSH, AC, KLIPPSTEIN, RN, AND KAPLAN, SD: *The Sodium Content of Your Food.* Home and Garden Bulletin No 233, US Government Printing Office, August, 1980.

ROBINSON, CH: *Basic Nutrition and Diet Therapy,* ed 4. Macmillan, New York, 1980. Chapter 27, *Diseases of the kidney.*

WILLIAMS, SR: *Mowry's Basic Nutrition and Diet Therapy,* ed 6. CV Mosby, St Louis, 1980. Chapter 18, *Diseases of the urinary tract.*

18

DIET IN GLANDULAR DISTURBANCES

OBJECTIVES

Upon completion of this chapter the student should be able to:

- Discuss the etiology, signs and symptoms, and diet therapy for Addison's disease, hyperthyroidism, hypothyroidism, tetany, and hypoglycemia and choose foods for the appropriate diet for each.
- Give the predisposing factors and signs and symptoms for diabetes mellitus.
- Trace the metabolism of carbohydrates in the body and the sources of glucose.
- Discuss diet therapy for diabetes mellitus, the effect of the type of insulin or hypoglycemic drug upon eating patterns, and the objectives of the dietary prescription.
- Select a day's menu for a diabetic patient from the food exchange lists and give the dietary prescription.

ADDISON'S DISEASE

Addison's disease is due to impaired function of the adrenal cortex. Signs and symptoms are loss of appetite, extreme weakness, dislike for fatty foods, fatigue, and a tan to bronze pigment deposit on the skin. There is an inability to retain sodium in this condition. Before the use of synthetic adrenal cortex hormones, the diet prescribed was a *high-sodium diet.* Patients are also subject to hypoglycemia if meals are too far apart. Frequent feedings high in protein help to prevent this. Some patients are treated by giving them adrenal cortex hormones. This treatment causes potassium loss and some sodium and fluid retention. Foods high in potassium should be included in the diet.

HYPERTHYROIDISM

Hyperthyroidism is overactivity of the thyroid gland. As the thyroid gland secretion, thyroxine, increases metabolism, there is an excessive energy output. These patients are hyperactive, usually thin, and do not gain weight no matter how much they eat. Because of the tremendous energy output, it is difficult to provide enough dietary carbohydrate and fat so that their body proteins will not be used for energy. The dietary prescription is a *high-calorie, high-protein diet.* Stimulants such as coffee are to be avoided.

HYPOTHYROIDISM

Hypothyroidism, or *myxedema,* is underactivity of the thyroid gland. Usually these patients are lazy and sleepy. Many have a tendency to be obese. A *low-calorie diet* is indicated.

TETANY

When the blood is low in calcium, a condition called tetany results, in which there may be muscular cramps or convulsions. Tetany can be caused by the lack of the hormone from the parathyroid glands, inadequate ingestion or absorption of calcium, or alkalosis after excessive vomiting. A *high-calcium, high-vitamin D diet* is usually prescribed.

HYPOGLYCEMIA

In hypoglycemia, or *hyperinsulinism,* more insulin is produced than is needed to metabolize the available carbohydrate. When carbohydrate is ingested, the islands of Langerhans are triggered to produce insulin. Normally, only the amount of insulin necessary to metabolize the amount of carbohydrate is produced. In hypoglycemia, too much insulin is produced each time.

The *hypoglycemic diet* is designed to make the body use some fat and protein for energy in place of the usual carbohydrates. A *high-protein diet* is usually prescribed.

Patients with hypoglycemia usually show symptoms within two hours after eating. They are nervous, perspire freely, tremble, and may lose consciousness. They complain of weakness and may have mental disturbances.

The diet prescription is similar to the diabetic diet with carbohydrate restriction. It is usually divided into three equal portions for the three daily meals. Occasionally, a patient may do better with five or six meals per day.

Complete the following exercises:

1. In Addison's disease, there is an inability to retain ____________ .

2. Plan a day's menu for a patient with Addison's disease.
   Breakfast:

   Lunch:

   Dinner:

3. What is the difference between the metabolism of a patient with hyperthyroidism and one with hypothyroidism?

4. What diet is used for the patient with hyperthyroidism?

5. What diet is frequently prescribed for the patient with hypothyroidism?

6. Plan a low-calorie diet menu for one day.
   Breakfast:

   Lunch:

   Dinner:

7. Using the same basic menu as in the low-calorie diet above, plan a high-calorie diet for one day. For example, if a broiled steak was planned for dinner on the low-calorie diet, a Swiss steak could be used on the high-calorie dinner.
   Breakfast:

   Lunch:

   Dinner:

DIABETES MELLITUS

Diabetes mellitus is a disease in which the patient has difficulty metabolizing carbohydrates due to deficiency of, or complete absence of, the secretion of insulin by the islands of Langerhans. Insulin is one of the hormones necessary for utilization of carbohydrates by the body.

Heredity and obesity are the most important predisposing factors. The diabetic gene is recessive; that is, it is not strong enough to overcome a nondiabetic gene in a normally healthy, well-nourished person. However, if conditions exist that predispose to diabetes, such as obesity or an excessive intake of carbohydrates, the recessive gene can lead to diabetes. Recent studies have indicated that viral infections, stress from certain diseases, and zinc and chromium deficiencies may be factors in the acquisition of diabetes.

Symptoms and Clinical Findings

POLYURIA. A frequent and abnormally large amount of urine results when glucose passes through the kidneys in excessive amounts.

POLYDIPSIA. The loss of fluid through polyuria causes excessive thirst.

DEHYDRATION. When polyuria exists and fluid replacement is insufficient, the body becomes "dry."

POLYPHAGIA. When carbohydrates are not metabolized properly, the body cells do not receive normal nourishment. They are "hungry," and the individual continually eats without satisfying the body.

GENERAL WEAKNESS AND WEIGHT LOSS. Carbohydrates are energy foods. When they cannot be metabolized, fats and proteins must be used for energy. This leads to tissue breakdown.

DECREASED ABILITY OF TISSUE TO HEAL. The abnormally high sugar content of the blood is an excellent breeding ground for bacteria, and the "starved" cells cannot function properly to throw off infection or to repair injuries.

DEGENERATIVE CHANGES. Changes especially prevalent in uncontrolled diabetes are peripheral neuritis, retinitis, disease of coronary arteries, and arteriosclerosis.

KETOSIS (also known as acidosis). When the body must use fats instead of carbohydrates for energy, fatty acids (ketones) accumulate in the blood, as fat does not metabolize completely when great amounts are used for energy. Body tolerance for ketones is limited, and excessive ketones result in coma.

GLYCOSURIA. When the blood sugar level is above normal, there is a spillage of some of the excess into the urine.

HYPERGLYCEMIA. This is the elevation of blood sugar above the normal of 120 milligrams per 100 milliliters of whole blood after 12 hours of fasting.

KETONURIA. When fatty acids are incompletely oxidized or used by the body, ketones are excreted in urine. Acetone is one of the ketones and its presence gives a positive Acetest.

Metabolic Pattern

Glucose in the body can originate from all three nutrients—carbohydrate, protein, or fat. When dietary carbohydrates are lacking or cannot be utilized as in diabetes mellitus, the body converts fat to glucose for use as energy. When fat is insufficient, protein can then be converted.

When the liver utilizes fat for energy, ketone bodies are released in larger than normal amounts. These fatty acids (ketones) disturb the acid-base balance of the body, causing acidosis.

About 58 percent of ingested protein can be converted to glycogen and thus to glucose. However, use of protein for energy leads to weight loss and tissue damage.

Treatment With Insulin

In diabetes mellitus, the body must be provided with insulin. The type of insulin necessary is determined by the physician; it may be regular insulin, which must be given 30 minutes before each meal, or one of the long-acting insulins. (Review insulin in your pharmacology text.) It is important to know which type of insulin the patient is getting in order to anticipate the time of greatest danger from an insulin reaction.

Treatment With Hypoglycemic Drugs

For the patient with a partially functioning pancreas, hypoglycemic drugs may be used instead of insulin. These drugs cause the functional cells of the pancreas to produce more insulin. The drugs cannot be used if there are no functional cells or during periods when the body's need for insulin fluctuates, such as during infection, surgery, or periods of rapid growth. For the older diabetic who developed mild diabetes late in life, the oral hypoglycemic drugs work very well and are less difficult for the patient to learn to use. The nurse should learn the expected and untoward reactions to these drugs.

Treatment With Diet Therapy

Milder types of diabetes can be controlled by dietary management alone. However, this can be done only if the patient is secreting sufficient insulin.

The objectives of diet therapy in diabetes are to:

1. Adjust the diet to the amount of insulin available
   A. Preventing sugar spillage into the urine.

B. Allowing the blood sugar level to rise only slightly above normal (80 to 120 milligrams per 100 milliliters of fasting whole blood).

2. Furnish an adequate diet for good health and normal activity.

Generally speaking, the diabetic person requires the same nutrients as the normal individual, and the same procedure is used to plan the diabetic diet with the following modifications:

1. Caloric requirements are determined, based upon height, weight, age, sex, activity, and so forth.
2. Most physicians recommend keeping the diabetic patient's weight slightly below normal.
3. Additional protein is frequently allowed as a preventive measure against degenerative diseases, which are prevalent among diabetic individuals.
4. Carbohydrate allowances are determined by examining the blood for sugar, by urinalysis, and by an estimate of available insulin.
5. The remaining dietary calories consist of fat.

There are several methods of dividing the daily food allowance between the meals. With quick-acting insulins that are given before each meal, the usual division is 1/3 of the carbohydrate level at breakfast, 1/3 at noon, and 1/3 at supper. If one of the longer-acting insulins is given, the diabetic patient may receive 1/5 of the carbohydrate allowance at breakfast, 2/5 for lunch, and 2/5 for supper. With the intermediate type of insulin, the division may be 1/6 at breakfast, 2/6 (1/3) at lunch, 2/6 (1/3) at supper, and the remaining 1/6 for an afternoon snack. When the time of greatest action for the insulin occurs in the evening, a supplementary feeding may be necessary. Supplementary feedings, whether between meals or at bedtime, must be deducted from the allowance for the meal nearest the feeding.

However the food allowance is divided, the diabetic patient must eat only the amount of food that is allowed, and *all* of the food must be consumed. If the diabetic patient eats more than has been planned, there will be a shortage of insulin to take care of it. Thus the patient is risking acidosis. If the diabetic patient does not eat all of the food planned on the diet, there will be an excess of insulin, which could result in insulin shock. The diabetic patient must always remember that the amount of food taken in must be in balance with the amount of insulin available to take care of it. This also means that the allowance for each meal must remain constant, as the carbohydrates must be available when the insulin is active. If diabetic patients do not consume all of the food allotted for a meal, they may be required to take orange juice or grapefruit juice to replace the unconsumed calories.

The physician will write the diet prescription for the exact amounts of carbohydrate, fat, and protein. In order to follow the prescription, the patient will either have to weigh the food or measure its volume using household implements. Weighing food is difficult, as the scale used is in the metric system with which many patients are unfamiliar. Weighing food is also a great deal of trouble and impossible under some conditions. Most patients understand the measured diet better. Measured diets are less trouble to prepare, and specially prepared diabetic food is not always necessary. Diabetic patients can even eat in public places if they choose their foods carefully.

Food Exchange List

Use of a food exchange list has made meal planning for the diabetic patients much easier. It is not necessary to prepare specially weighed foods when using the exchange lists. Measurements are simple household measurements. A wider variety of foods is available to patients, and they can plan a menu of foods they are accustomed to in most cases.

Within the exchange lists, foods are grouped according to the amounts of carbohydrate, fat, and protein they contain. While the ratio of the three nutrients may be the same in various foods of one group, one food may contain a larger amount of each. For example, oranges, bananas, and raisins are all essentially carbohydrate foods with negligible amounts of fat and protein; therefore, they are grouped in one "exchange." However, since the amount of carbohydrate varies among the three fruits, the amount of each fruit allowed as one "exchange" is limited to that which will produce 10 grams of carbohydrate. One small orange, half a medium banana, or 1 full tablespoon of raisins will yield 10 grams of carbohydrate. Diabetic patients who are allowed one "fruit exchange" may choose any of the fruits listed under "fruit exchange" *in the amount listed.* If two fruit exchanges are allowed for a meal, they may choose two of the fruits in the amounts listed or they may double the portion of one fruit.

There is an exchange list for each of the following: milk, meat and other high-protein foods, fruit, bread or carbohydrates, vegetables, and fats. Exchange lists are given in the Appendix.

Most foods are easily placed in the proper category, but there are several exceptions. An avocado is a fruit, but its fat content is so high that it is in the fat exchange. Cream is in the fat exchange, while cheese, also a milk product, is found in the meat exchange. Although a meat product, bacon is in the fat exchange because it is deficient in protein and has an excess of fat. Olives and nuts are also found in the fat exchange. Corn, dried beans, peas, and certain cereals are found in the bread exchange.

In addition to the above deviations, several "odd" foods cannot be placed in an exchange list without modifications. Whole milk is one of these. Skim milk has the same amount of protein and carbohydrate as whole milk, but it lacks the fat. When diabetic patients use whole milk, they have to use two of their fat exchanges. These must be deducted from their allowed fat exchanges for that meal in order to stay within their dietary prescription. Ice cream is listed in the bread exchange, but when it is chosen, two fat exchanges must be available for use. Ice cream then takes one bread exchange and two fat exchanges.

Vegetables are divided into two groups, according to the amount of carbohydrate found in them. The raw vegetables group contains so little carbohydrate that when they are served the carbohydrate is not counted. These vegetables make good "fillers."

There are also a number of condiments, seasonings, and very low-calorie foods that the diabetic patient may use without restriction.

In using the food exchange lists to plan the daily menu, the patients choose the way they "spend" their exchanges. For example, the three breakfast menus below have been planned with the same number of exchanges—two bread exchanges, two meat exchanges, one fruit exchange, one milk exchange, and three fat exchanges.

Breakfast #1

Orange juice, 1/2 cup	1 Fruit exchange
Broiled bacon, 1 slice	1 Fat exchange
Boiled eggs, 2	2 Meat exchanges
Small biscuits, 2	2 Bread exchanges
Skim milk, 1 cup	1 Milk exchange
Butter, 2 pats	2 Fat exchanges
Black coffee, ad lib.	

Breakfast #2

Shredded wheat biscuit, 1 small	1 Bread exchange
with	
Medium banana, 1/2	1 Fruit exchange
and	
Whole milk, 1 cup	2 Fat exchanges 1 Milk exchange
Ham, 1 slice,	1 Meat exchange
Poached egg, 1	1 Meat exchange
Toast, 1 slice	1 Bread exchange
Butter, 1 pat	1 Fat exchange
Tea with artificial sweetener, ad lib.	

Breakfast #3

Grapefruit, 1/2 small	1 Fruit exchange
Creamed dried beef on toast made with	
Butter, 1 pat	1 Fat exchange
Whole milk, 1 cup	1 Milk exchange 2 Fat exchanges

Flour, $2\frac{1}{2}$ tbsp. . . . . 1 Bread exchange
Dried beef, 2 slices . . . . 2 Meat exchanges
Toast, 1 slice . . . . 1 Bread exchange

Black coffee, ad lib.

Complete the following exercises:

1. In diabetes mellitus ________________ are not properly utilized by the body. This is due usually to a deficiency of a hormone called ________________ .

2. The two most important factors in the development of diabetes are ________________ and ________________ .

3. When the blood sugar is in excess of 120 milligrams per 100 milliliters of whole fasting blood, the condition is called ______________ . This condition leads to an excessive overflow of urine called ________________ . This in turn leads to excessive thirst, or ________________, and a loss of body fluids, leaving the body in a state of ________________. When carbohydrates are not properly metabolized, the cells do not receive proper nourishment, and the patient is constantly hungry. Excessive eating is called ________________ . When carbohydrate is not used for energy, fat must be substituted. Excessive use of fat for energy leads to an excess of fatty acids and ________________ in the blood. These fatty acids disturb the acid-base balance of the body, causing the coma-like condition known as ________________ or ________________ . This condition can be determined by two tests on urine; when the urine tests are positive for acetone, the condition is known as ________________ .

4. Diabetes mellitus is treated by:

   A.

   B.

5. In writing the diabetic dietary prescription, the doctor determines:

   A. The caloric requirement by:

B. The carbohydrate allowance by:

C. The fat allowance by:

6. How the daily food allowance is to be divided depends upon:

7. Using the food exchange list, plan menus based upon the exchanges given and staying within a 1000-calorie daily allotment.

Breakfast:

1 Fruit exchange
1 Bread exchange
2 Meat exchanges
1/2 Milk exchange
Coffee or tea, ad lib.

Lunch:

2 Meat exchanges
1 Bread exchange
Vegetables, raw, ad lib.
1 Fruit exchange
1/2 Milk
1 Fat exchange
Coffee or tea, ad lib.

Dinner:

2 Meat exchanges
1 Bread exchange
Vegetables, raw, ad lib.
1 Vegetable
1 Fruit exchange
Coffee or tea, ad lib.

8. There are 10 grams of carbohydrate in one fruit exchange. How many calories are there in one fruit exchange?

9. There are 12 grams of carbohydrate, 8 grams of protein, and a trace of fat in one milk exchange. How many calories are there in one milk exchange?

10. In one meat exchange, there are 7 grams of protein and 3 grams of fat. How many calories?

11. There are 5 grams of fat in one fat exchange. How many calories?

12. In one bread exchange, there are 15 grams of carbohydrate and 2 grams of protein. How many calories?

13. If there are 5 grams of carbohydrate and 2 grams of protein in each vegetable exchange, how many calories are in one cup of vegetables?

14. Plan a menu based upon the exchanges given and compute the number of calories allowed for the day.

Breakfast:	Calories
2 Fruit exchanges	________
2 Bread exchanges	________
2 Meat exchanges	________
1 Milk exchange	________
1 Fat exchange	________
Coffee or tea, ad lib.	________

Lunch:

	Calories
2 Meat exchanges	________
2 Bread exchanges	________
Vegetables, raw, ad lib.	________
1 Vegetable	________
1 Fruit exchange	________
1 Milk exchange	________
1 Fat exchange	________
Coffee or tea, ad lib.	________

Dinner:

2 Meat exchanges	________
2 Bread exchanges	________
Vegetables, raw, ad lib.	________
1 Milk exchange	________
1 Fat exchange	________
Coffee or tea, ad lib.	________
TOTAL:	

15. The following menu is one used for a diabetic patient who had to carry lunch to work. Decide which exchanges the patient had to have and then find out how many calories were allowed each day.

Breakfast:

	Exchange	Calories
Orange juice, 1 cup	________	________
Cooked cereal, 3/4 cup	________	________
Toast, 1 slice	________	________
Egg, poached, 1	________	________
Ham, boiled, 1 slice, $3 \times 2 \times 1/3$ in.	________	________
Butter, 2 tsp.	________	________
Milk, skim, 1 cup	________	________
Black coffee, 1 cup	________	________

Lunch:

Egg, hard boiled and chopped, 1,	________	________
mixed with mayonnaise, 1 tsp.	________	________
Bread, 2 slices	________	________
Lettuce, 1 leaf	________	________
(Made into a sandwich)	________	________

	Exchange	Calories
Lunch—*continued*		
Dill pickles and radishes, 3 each	______	______
Orange, small, 1	______	______
Apple, small, 1	______	______
Milk, skim, 1 cup	______	______
Mid-afternoon snack:		
American cheese, 1 slice	______	______
Soda crackers, 3	______	______
Butter, 1 tsp.	______	______
Coffee, 1 cup	______	______
Dinner:		
Grapefruit juice, 1/2 cup	______	______
Tuna fish, 3/4 cup	______	______
Potato, baked, 4 in. diameter	______	______
Butter, 1 tsp.	______	______
Peas, 1/2 cup	______	______
Lettuce salad, 1 cup with tarragon vinegar	______	______
Bread, 2 slices	______	______
Pear, 1 small	______	______
Milk, whole, 1 cup	______	______
Bedtime snack:		
Sandwich made from:		
Rye bread, 2 slices	______	______
Ham, 2 slices	______	______
Mayonnaise, 1 tsp.	______	______
TOTAL:	______	______

16. Would the patient above be on regular or long-acting insulin? ________ Why do you think so?

17. In what exchange do we find avocado?

18. Bacon is in the ____________ exchange. Ice cream is in the ____________ exchange. If you wish ice cream, what other exchange must you have?

19. If you serve whole milk for one milk exchange, you must have ________________________ exchanges to stay within the dietary prescription.

20. May J., a diabetic, refused to eat one slice of her bread at lunch. What should she do?

21. How many calories are in 1 slice of bread? ________ How much orange juice would it take to make up the same number of calories? ________

22. Orange juice contains glucose, which does not need digesting and can be absorbed immediately. Which of the following is best to give a patient in insulin shock who is still able to swallow? Orange juice, crackers, or bread and butter?

23. Sugar can be given to patients in insulin shock. What ways are there to give sugar other than by mouth?

24. Why is glucose the best form of sugar to give by mouth to the patient in shock?

OPTIONAL ACTIVITY TO ENHANCE LEARNING

ACTIVITY 1

Case Study

Mr. K. is a 45-year-old carpenter admitted to the hospital with gangrene of the left big toe. His father was a diabetic and Mr. K.'s blood sugar was 248 on admission. He weighs 230 pounds and is six feet tall. Mr. K. usually has two eggs, bacon, toast, and coffee for breakfast. He carries two sandwiches, a pickle, and a piece of cake for lunch. For supper, his wife usually prepares a meat, potatoes, cornbread, green beans or peas, and a dessert. Mr. K.'s bedtime snack consists of a glass of milk and another helping of dessert. Upon questioning Mr. K., the physician learned that he had been voiding an increasing amount of urine, which he attributed to the fact that he was drinking large amounts of water during the hot weather. The physician prescribed a 1200-calorie diabetic diet with 85 grams of protein, 30 grams of fat, and 150 grams of carbohydrate. Fats are to be mostly polyunsaturated. Regular insulin would be given until such time that Mr. K. could be maintained on diet alone. The dietitian visited Mr. K. and the following meal plan was chosen.

Breakfast—1 fruit exchange, 2 bread exchanges, 2 lean meat exchanges, 1 skim milk exchange.

Lunch—3 lean meat exchanges, 2 bread exchanges, 1 vegetable exchange, 1 fruit exchange, 1 skim milk exchange.

Dinner—3 meat exchanges, 1 vegetable exchange, 1 bread exchange, 1 fat exchange, 2 fruit exchanges.

Bedtime snack—May take 1 or 2 exchanges from the dinner allowance to use in addition to foods from those allowed as desired.

Prepare a nutritional care plan.

BIBLIOGRAPHY

BIERMAN, EL: *Diabetes mellitus.* Contemporary Nutrition 2(12), December, 1977.

CALIENDO, MA: *Nutrition and Preventitive Health Care.* Macmillan, New York, 1981. Chapter 11, *Diet, nutrition and other diseases (diabetes, hypertension, alcoholism).*

DANOWSKI, TS: *Sugar and disease.* Contemporary Nutrition 3(12), December, 1978.

HALPERN, SL ET AL: *Quick Reference to Clinical Nutrition: A Guide for Physicians.* JB Lippincott, Philadelphia, 1979. Chapter 16, *New concepts of the diet therapy of diabetes mellitus.*

HODGES, RS: *Nutrition in Medical Practice.* WB Saunders, Philadelphia, 1980. Chapter 7, *Nutrition and the endocrine system.*

HOFMANN, L: *The Great American Nutrition Hassle.* Mayfield, Palo Alto, California, 1978. Chapter 24, *Sugar doctors push hypoglycemia.*

KRAUSE, MV AND MAHAN, LK: *Food, Nutrition and Diet Therapy,* ed 6. WB Saunders, Philadelphia, 1979. Chapter 25, *Nutritional care for patients with disorders of the endocrine pancreas: Diabetes mellitus and hypoglycemia.* Chapter 26, *Nutritional care for patients with diseases of the adrenal cortex and thyroid gland and other diseases of metabolism.*

LORICH, ML AND KAISER, SA: *A diabetic child is still a child—with diabetes.* RN 38 (10), October, 1975.

MARSH, AC, KLIPPSTEIN, RN, AND KAPLAN, SD: *The Sodium Content of Your Food.* Home and Garden Bulletin No 233, US Government Printing Office, August, 1980.

MARTIN, MM: *Insulin reaction.* American Journal of Nursing 67(2), February, 1967.

ROBINSON, CH: *Basic Nutrition and Diet Therapy,* ed 4. Macmillan, New York, 1980. Chapter 23, *Diabetes mellitus.* Chapter 24, *Various metabolic disorders.*

SERVUCE, FJ: *Hypoglycemia.* Contemporary Nutrition 2(7), July, 1977.

SUITOR, CW AND HUNTER, MF: *Nutrition: Principles and Application in Health Promotion.* JB Lippincott, Philadelphia, 1980. Chapter 30, *Alteration in blood sugar.*

WILLIAMS, SR: *Mowry's Basic Nutrition and Diet Therapy,* ed 6. CV Mosby, St Louis, 1980. Chapter 21, *Diabetes.*

19

DIET IN FEVERS AND INFECTIONS

OBJECTIVES

Upon completion of this chapter the student should be able to:

- State the changes that occur in the body when its temperature is elevated.
- Plan the diet for a patient with a fever or infection, selecting foods appropriate to the stage of the infection.

Infection frequently makes itself known by causing an increase in body temperature known as fever. Several bodily changes occur during a fever:

1. The body produces more heat than it can dissipate.
2. Metabolism and energy output increase.
3. Nitrogen, an element of protein, is lost.
4. Resistance to disease and further infection is lowered.
5. Toxic material may accumulate in the body.
6. Water balance may be disturbed, and dehydration usually occurs.

There are three types of infection:

1. *Acute* infections are usually caused by colds, pneumonia, influenza, and typhoid fever.
2. *Chronic* infections may be caused by diseases such as tuberculosis.
3. *Recurrent* infections may be caused by diseases such as malaria.

The general principles of dietary treatment in each type of infection are the same while there is fever. In the subacute, or afebrile, phase of the infection, less protein and fewer calories are necessary.

A *high-calorie diet* is given to patients with fever to replenish the energy used by increased metabolism and patient restlessness. For each degree Farenheit that the temperature is elevated, the body needs an 8 percent increase in calories. The diet should be *high in protein* to counteract the loss of nitrogen.

Foods chosen should be easily digested and offered in small quantities at two- to three-hour intervals rather than in three large meals. Milk and egg dishes are the most easily digested proteins. For ease of digestion and for quick energy, glucose, corn syrup, and cane sugar are used to sweeten the food as necessary. The use of emulsified fats aids in digestion, but if the patient is nauseated, even emulsified fats are omitted. There is an increased need for vitamin B complex and vitamin C.

Fluids are an important part of the dietary prescription. The patient should receive 3000 to 5000 milliliters of fluids per day. This amount is needed to replenish fluids lost in perspiration. Fluids are also needed to provide water for removal of toxic materials through the kidneys.

When milk is given to patients having difficulty breathing due to excess mucus in the throat, the nurse should use suction or other means to clear the throat after the milk is taken. Salt balance can be maintained by using salty broths, consommes, and bouillon as part of the fluid intake. Liquids that have a slightly tart flavor rather than very sweet ones should be served, as sweet liquids may cause digestive upsets.

In the subacute, or afebrile, phase of the infection, less protein and fewer calories are necessary. As the patient with fever improves, the diet can progress from a *full liquid diet* to a *soft bland diet of low fiber content.* The patient will still need extra protein daily for a while. Consideration should be given to the patient's need to conserve energy and the food should be easy for the patient to eat.

Complete the following:

1. Plan a day's full liquid menu for a patient with fever. Give the hour and the amount of each feeding.

2. Plan a soft bland diet for a patient with fever and include between meal feedings:

Breakfast:

Mid-morning:

Lunch:

Mid-afternoon:

Dinner:

Bedtime:

3. How many milliliters of fluid does your soft diet menu have?

4. What foods that are high in vitamin B complex could the patient on a soft bland diet have?

5. What foods that are high in vitamin B complex could the patient on a full liquid diet have?

6. What foods that are high in vitamin C could the patient on a full liquid diet have?

7. Why is extra protein necessary for a patient with an infection and fever?

8. Why are more calories necessary for a patient with an infection and fever?

9. If there is increased perspiration and loss of salts through perspiration, what happens to the water balance of the body?

10. How can water balance be maintained?

11. What foods contain emulsified fats?

OPTIONAL ACTIVITY TO ENHANCE LEARNING

ACTIVITY 1

Case Study

Mr. L. is a 65-year-old recluse who lives alone on a farm several miles from his nearest neighbor. Mr. L. was discovered in his small house when one of the neighbors went to ask him if he had seen a lost horse. Mr. L. was very ill, burning with fever, and had apparently been ill for some time. Upon admission to the hospital his temperature was 105°F. His skin was flushed and dry. His eyes were sunken and he showed signs of photophobia. His lips were cracked; his tongue coated. When Mr. L. awakened, he complained of headache and weakness. His usual weight was 145 pounds; on admission Mr. L. weighed 132 pounds. A nutritional history could not be obtained on admission because Mr. L. had difficulty concentrating on the questions. The diagnosis on admission was fever of undetermined origin. Because Mr. L. refused to eat, his physician ordered that he be given fluids, as much as can be forced without adverse reactions. The physician wants to avoid giving intravenous feedings after the bottle that was started on admission has been completed.

Prepare a nutritional care plan.

BIBLIOGRAPHY

ANDERSON, TW: *Vitamin C and the common cold.* Contemporary Nutrition 3(10), October, 1978.

HODGES, RE: *Nutrition in Medical Practice.* WB Saunders, Philadelphia, 1980. Chapter 9, *Nutrition and Infection.*

KRAUSE, MV AND MAHAN, LK: *Food, Nutrition and Diet Therapy,* ed 6. WB Saunders, Philadelphia, 1979. Chapter 35, *The metabolic stress response and methods for providing nutritional care to stressed patients.*

PALOMBO, JD AND BLACKBURN, GL: *Human protein requirements.* Contemporary Nutrition 5(1), January, 1980.

ROBINSON, CH: *Basic Nutrition and Diet Therapy,* ed 4. Macmillan, New York, 1980. Chapter 24, *Various metabolic disorders.*

SUITOR, CW AND HUNTER, MF: *Nutrition: Principles and Application in Health Promotion.* JB Lippincott, Philadelphia, 1980. Chapter 27, *Diet changes and stress.*

WATSON, RR: *Nutrition and immunity.* Contemporary Nutrition, 6(5), May, 1981.

20

DIET IN ALLERGIES

OBJECTIVES

Upon completion of this chapter the student should be able to:

- Explain how substances that cause allergic reaction enter the body and give some methods of identifying the causative agents.
- Explain the procedure used in the Rowe elimination diet.
- Identify the foods that most commonly cause allergic reactions.

ALLERGY

Allergy is a condition of exaggerated specific reaction to a substance to which the majority of people will not react. Substances that cause allergic reactions may be taken in by mouth, by inhaling into the lungs, by direct contact with the skin, and by injection. Although more adults than children have allergies, children most often have food allergies. It has not been proved that allergies are inherited, but it is known that the tendency toward allergies occurs in families. An individual usually has more than one allergy.

Diagnosis of allergies (actually identifying the causative agent) is made by:

1. Skin tests.
   A. The suspected agent is taped to the skin for a period of time to see if a reaction will occur.
   B. The skin is scratched and a little of the suspected substance is rubbed into the scratch.
   C. The substance is injected intradermally, between the layers of skin.
2. Elimination of a possible agent's contact with the patient.

ROWE'S ELIMINATION DIET. This is frequently used when food is suspected of causing the allergic reaction. The diet consists of five specific items: one meat, two vegetables, one cereal, one fruit. If the first five foods cause no reaction symptoms, other foods are gradually added. This is tedious and very discouraging to the patient, especially as most allergies do not occur singly. If one is present, there is usually another that may cause reactions.

Protein foods seem to cause more food allergies than fats or carbohydrates. The most frequent offenders are eggs, milk, chocolate, wheat, fish, tomatoes, and strawberries. If an infant is allergic to strawberries, oranges, shellfish, eggs, or milk, the infant may have an allergic reaction when breastfed if the mother has had these foods in her meals. The dietary treatment of a food allergy is to avoid the offending agent. However, when the food is important in furnishing essential nutrients, other foods that will supply the need must be substituted.

Occasionally, if the allergic reaction is mild, *desensitization* is attempted. After prolonged abstinence, small amounts of the offending food are gradually introduced into the diet. Desensitization is usually tried when the allergy is to an important food such as milk.

OPTIONAL ACTIVITY TO ENHANCE LEARNING

ACTIVITY 1

Case Study

Miss T. is a 17-year-old student. She has just been diagnosed as being allergic to eggs. Several months ago she developed diarrhea and abdominal cramps at intermittent intervals. She was seen in the gastrointestinal clinic where the workup revealed no pathologic reasons for her discomfort. She was referred to the allergy clinic for testing. She lives with her mother; her parents obtained a divorce a month before her first clinic visit. She is an only child and has been close to both parents. Prior to the

OPTIONAL ACTIVITIES—*Continued*

recent episodes of diarrhea, Miss T. has never had any major illnesses. She usually eats cereal with milk for breakfast, occasionally having waffles. She weighs 105 pounds and is 5 feet 2 inches tall. Because her peers are weight conscious, she has gotten into the habit of joining them in their diet luncheon consisting of a boiled egg, lettuce salad, and tea. Lately she has been nibbling at dinner time, as her mother works in the evening and Miss T. does not like to eat alone. She usually chooses cheese or luncheon meat and a piece of cake or cookie for dinner. Miss T. is being referred to the clinical psychologist for counseling and has been placed on an egg-free diet.

Prepare a nutritional care plan.

BIBLIOGRAPHY

BRENEMAN, JC: *Food allergy.* Contemporary Nutrition 4(3), March, 1979.

FOMON, SJ: *Infant Nutrition.* WB Saunders, Philadelphia, 1974. Chapter 17, *Food allergy.*

KRAUSE, MV AND MAHAN, LK: *Food, Nutrition and Diet Therapy,* ed 6. WB Saunders, Philadelphia, 1979. Chapter 31, *Nutritional care for patients with food allergy.*

PARKER, C: *Food allergies.* American Journal of Nursing 80(2), February, 1980.

ROBINSON, CH: *Basic Nutrition and Diet Therapy,* ed 4. Macmillan, New York, 1980. Chapter 33, *Food allergies and skin disorders.*

SUITOR, CW AND HUNTER, MF: *Nutrition: Principles and Application in Health Promotion.* JB Lippincott, Philadelphia, 1980. Chapter 9, *Promoting sound eating habits during childhood and adulthood.*

WILLIAMS, SR: *Mowry's Basic Nutrition and Diet Therapy,* ed 6. CV Mosby, St Louis, 1980. Chapter 24, *Allergy.*

21

DIET IN DISEASES OF THE MUSCULOSKELETAL SYSTEM

OBJECTIVES

Upon completion of this chapter the student should be able to:

- Give the dietary objectives and dietary prescription for arthritis, gout, lead poisoning, fractures, and dental caries.
- Select food for a day's menu for a low-purine diet and a high-calcium diet.

ARTHRITIS

Arthritis is inflammation of the joints. There are several types of arthritis, but in each the dietary objective is usually to prevent obesity, which adds to the work of the joints and to maintain good nutritional status. Unfortunately, many arthritic patients have poor eating habits. If malnutrition exists, it should be corrected. To prevent obesity, a *low-calorie diet* may be indicated as the arthritic patient usually cannot be as active as other individuals.

GOUT

Gout is an arthritic-like condition of metabolic origin in which the joints may be swollen and painful. Uric acid is the end product of metabolism of certain proteins called purines and normally is excreted through the kidneys. For some unknown reason, in gout, uric acid is not excreted normally. Deposit of uric acid salts in the joint causes the swelling and pain.

The dietary treatment during the acute stage of gout is a *low-purine diet.* Fats should be kept to a low-normal level because they interfere with the body's ability to excrete uric acid products. All animal proteins are high in purine, and glandular meats, such as liver and kidney, are especially high. The patient is allowed only two servings of meat per week, and broths, gravies, and soups of meat extracts should not be served. Eggs and cheese are served as meat substitutes. Vegetables high in protein, such as dried beans, dried peas, and lentils, are avoided. Milk is used to make up the protein needed. All stimulants, such as coffee, tea, or alcoholic beverages, are omitted. All fruits and cereals except oatmeal are permitted. This is a difficult diet to maintain.

Because there are drugs available today that aid in removal of excessive uric acid, the subacute phase of gout no longer requires a rigid dietary regimen. High-purine foods should be avoided. A weight-reduction diet may be ordered for obese patients.

LEAD POISONING

Lead poisoning can occur when there is contact with lead through the skin, the gastrointestinal tract, or the respiratory tract. Lead poisoning is accumulative. Lead is stored in the bones, and the patient may have anemia with degeneration of red blood cells. Early symptoms are abdominal pains, vomiting, irritability, weakness, and loss of appetite. The patient may complain of pains in the joints. Children frequently are poisoned by the lead in paint on, or chipping off, furniture or walls.

During the acute phase of lead poisoning, the patient is given a diet high in calcium to prevent release of lead from the bones in large doses, which would destroy red blood cells. After the acute phase, a diet low in calcium may be given to permit the slow withdrawal of lead from the bone. The anemia is treated by extra proteins and iron. In the *high-calcium diet,* the patient is encouraged to drink one to two quarts of milk a day and to eat cheese three or four times a week.

FRACTURES

Although calcium and phosphorus are necessary for bone repair, recent research has shown that there is a tendency for large amounts of calcium and phosphorus to be excreted when bone is immobilized and stress is not placed upon it. If excessive amounts of calcium are ingested, this calcium and the calcium released by the bones causes a problem for the kidneys because renal calculi form when excessive minerals are excreted.

The patient with a fracture is now placed on a *high-protein diet* to aid in tissue repair. If the fracture is in a weight-bearing area, reduction of the caloric content of the diet may be necessary to discourage obesity.

DENTAL CARIES

Ninety-eight percent of all the people in the United States have a problem with dental caries. This is an infectious disease caused by bacteria that grow on teeth and destroy the enamel with acids they produce from starches and sugars. The longer sugars remain in the mouth the more quickly caries form.

Tooth formation begins before birth and the teeth are completely set by age 12. Poor nutrition during the formative stages can never be overcome. A diet adequate in calcium, phosphorus, and vitamins A and C is recommended at all stages. Fluorides added to drinking water and dentrifices are effective in increasing resistance to caries but fluorides do not pass the placental barrier.

Good dental hygiene is absolutely necessary to prevent caries and should be carried out after each meal or snack. Foods that are high in sugar and that are sticky are the worst offenders in causing caries.

Oral hygiene is also important for infants. Milk and other liquids should be cleansed from the mouth. Infants and small children who are allowed to go to sleep with a bottle in their mouths are prone to decay of the teeth. This is called "nursing bottle syndrome" and can be quite severe, especially when sweet liquids are given.

Complete the following exercises:

1. What foods metabolize into uric acid?

2. What foods should the patient with gout avoid?

3. How does the patient with gout obtain the necessary dietary protein?

4. Why are dried beans, dried peas, and other legumes to be avoided by the patient with gout?

5. Plan a day's menu for a patient with gout.
Breakfast:

Lunch:

Dinner:

6. Plan a low-calorie diet for a patient with arthritis.
Breakfast:

Lunch:

Dinner:

7. Plan a day's menu for a diet high in calcium for the patient with lead poisoning.
Breakfast:

Lunch:

Dinner:

8. Why isn't a patient with a fracture given extra calcium?

9. If a patient with a fractured leg is in a walking cast, why may the physician want the patient to reduce caloric intake?

10. Dental caries are caused by:

11. To prevent tooth malformations, the diet should be adequate in:

12. The "nursing bottle syndrome" is caused by:

13. How is fluoride ingested?

14. What can you do to prevent dental caries?

OPTIONAL ACTIVITY TO ENHANCE LEARNING

ACTIVITY 1

Case Study

Mr. P. has been having pain in his right knee and in the joint of his left big toe. The joint appears to be swollen and is warmer than the surrounding tissues. Blood work showed that Mr. P. had a sharply elevated uric acid level. Mr. P. owns a farm and complains that his knee and toe make it uncomfortable to do his chores. The P. family butcher their own meat and keep their deep freeze filled with beef and pork. They seldom eat fish and Mr. P. reported that strawberries make him itch. The family milk their own cows and use the cream on their breakfast oatmeal. Skim milk is drunk at every meal. Mr. P. drinks two cups of coffee at breakfast. Mr. and Mrs. P. belong to a dance club and Mr. P. usually drinks five or six beers at every dance. Mrs. P. frequently makes homemade soup for lunch based on her own meat broth. Although the physician ordered medication to remove excess uric acid from Mr. P.'s body, the physician has suggested that Mr. P. stay on a low-purine diet until the next visit.

Prepare a nutritional care plan.

BIBLIOGRAPHY

BRIGGS, GM AND CALLOWAY, DH: *Bogert's Nutrition and Physical Fitness*, ed 10. WB Saunders, Philadelphia, 1979. Chapter 23, *Dental health, nutrition and diet.*

BOWEN, WH: *Dental caries.* Contemporary Nutrition 2(8), August, 1977.

CALIENDO, MA: *Nutrition and Preventitive Health Care.* Macmillan, New York, 1981. Chapter 10, *Diet, nutrition and dental caries.*

COLLIER, DR: *Fluorine: An essential element for good dental health.* Contemporary Nutrition 4(10), October, 1979.

DELUCA, HF: *Modern view of vitamin D.* Contemporary Nutrition 6(2), February, 1981.

HALPERN, SL ET AL: *Quick Reference to Clinical Nutrition: A Guide for Physicians.* JB Lippincott, Philadelphia, 1979. Chapter 22, *Nutrition in dental health.*

HODGES, RE: *Nutrition in Medical Practice.* WB Saunders, Philadelphia, 1980. Chapter 6, *Nutrition and the musculoskeletal system.*

KRAUSE, MV AND MAHAN, LK: *Food, Nutrition and Diet Therapy*, ed 6. WB Saunders, Philadelphia, 1979. Chapter 33, *Nutritional care for patients with diseases of the musculoskeletal system.*

RIPA, LW: *Nursing habits and dental decay in infants: 'Nursing bottle caries.'* Contemporary Nutrition 3(5), May, 1978.

SUITOR, CW AND HUNTER, MF: *Nutrition: Principles and Application in Health Promotion.* Chapter 17, *The role of nutrients in dental health.*

WORTHINGTON-ROBERTS, BS: *Contemporary Developments in Nutrition.* CV Mosby, St Louis, 1981. Chapter 14, *Nutrition, diet, and oral health.*

22

DIET IN PSYCHIATRIC CONDITIONS AND DISEASES OF THE NERVOUS SYSTEM

OBJECTIVES

Upon completion of this chapter the student should be able to:

- Discuss nutritional needs in psychiatric conditions, anorexia nervosa, alcoholism, and drug addiction.
- State why megavitamin therapy can be dangerous.
- Define and give the signs and symptoms and diet therapy for neuritis, epilepsy, multiple sclerosis, and hyperkinesis.
- Select foods for a ketogenic diet.

Although it is known that certain nutritional deficiencies affect the brain and nervous system (and thus mental functioning), it is questioned that diet therapy is effective in conditions in which there is no deficiency. The brain and nervous system metabolize nutrients at a greater rate than any other tissue. Glucose is metabolized so quickly that convulsions and coma occur when high levels of insulin induce severe hypoglycemia. The synthesis of *neurotransmitters,* substances that transmit signals across the synapses of nerve cells, is affected by the diet; a high protein intake alters the effect of the drug L-dopa, given for parkinsonism. Tryptophan, an amino acid found in milk, is useful for inducing sleep. B-complex deficiency can cause depression, irritability, and mental confusion.

Recent studies have shown that there is probably a chemical basis for schizophrenia. This has led to the use of *megavitamin therapy*, a questionable practice. The use of excessive vitamins can result in toxicity with the fat-soluble vitamins and rebound deficiency conditions if the megavitamin therapy is suddenly stopped. Even the water-soluble vitamins, which have limited storage in the body, can be detrimental in excessive doses. Niacin in large doses causes flushing and itching, liver damage, and hyperglycemia. Ascorbic acid in massive doses may precipitate gout or hemolytic anemia in susceptible persons. Megadoses of pyridoxine can produce liver disease. Megavitamin therapy can be a dangerous practice, especially in the hands of a layman.

MENTAL ILLNESS

It is estimated that 50 percent of hospitalized patients have mental or emotional problems. Many of these are in a poor nutritional state because their anxieties have caused them to neglect their physical health. Some have used food to overcome anxieties and are overweight; others have neglected to eat properly, or at all, and are underweight. It is the nurse's responsibility to encourage the patient to accept a well-balanced diet. Mealtime is a time of social interaction and the rituals of eating can be utilized as a part of psychiatric therapy.

Mealtimes for mental patients should be especially pleasant and non-threatening. The likes and dislikes of the patient must be taken into consideration, as well as the diagnosis. Patients in half-way houses can be helped by the nurse with problems of selecting, purchasing, and preparing meals, activities that may be overwhelming to the patient at first.

ANOREXIA NERVOSA

Anorexia nervosa, a condition found mostly in teenage girls (although it can occur in men and older persons), is a psychologic problem in which the patient refuses to eat. The patient becomes emaciated and overactive. Cessation of the menstrual period occurs and the basal metabolism rate falls. Basically, these patients think they are grossly overweight and start dieting drastically. They do not feel hungry or fatigued. Some have episodes of overeating followed by guilt and may induce vomiting or use strong cathartics to rid their bodies of the food ingested.

The treatment for anorexia nervosa involves both psychotherapy to uncover emotional problems and diet therapy to remedy the nutritional deficits. In starvation, there comes a time when there is no desire to eat. This makes it even more difficult to obtain the cooperation of a patient with severe anorexia nervosa. The patients' menus are selected for them to relieve the patients of decision-making. A *high-calorie, high-protein, liquid diet* is usually offered first, in small amounts and at frequent intervals. As fluid intake is increased, there may be edema at first and consequent weight gain. This initial weight gain may be lost when the edema subsides. As the patient makes progress, small frequent feedings of highly nutritious solid foods are added to the diet. The patient should be closely observed during and after meals to be sure that the feedings are retained.

ALCOHOLISM

It is estimated that 5 to 10 percent of the people in the United States are alcoholics. A growing number of these are teenagers and women. Alcoholism in women is of great concern because alcohol can cause birth defects. Most physicians now forbid any alcoholic beverages for the pregnant woman.

Alcoholics frequently neglect to eat a well-balanced diet. Alcohol curbs the appetite with its "empty calories," interferes with absorption in the intestines, and damages the liver and pancreas. There is altered metabolism of fats, sugars, and vitamin B complex. Increased urinary output leads to loss of some minerals and electrolytes. Alcohol is a toxic agent and the ability of the body to withstand its effect is diminished by the changes due to liver damage and poor nutrition.

The dietary prescription depends upon the physical condition of the alcoholic. When there is liver damage, a *high-calorie, high-protein, high-vitamin diet* is needed. In less severe cases, a diet based on the basic four food groups may be sufficient. In all cases, continuing to ingest alcohol reduces or negates the effectiveness of a diet and continues body damage.

DRUG ADDICTION

Drug addiction usually results in malnutrition because food money is used to support the habit—a habit that often adds to the problem by suppressing the appetite. Amphetamines and other "uppers" increase the energy output, change taste sensations, and are often used by dieters to suppress appetite. Heroin not only interferes with appetite but also causes a craving for sweet-tasting foods. Both heroin and methadone alter gastrointestinal motility. One of the side effects of cocaine is nausea and vomiting.

As with alcoholism, there is damage to gastrointestinal functioning, the liver, and pancreas during addiction. There is an increased loss of nutrients due to vomiting, diarrhea, fever, and urinary output.

Diet therapy has to be individualized, taking into consideration the state of health of the patient. Hepatitis, for example, is common among addicts who inject drugs. Working with the psychotherapist, the dietitian plans meals to tempt the patient and to overcome nutritional deficiencies.

Complete the following:

1. What nutrient is especially needed by the central nervous system?

2. What are the dangers in using megavitamin therapy?

3. Draw up a nutritional care plan for a mental patient in a half-way house for one week.

4. Anorexia nervosa is a condition in which:

5. Your patient has anorexia nervosa. What can you put in your nutritional care plan to help improve this patient's nutritional status?

6. Alcoholism affects the body by:

7. You are instructing an alcoholic patient about diet. What would you tell the patient?

8. Some of the effects of various drugs on nutrition are:

9. What is the objective of diet therapy for drug addicts?

NERVOUS SYSTEM

The nervous system seems peculiarly susceptible to malnutrition. When nutritional status is poor, the individual is usually irritable, and may exhibit a poor memory, anxiety, and signs of mental disease.

NEURITIS

Neuritis is inflammation of a nerve, which may be caused by infection, injury, tumor, or deficiency. *Polyneuritis* involves a number of nerves and usually involves a vitamin deficiency. The patient's diet is often deficient in vitamins, particularly thiamin, niacin, pyridoxine, and riboflavin. Dietary treatment consists of an *adequate diet high in vitamin B complex.*

EPILEPSY

Epilepsy is a functional disease of the nervous system characterized by convulsive seizures. Today, there are many drugs available to control the seizures, but some physicians still use the *ketogenic diet* on occasion. Some cases of epilepsy can be controlled by producing a state of ketosis in the blood. The patient is given a *high-fat, low-carbohydrate diet,* which forces the body to use fats instead of carbohydrates for sufficient energy and produces ketones. Excessive ketones change the acid-base balance of the blood, making it acid.

On the *ketogenic diet,* the carbohydrate intake is reduced gradually and the fat intake increased gradually to maintain the necessary number of calories. Because fat satisfies the appetite quickly, foods should be chosen carefully. Forty percent cream, oils, and fat meat are used extensively. To keep the carbohydrate intake low, fruits and vegetables from the 3 to 6 percent carbohydrate groups are chosen. Coffee, tea, and alcoholic beverages are restricted as they may precipitate seizure. Since it has been found that patients have less of a tendency to seizures when slightly dehydrated, they are not encouraged to drink many fluids.

Complete the following exercises:

1. Plan a day's menu high in vitamin B complex for a patient with neuritis.
   Breakfast:

   Lunch:

   Dinner:

2. The diet of the neuritis patient is usually found to be deficient in which three vitamin B complex vitamins?

3. Plan a diet high in fats and low in carbohydrates for an epileptic patient.
   Breakfast:

   Lunch:

   Dinner:

OPTIONAL ACTIVITY TO ENHANCE LEARNING

ACTIVITY 1

Case Study

The medical ward of the county hospital admitted Mr. S., age 59, complaining of severe pain in his legs. Mr. S. is a transient with no visible means of support. He had been living under the railroad bridge on the edge of town. Physical examination revealed a dry scaly skin, cracks at the corner of his mouth, and a sore tongue. The muscles of his legs, arms, and face occasionally twitch. Mr. S. stated that he had frequent bouts of indigestion. His diet consists of whatever he can get. He is 5 feet 8 inches tall and weighs 120 pounds. He admits that he drinks heavily, usually wine, and will spend his money on that rather than purchasing food. Most of his diet at present consists of oranges he "borrows" from nearby orchards. Certain cheeses give him a headache; he is not sure of the names of the cheeses. The admitting physician placed him on a high-calorie, high-vitamin, high-vitamin B-complex diet.

Prepare a nutritional care plan.

BIBLIOGRAPHY

CALIENDO, MA: *Nutrition and Preventitive Health Care.* Macmillan, New York, 1981. Chapter 11, *Diet, nutrition and other diseases (diabetes, hypertension, alcoholism).*

GROWDON, JH AND WURTMAN, RJ: *Nutrients and neurotransmitters.* Contemporary Nutrition 4(12), December, 1979.

HALPERN, SL ET AL: *Quick Reference to Clinical Nutrition: A Guide for Physicians.* JB Lippincott, Philadelphia, 1979. Chapter 27, *The nutritional management of alcoholism, drug addiction and acute toxicity syndromes.*

HARLEY, JP AND MATTHEWS, CG: *The Feingold hypothesis: Current studies.* Contemporary Nutrition 3(4), April, 1978.

HERBERT, VD: *Megavitamin therapy.* Contemporary Nutrition 2(10), October, 1977.

HODGES, RE: *Nutrition in Medical Practice.* WB Saunders, Philadelphia, 1980. Chapter 5, *Nutrition and the nervous system.*

HOFMANN, L: *The Great American Nutrition Hassle.* Mayfield, Palo Alto, California, 1978. Chapter 18, *Megavitamin therapy cures mental and emotional disorders.* Chapter 19, *Diet and hyperactivity: Any connection?* Chapter 22, *Drug-vitamin interrelationships.*

HUTCHENS, C: *Hyperkinetic children and the Feingold diet.* Journal of Practical Nursing Vol 28, July, 1979.

KRAUSE, MV AND MAHAN, LK: *Food, Nutrition and Diet Therapy,* ed 6. WB Saunders, Philadelphia, 1979. Chapter 32, *Nutritional care for patients with diseases of the nervous system and mental illness.*

LIEBER, CS: *Alcohol-nutrition interaction.* Contemporary Nutrition 3(9), September, 1978.

LUCAS, AR: *Anorexia nervosa.* Contemporary Nutrition 3(8), August, 1978.

SUITOR, CW AND HUNTER, MF: *Nutrition: Principles and Application in Health Promotion.* JB Lippincott, Philadelphia, 1980. Chapter 35, *Care of clients with other special nutritional needs.*

23

DIET IN DEFICIENCY CONDITIONS

OBJECTIVES

Upon completion of this chapter the student should be able to:

- Correlate deficiency conditions with the nutrients that are lacking in the diet.
- Select foods that are good sources of those nutrients lacking in the diet.

In a *deficiency disease,* the body cannot obtain or utilize an essential nutrient. It may be due to an inadequate diet or a condition that interferes with the body's ability to digest, absorb, or metabolize the nutrient.

Nutritional status has a tremendous effect upon the body's ability to:

1. Adjust to new situations.
2. Resist infections.
3. Repair wear and injury of tissues.
4. Maintain emotional equilibrium.

Deficiencies are seldom singular; they appear in groups. A *well-balanced, adequate diet* is the basis for treatment of most deficiency conditions. In addition, supplementary doses of the nutrient in which the diet has been deficient are given.

VITAMIN A DEFICIENCY

NIGHT BLINDNESS. As vitamin A is necessary for the regeneration of visual purple in the rods of the retina, the individual deficient in vitamin A has difficulty in distinguishing objects in the dark or in dim light.

HYPERKERATOSIS. The skin shows "gooseflesh" and becomes dry and scaly. The forearms and thighs are particularly susceptible.

THIAMIN DEFICIENCY

BERIBERI. There are two types of beriberi. In "dry" beriberi, there is polyneuritis and paralysis. In "wet" beriberi, the patient is edematous, has cardiac symptoms, and is also emaciated.

RIBOFLAVIN DEFICIENCY

ARIBOFLAVINOSIS. Ariboflavinosis manifests itself by lesions (cracks) at the corners of the mouth, a purple tongue, and greasy skin. It is thought to be one of the most common deficiency conditions in the United States.

NIACIN DEFICIENCY

PELLAGRA. This condition is commonly found in poor people whose diets are often deficient in niacin. These individuals become weak and lazy, have no appetite, and complain of indigestion. Typically, they develop a sore tongue and dermatitis, which is aggravated by sunlight.

VITAMIN C DEFICIENCY

SCURVY. The classic symptoms of scurvy are sore, swollen gums and, in severe cases, loss of teeth. The individual bruises easily and complains of pain in the joints of the arms and legs. The general condition is usually poor, and the individual lacks an appetite.

VITAMIN D DEFICIENCY

RICKETS. Rickets occurs during the periods of growth and development, infancy and childhood. Due to vitamin D deficiency, the bone cannot hold calcium and becomes soft and deformed. Bowlegs and pigeon chest are common deformities. The legs bow as the weight of the child becomes too much for the softened bone to support. Infants also develop small knots on the ribs known as a "rachitic rosary." The pelvis becomes deformed; in girls this may later prevent normal deliveries.

OSTEOMALACIA. Osteomalacia is marked by increased softening of the bones. The bones become deformed and the individual complains of pain. This deficiency condition is found in adults, especially the elderly, who have an inadequate diet and not enough sunlight.

CALCIUM DEFICIENCY

Because calcium and phosphorus function together, a deficiency of either will cause rickets or osteoporosis.

RICKETS. See section under Vitamin D Deficiency above. This condition can also be due to an inadequate intake of calcium.

OSTEOPOROSIS. Osteoporosis is usually found in women past menopause and in elderly men. Calcium is lost from bone when the body needs the calcium elsewhere. Prolonged immobilization tends to increase calcium loss. The bones weaken and are easily fractured by only a small stress. There may be pain and cramping before the bone becomes weak enough to fracture.

IRON DEFICIENCY

IRON DEFICIENCY ANEMIA. This type of anemia is most common among infants, pregnant women, and adolescents with inadequate diets. There may be a sufficient number of erythrocytes, or there may be fewer than normal. In all cases, the percentage of hemoglobin is less than normal.

IODINE DEFICIENCY

SIMPLE GOITER. When the thyroid gland receives less iodine than it needs to produce thyroxine, it enlarges in an attempt to overcome the deficiency. As the thyroid gland normally becomes more active at puberty, deficiency of iodine is felt most acutely by adolescents. The adolescent most often develops simple goiter.

MAGNESIUM DEFICIENCY

MAGNESIUM DEFICIENCY TETANY. This condition occurs during renal disease, diuretic therapy, persistent vomiting, and continuous gastrointestinal suctioning. The patient exhibits symptoms of depression, muscular weakness, and dizziness, and may convulse.

ZINC DEFICIENCY

Zinc deficiency is manifested by underdevelopment of the sex organs and failure to grow tall. Often the individual is bald and has skin lesions. Zinc deficiency is usually found in a child who eats little meat while drinking large amounts of cow's milk.

PROTEIN DEFICIENCY

Protein deficiency is serious at any age but is particularly dangerous in childhood. Inadequate protein consumption during early childhood usually leads to a dulling or slowing of mental activity.

NUTRITIONAL EDEMA. Nutritional edema occurs most often in the legs and feet but can involve all of the body if it is severe. It is preceded by hypoproteinemia and may mask true weight loss due to tissue loss. Protein deficiency can occur when the diet lacks any of the essential amino acids.

KWASHIORKOR. Kwashiorkor results from protein-calorie deficiency in children who are fed a high-carbohydrate, low-protein diet with the proteins often being incomplete proteins. The child is usually potbellied and does not grow or develop normally. Nutritional edema may be present, and the skin has a reddish color.

DEFICIENCIES OF UNCERTAIN CAUSES

SPRUE. Symptoms of sprue are sore mouth, anemia, weight loss, and loss of appetite. The patient has frequent, frothy, foul-smelling stools. The dietary treatment is a *high-protein, low-carbohydrate, low-fat diet.* Fats are not well absorbed by these patients, and carbohydrates have to be chosen according to individual tolerance. Usually strawberries, bananas, orange juice, and tomato juice can be taken by the patient.

Complete the following exercise:

1. What foods are good sources of:

   Vitamin A:

   Vitamin B_1:

   Vitamin B_2:

   Niacin:

   Vitamin C: ORANGE

   Vitamin D:

   Calcium: MILK & MILK PRODUCTS

   Iron: LIVER

   Iodine:

   Magnesium:

   Zinc:

   Proteins with all the essential amino acids:

OPTIONAL ACTIVITY TO ENHANCE LEARNING

ACTIVITY 1

Case Study

Twenty-one-year-old Miss P. has been feeling tired lately and, when she exerts herself, she gets short of breath and her heart pounds. She works as a salesclerk in a local department store. Examination revealed pallor around her mouth and a pale conjunctiva. She gets headaches easily. She does not eat breakfast and usually has a bowl of soup for lunch. She is allergic to fish and dislikes milk intensely. Her dinner often consists of a fruit or vegetable salad because she has to cook on a hotplate and finds it difficult to prepare a full meal. She has a small refrigerator but no freezer to store foods. She is eligible for food stamps because her salary as a salesclerk in a department store is so small, but she has never applied for them. Her urinalysis was within normal limits. Her hematocrit was 37.5; all other blood tests were within normal limits. (The red blood cell count was not made at this time.) A provisional diagnosis of iron deficiency anemia was made at this time. Ferrous sulfate and a high-iron diet were ordered until the red blood cell count and a gastric analysis could be made to rule out other types of anemia.

Prepare a nutritional care plan.

BIBLIOGRAPHY

GILLIE, RB: *Human Nutrition: Readings from Scientific American.* WH Freeman & Company, San Francisco, 1978, p 213. *Endemic goiter.*

HODGES, RE: *Nutrition in Medical Practice.* WB Saunders, Philadelphia, 1980. Chapter 8, *Nutrition and hematopoiesis.*

KRAUSE, MV AND MAHAN, LK: *Food, Nutrition and Diet Therapy,* ed 6. WB Saunders, Philadelphia, 1979. Chapter 12, *Nutritional deficiency diseases.*

LOOMIS, WF: *Human Nutrition: Readings from Scientific American.* WH Freeman & Company, San Francisco, 1978, p 193. *Rickets.*

LOWENBERG, ME, ET AL: *Food and People,* ed 3. John Wiley & Sons, New York, 1979. Chapter 8, *Chronic hunger.* Chapter 9, *Malnutrition.* Chapter 10, *Programs to improve nutrition.*

PALOMBO, JD AND BLACKBURN, GL: *Human protein requirements.* Contemporary Nutrition 5(1), January, 1980.

24

DIET IN SURGICAL CONDITIONS AND CANCER TREATMENT

OBJECTIVES

Upon completion of this chapter the student should be able to:

- Discuss the role of nutrition in surgery.
- Compare the various diets used before and after surgery.
- Discuss total parenteral nutrition and give the conditions in which it may be used, the composition of the nutrient solutions, the nursing care involved, and the complications that can occur.
- Describe tube feeding formulas and give the procedure for feeding by nasogastric tube.
- Discuss the nutritional problems, diet therapy, and precautions to observe in gastric surgery; intestinal surgery; head, neck, and mouth surgery; cholecystectomy; hemorrhoidectomy; tonsillectomy; and severe burns.
- List the recommendation of the National Cancer Institute and the ways in which cancer causes malnutrition.
- Discuss diet therapy of cancer patients, listing problems encountered during treatment by surgery, chemotherapy, and radiation therapy and define the nurse's role.

Good nutritional status in the surgical patient helps prevent infections, hastens healing, prevents complications, and makes the convalescent periods shorter and more pleasant. If there is sufficient time before surgery, the physician will attempt to bring the nutritional status to the optimum level. Special conditions, such as diabetes, may have to be brought under dietary control.

Generally, the following practices are instituted by the physician prior to surgery:

1. Extra protein and carbohydrates are added to the diet. The proteins are necessary to prevent tissue loss. The extra carbohydrates insure an adequate storage of glycogen, which aids in preventing postoperative ketosis and vomiting.
2. Vitamins are added to the diet. Vitamin C promotes wound healing. Vitamin K promotes normal blood clotting.
3. Fluid intake should be slightly above normal so that body wastes are properly disposed of and dehydration is prevented.

In emergencies, there is no time to prepare the patient nutritionally for the stress of the operation. For these cases, the physician may need to give glucose, salts, vitamins, amino acids, or fat emulsions by intravenous injections. The stomach should be empty at the time of surgery to prevent possible vomiting and aspiration of stomach contents into the lungs.

Postoperative diets vary according to the patient's condition and the type of surgery. As soon as the patient can tolerate food without nausea and vomiting, the doctor will order a diet. Many doctors are much more liberal with postoperative diets now than formerly. It is realized that the sooner the patient receives an adequate diet the sooner the patient gets well. Some physicians still prefer to start the patient on a *surgical liquid diet* at first and progress through the *full liquid* and *soft diets* to the *general diet,* usually in five days. Even with a surgical liquid diet (which is very inadequate nutritionally), the patient will be receiving some fluids and electrolytes, and the ability to retain fluids will be tested and the surgeon will be able to find out if peristaltic action has resumed. Again, as with the preoperative diet, proteins, carbohydrates, vitamins C and K, and fluid intake are increased, unless contraindicated by the diagnosis.

Even before the surgical liquid diet is ordered, the patient is often given chips of ice to relieve thirst. Milk and orange juice are often withheld from the liquid diet because of their tendency to cause distention. Milk should not be given to patients who are having difficulty in breathing as it encourages the collection of mucus in the throat.

TOTAL PARENTERAL NUTRITION (TPN)

Total parenteral nutrition (TPN), also known as *hyperalimentation,* is indicated whenever the patient can not obtain nutrients normally through the digestive tract. It is used after major surgery of the gastrointestinal system; when there are tumors or other obstructions in the throat, esophagus, or stomach; and when malnutrition is severe. It can also be used when it is desirable to alter blood chemistry in conditions of kidney, liver, or brain damage.

Intravenous solutions are given through catheters in the veins of the neck, arms, or legs. The catheter ends in the vena cava. The solutions contain concentrated nutrients and the patient must be monitored closely with laboratory tests to prevent fluid and electrolyte imbalances. Nutrients most frequently given are dextrose, amino acids, minerals, and vitamins. Occasionally, essential fatty acids are needed. The tubing for TPN must not be used for other purposes, such as taking blood or giving medication.

Because the tip of the TPN catheter is in the vena cava, a major blood vessel, extreme caution in caring for the entry site is necessary to prevent infection. Complications of TPN include infection, emboli, lung congestion, hyperglycemia, and electrolyte imbalances. The TPN tubing and catheter are not usually changed and care must be used not to displace them.

TUBE FEEDING

Tube feedings must be ordered individually by the physician. In some cases, there is no difficulty with the digestive process, the patient simply cannot swallow due to paralysis. A *pureed diet* prepared by putting regular solid foods through a blender will provide an adequate diet for these patients. There is less diarrhea than when the patient receives a formula tube feeding. If the patient is conscious, preparing each food separately in the blender so that the patient can see the different colors adds pleasure to the feeding time.

The typical tube feeding formula includes 2500 calories per day, divided into 65 grams protein, 125 grams fat, and 275 grams carbohydrate. Usually, this is obtained from milk, eggs, and sugar. Occasionally, soybean mixtures provide the protein.

Many commercial formulas are available, which can be given as tube feedings. Often these are prepared to specific electrolyte needs as well as protein, carbohydrate, and fat levels.

To tube feed a patient:

1. Allow the feeding to warm to room temperature. Putting a cold formula directly into the stomach results in constriction of the blood vessels in the stomach and cramping pains.
2. Check the gastric tube to be sure it is still in the stomach before starting the feeding. One method of checking the gastric tube is to withdraw a small amount of stomach contents with an asepto syringe. Another method is to place the open end of the gastric tube under water. If bubbles appear, the tube is in the lungs. A small amount of

air can be injected into the gastric tube while the nurse listens with a stethoscope at the apex of the stomach. A gurgling sound can be heard if the tube is in place.

3. Being careful not to allow air to get into the tube, allow the formula to enter the stomach *by gravity.* Too sudden distention of the stomach is a shock to the system and can cause pain.
4. After the formula has completely run in, allow a small amount of water (room temperature) to flow into the tubing to wash it out so that the formula will not have a chance to coagulate and occlude the tube.

GASTRIC SURGERY

Following surgery on the stomach, a gastric tube may be in place. When it is removed and the patient is allowed to eat a *small bland diet,* the patient must be observed for the "dumping syndrome." About 15 minutes after eating, the patient complains of nausea, abdominal cramps, and fullness and may exhibit symptoms of shock and stress. This is due to the sudden release of food from the stomach into the small intestines. The entire meal is "dumped." Gastric surgery patients should be encouraged to eat slowly and to chew their food well. Lying down immediately after eating is also helpful as it tends to keep the meal in the stomach. Feedings are usually small and at frequent intervals.

Some surgeons prefer a *high-protein, high-fat, low-carbohydrate diet* as the fat normally is retained by the stomach longer than other foods. Liquid foods may be restricted as they leave the stomach faster than solids.

INTESTINAL SURGERY

Often the patient is prepared for intestinal surgery with an antibiotic to destroy bacteria in the intestines and prevent postoperative infections. These patients may need supplementary vitamin K until the normal bacteria have had a chance to grow again.

After severe surgery, the patient may be on gastric suction and have to be on *TPN* for a period of time. The patient will progress to a *liquid diet* and then to a *soft, low-residue diet.* Fruits are limited to banana and scraped apple. These patients do not tolerate milk well. Six small feedings are accepted better than three large meals.

Following resection of the small intestine, the patient may have problems with the absorption of nutrients, depending upon the amount and location of the intestine that was removed. *TPN* or a *continuous nasogastric drip* may be necessary. After resection of the small intestine, the patient will probably be more comfortable with six small meals per day.

Some excessively overweight individuals have had small intestine resection as a means to control weight. Because malabsorption can be so severe in some cases that the patient is hospitalized, this is a dangerous practice.

CHOLECYSTECTOMY

Following removal of the gallbladder, a *surgical liquid diet* is usually given as soon as possible. The diet is advanced to a *general diet* as the patient is able to tolerate other foods. Some patients may not be able to ingest many fats at first and the surgeon may order a *low-fat diet.*

HEMORRHOIDECTOMY

After surgery on the rectum and anus, the patient usually finds a *low-residue diet* more comfortable during the earliest postoperative phase. If a *general diet* is given, stool softeners or lubricating medications are usually ordered to prevent painful defecation.

HEAD, NECK, AND MOUTH SURGERY

Following surgery on the head, neck, or mouth, the patient may be on *TPN* or *tube feedings* for a period of time. When the time comes to try oral feedings, the patient may be afraid to eat because of pain. A *full liquid diet* or a *pureed diet* may be given at first. Liquids should be nonirritating and milk should be avoided as it increases the problem of phlegm in the throat. Some patients find that the thick consistency of the pureed diet assists them in swallowing.

When the patient has progressed to a *soft diet,* small frequent feedings are preferable. To help the patient swallow solids, all foods should be moist. Sauces and gravies can be utilized for moistening food and the patient should be encouraged to dip breads and other suitable items in soups and drinks to soften them. Because the patient may be eating limited quantities due to pain and fatigue, nutritional intake is improved by excluding "empty calories" from the diet.

TONSILLECTOMY

Tonsillectomy patients have a short convalescence. To prevent pain and possible hemorrhage, *very cold* and *very bland foods* are given.

SEVERE BURNS

Because severe or extensive burns cause a tremendous loss of protein, fluids, and electrolytes, diet alone cannot replace these nutrients and intravenous therapy is necessary. Tube feedings are given if the injured area includes the face and throat and the patient cannot swallow. A *high-protein, high-calorie, high-vitamin diet* or *tube feeding* is necessary. The protein is needed for tissue repair. If calories from carbohydrates and fats are insufficient, the protein will be used for energy. Vitamins also promote tissue repair.

Complete the following exercises:

1. What foods are allowed on a surgical liquid diet?

2. What can be added to the surgical liquid diet to increase the protein?

3. What foods are added to a regular diet to increase the protein intake?

4. The symptoms of the "dumping syndrome" are:

5. How can the "dumping syndrome" be prevented?

6. If you needed a variety of pureed foods for a patient at home, how could you obtain them easily without going through the process of chopping, mashing, and straining?

7. Plan a tray for a one day postoperative tonsillectomy patient.

8. After a tube feeding, the patient complained of pain and cramps. What did the nurse forget to do?

9. How fast should a tube feeding be given?

10. Plan a low-residue breakfast menu for a patient who has had a hemorrhoidectomy.

11. List at least three nursing actions you think would be appropriate in caring for a patient receiving TPN.

12. Plan a day's menu for a patient who is convalescing from an intestinal resection.

13. Plan a day's menu for a patient who has had neck or mouth surgery and has had a soft diet ordered.

CANCER

Cancer is the second most common cause of death in the United States. Studies into the effect of diet on development and growth of cancer have been conducted, but at this time what is known is not conclusive. However, the Diet, Nutrition and Cancer Program of the National Cancer Institute recommends the following:

1. Keep the calorie count down and avoid high-fat foods and "empty calories."
2. Eat fewer foods with additives.
3. Increase intake of unrefined foods.
4. Get sufficient exercise.
5. Reduce stress in daily life.

Cancer causes malnutrition in several ways. Cancer cells themselves take the nutrients before the normal cells because they metabolize more rapidly than normal cells. Many patients find that appetite changes occur and that they often "feel full" after eating only a small amount. The emotional state of the patient also has a great effect upon appetite. If the gastrointestinal tract is involved in the disease, there is impaired digestion and absorption. When there is vomiting, "weeping" lesions, or bleedings, there is loss of proteins and other substances. And, of course, the treatment of cancer can cause nutritional problems.

Because the diagnosis of cancer is so frightening to patients and their loved ones, many grasp desperately at any hope of cure. It has never been proved that cancer can be cured with any special diet or nutrient.

Diet therapy depends upon the type and location of the tumor. It is known that some tumors can be affected by certain nutrients but cancer nutrition studies are still inconclusive. Protein, carbohydrate, and fat metabolism are disturbed in all cancers and fluids and electrolytes may be imbalanced. The objective of diet therapy in cancer is to overcome deficiencies and provide nutrients necessary for healing.

Treatment of cancer includes surgery, chemotherapy, and radiation therapy. Often, more than one method of treatment is used. Unfortunately, each method has side effects.

When cancer and the *surgery* to remove it involve the digestive tract and the accessory organs, such as the liver and pancreas, digestion, absorption, and metabolism are severely impaired. There is interference with ingestion of food when the surgery is on the face, mouth, or neck.

Drugs used in *chemotherapy* can cause loss of appetite, diarrhea, nausea, and vomiting. Some cause fevers with loss of fluid and electrolytes and others cause taste changes. Still others lead to deficiencies of protein, minerals, and vitamins.

Radiation therapy does not affect only cancer cells; normal cells in the field are also damaged. When the gastrointestinal system is treated, there is nausea, vomiting, poor absorption of nutrients, and possibly diarrhea. Radiation of the mouth not only destroys taste but also decreases the production of saliva and causes gum and tooth problems. The patient will have tender gums and may lose some teeth.

After the physician has decided upon the dietary prescription, the nurse and dietitian can help the patient accept the diet. The patient can be encouraged to eat by being offered a wide choice of foods prepared in many different ways. By intensifying flavors and increasing the amount of seasoning, the patient with altered taste perception can enjoy more foods. When the patient's condition allows, permission to take meals in the cafeteria or to choose tidbits from the ward refrigerator will help to increase intake. Sometimes changing food temperature will help. At all times, the nurse and dietitian should teach patients about their nutritional needs and how they can be met.

Complete the following exercises:

1. The recommendations of the National Cancer Institute are:

2. How does cancer cause malnutrition?

3. What is the objective of diet therapy in cancer?

4. List some of the nutritional problems encountered in treating cancer by:
   Surgery:

Chemotherapy:

Radiation therapy:

5. What is the role of the nurse in diet therapy for cancer patients?

OPTIONAL ACTIVITY TO ENHANCE LEARNING

ACTIVITY 1

Case Study

The gastric tube was removed from Mr. P. three days after his subtotal gastrectomy and vagotomy. Mr. P., a school principal, had been admitted due to hemorrhaging from a gastric ulcer. For 12 hours after the removal of the tube, all oral fluids had been restricted and then Mr. P. was given small sips of water, which he tolerated well. Today, the surgeon ordered a bland diet. Mr. P. is allergic to fish and tells the nurses he is tired of milk, as he was on a Sippy diet for a long time before he started hemorrhaging. He appears to be recuperating well from the surgery and wants to be cooperative about his diet.

Prepare a nutritional care plan.

BIBLIOGRAPHY

BORGEN, L: *Total parenteral nutrition in adults.* American Journal of Nursing 78(2), February, 1978.

BUTTERWORTH, CE, JR: *New concepts in nutrition and cancer: Implications for folic acid.* Contemporary Nutrition 5(12), December, 1980.

CALIENDO, MA: *Nutrition and Preventitive Health Care.* Macmillan, New York, 1981. Chapter 8, *Diet, nutrition and cancer.*

DAVENPORT, RR: *Tube feeding for long-term patients.* American Journal of Nursing 64(1), January, 1964.

DONOVAN, L: *Is the doctor starving your patient?* RN Vol 41, July, 1978.

DUDRICK, SJ AND RHOADS, JE: *Human Nutrition: Readings from Scientific American.* WH Freeman & Company, San Francisco, 1978, p 171. *Total intravenous feeding.*

ENNIS, CE ET AL: *Nutritional management of the surgical patient.* AORN Journal Vol 31, June, 1980.

FRIEDRICH, HN: *Oral feedings by food pump.* American Journal of Nursing 62(2), February, 1962.

GRIGGS, B AND HOPPE, MC: *Update: Nasogastric tube feedings.* American Journal of Nursing 79(3), March, 1979.

HALPERN, S ET AL: *Quick Reference to Clinical Nutrition: A Guide for Physicians.* JB Lippincott, Philadelphia, 1979. Chapter 11, *Surgical nutrition.* Chapter 18, *Nutrition in cancer.* Chapter 20, *Total parenteral nutrition and elemental diets.* Chapter 27, *The nutritional management of alcoholism, drug addiction and acute toxicity syndromes.*

HODGES, RE: *Nutrition in Medical Practice.* WB Saunders, Philadelphia, 1980. Chapter 15, *Feeding patients.*

THE INSTITUTE OF FOOD TECHNOLOGISTS EXPERT PANEL ON FOOD SAFETY AND NUTRITION AND THE COMMITTEE ON PUBLIC INFORMATION: *Dietary fiber.* Contemporary Nutrition 4(9), September, 1979.

KRAUSE, MV AND MAHAN, LK: *Food, Nutrition and Diet Therapy,* ed 6. WB Saunders, Philadelphia, 1979. Chapter 34, *Nutritional care for patients having surgery, trauma or burns.* Chapter 35, *The metabolic stress response and methods for providing nutritional care to stressed patients.* Chapter 36, *Nutrition, diet and cancer.*

METHENY, NA AND SNIVELY, WD, JR: *Perioperative fluids and electrolytes.* American Journal of Nursing 78(5), May, 1978.

ROBINSON, CH: *Basic Nutrition and Diet Therapy,* ed 4. Macmillan, New York, 1980. Chapter 31, *Nutrition and diet in cancer.* Chapter 32, *Nutrition in surgical conditions.*

ROSE, JC: *Nutritional problems in radiotherapy patients.* American Journal of Nursing 78(7), July, 1978.

SUITOR, CW AND HUNTER, MF: *Nutrition: Principles and Application in Health Promotion.* JB Lippincott, Philadelphia, 1980. Chapter 5, *Meeting nutrient needs by means of a prudent diet.* Chapter 35, *Care of clients with other nutritional needs.*

WORTHINGTON-ROBERTS, BS: *Contemporary Developments in Nutrition.* CV Mosby, St Louis, 1981. Chapter 12, *Diet and cancer.*

25

DIET IN COMPLICATIONS OF PREGNANCY

OBJECTIVES

Upon completion of this chapter the student should be able to:

- List the dietary changes in the diet of a pregnant woman with complications of anemia, heart condition, toxemia, or diabetes.
- Compare the dietary management of "morning sickness" and hyperemesis gravidarum.
- Discuss nutritional needs during labor and the reasons for the ways in which they are met.

The nutritional status of the pregnant woman is important not only to her but also to her baby. Her diet must be adequate for her own needs and the needs of the baby. However, often a condition is present or develops during pregnancy that requires that the usual diet for the pregnant woman be modified in some way.

ANEMIA

Anemia, characterized by either a low red blood cell count or a low hemoglobin rate, is somewhat common in pregnancy due to the increased amounts of iron and protein needed by the growing fetus. The fetus will take iron from the mother regardless of her needs. Also, during pregnancy, blood volume increases, but the number of red blood cells does not. Treatment consists of a *diet high in complete protein, iron, and vitamin B complex.* Many obstetricians give every pregnant woman an iron supplement to protect against iron deficiency anemia.

HEART CONDITIONS

A cardiac condition requiring a special diet before pregnancy will most certainly require careful dietary treatment during pregnancy. Sodium and fluids are usually restricted as the pregnant woman has a tendency to edema. Weight gain is limited to lessen the burden on the heart. In very severe cardiac conditions, low-sodium milk may be prescribed.

TOXEMIA

In toxemia of pregnancy, the blood pressure is elevated, the extremities become edematous, and albumin appears in the urine. When untreated, the patient goes into convulsions and coma leading to death. Because of the loss of body protein as albumin in the urine, a *high-protein diet* may be advocated. To relieve the edema and increased blood pressure, sodium and fluids may be restricted. Complete proteins are high in sodium so the physician may prescribe low-sodium milk to increase the protein intake without increasing the sodium intake.

In recent years, some physicians have found that it is not necessary to restrict sodium intake or increase the protein allowance on all toxemic patients.

DIABETES

The pregnant, diabetic patient must follow her physician's orders and keep her diabetic condition under control or risk losing her baby or developing toxemia. The diet and amount of insulin must be watched very carefully throughout the pregnancy, as the needs of her body change with the growth of the fetus. Even those diabetic patients who have always been controlled by diet alone may need insulin during pregnancy. The need for insulin rises sharply during the fifth month of pregnancy, and very frequent changes in the amount of insulin may have to be made from then on. Infants born to diabetic mothers are usually very large, and at least a fourth of these babies weigh over 10 pounds.

When the diabetic patient goes into labor, she undergoes more changes and should be watched closely for coma or insulin shock. In some cases, the baby is taken by cesarean section rather than risking the mother's life with labor.

The complications of pregnancy in the diabetic patient are in inverse proportion to the care she receives. The necessity for good medical care and for following the physician's directions as to diet and insulin must be stressed.

NAUSEA AND VOMITING

Although termed "morning sickness," nausea and vomiting during pregnancy can occur at any time of the day. The symptoms usually disappear after a few weeks. Although morning sickness is not an alarming condition, the patient can become deficient in proteins and electrolytes if vomiting is excessive. Taking a small snack of crackers or other simple carbohydrates before getting out of bed helps some women. Others find that restricting fluids at mealtime and just before and after meals helps. Still others prefer a midmorning meal of crackers, toast, or bread and jelly to keep them from becoming nauseated.

HYPEREMESIS GRAVIDARUM

Hyperemesis gravidarum is persistent vomiting during pregnancy, not the morning sickness experienced by so many pregnant women. Vomiting is so violent and persistent that the patient can retain very little food or fluids. Acute dehydration occurs, and the patient may require intravenous fluids until the vomiting is controlled.

In addition to a *dry diet* served in small amounts at frequent intervals, the physician will order drugs to control the vomiting. During the most severe stage of hyperemesis gravidarum, oral fluids are withheld. As improvement is shown, fluids may be taken one hour before and after meals but not with meals. Later, fluids and fats are gradually added to the *dry diet.*

The dry diet consists of Melba toast with jelly, saltine crackers, baked potato, and thickly cooked cereal (without cream or milk). After improvement is shown, hard-boiled eggs, broiled lean meats, and plain cakes made without butter are added.

PICA

Many pregnant women exhibit a craving for unusual foods. It is an enduring joke that the husband of a pregnant woman will be sent out in the middle of the night to locate sour pickles and ice cream or some other unlikely combination. But when the cravings become so intense they interfere with normal nutritive intake or involve the ingestion of nonfood substances (pica), they can be harmful. Some of the items ingested are cornstarch, clay, dirt, ice, and ashes. Often ingestion of these unusual items interferes with absorption of nutrients such as iron.

After the physician has ascertained whether or not the woman is craving because of some deficiency, the nurse must help her adjust to the diet as prescribed by the physician. The woman must understand what such a habit can mean to herself and the baby.

HEARTBURN

As the uterus grows and applies pressure to the stomach, the woman may complain of heartburn. Alcoholic beverages, coffee, tea, and cola increase heartburn and should be avoided. To relieve pressure on the stomach, small meals are suggested and the woman should not lie down immediately after eating.

LEG CRAMPS

Leg cramps at night are quite common during pregnancy. It is thought that this might be due to a temporary high level of phosphorus with a low level of calcium in the blood. Because milk contains a large amount of phosphorus, the woman may have to reduce milk intake and obtain her calcium through supplementary medications.

LABOR

Labor is a normal physiologic process. As soon as it starts, the woman's entire body concentrates upon the task of delivering the baby and the processes not directly concerned with delivery slow down. The digestive process stops almost completely, and the stomach does not empty itself. Solid foods should not be taken, and many obstetricians restrict even the taking of liquids after true labor starts. It is not uncommon during labor for a woman to vomit food that was eaten 24 to 48 hours previously. If the patient is unconscious or semiconscious, she may aspirate these stomach contents that are well saturated with gastric juices. Gastric juices are very irritating to lung tissue and may cause obstruction or pneumonia.

Complete the following:

1. In a pregnancy with complications, the basic diet is the same as for a normal pregnancy with modifications to meet the needs created by the complication. Thus, the anemic pregnant woman will need an adequate diet with increased ________________. The pregnant woman with a cardiac condition will receive a diet adequate in nutrients that may be restricted as to ____________________________ and ________________ if she shows edema.

2. Calcium need increases during pregnancy. If the pregnant woman with a cardiac condition cannot have milk because of its high sodium content, how is she to get the required amount of calcium?

3. Because she cannot have table salt (which is usually iodized) on a low-sodium diet, the pregnant woman with a cardiac condition may have to get her iodine in other ways. What foods are high in iodine?

Would she be able to have these foods on her sodium-restricted diet?

4. The diabetic pregnant woman will need to be watched closely for hyperglycemia and glycosuria, especially after the ____________ month.

5. When the diabetic patient is admitted to the hospital in labor, the nurse should immediately make sure there is an adequate supply of insulin and ________________ on hand because the patient may experience sudden changes in her blood sugar level.

6. What is the difference between "morning sickness" and hyperemesis gravidarum?

7. Usually a transitory condition, "morning sickness" responds to small frequent snacks of ______________________.

8. The patient with hyperemesis gravidarum is served a ____________ diet in small amounts at frequent intervals. Fluids are usually restricted ____________ and ____________ meals.

9. The dry diet consists of:

10. The patient with toxemia of pregnancy is usually placed on a ________________ diet with restricted ________________ and ________________. It is felt that edema is relieved and blood pressure is lowered by restricting ______________________ and ________________ intake.

11. As animal proteins have a high sodium content, dietary proteins are increased by giving the patient ______________________.

12. When instructing the patient about what to do when she goes into labor, the physician or nurse should inform her not to eat ________________.

13. What harm can pica cause?

14. Foods that stimulate acid production in the stomach can add to the problem of heartburn. List some foods that start the digestive juices to flowing.

15. If the pregnant woman wishes to increase calcium intake without ingesting milk and milk products, what foods do you suggest?

Do these foods increase the ratio of calcium to phosphorus in the diet?

OPTIONAL ACTIVITY TO ENHANCE LEARNING

ACTIVITY 1

Case Study

Mrs. B., 30 years old and a primagravida, has been admitted with a diagnosis of hyperemesis gravidarum. She was started on intravenous fluids to overcome dehydration and placed on drugs to relieve nausea. The obstetrician wants to discontinue these as quickly as possible and has left an order for a dry diet. Mrs. B. has been trying to get pregnant for five years and is very apprehensive at this time. She is well nourished and has eaten a diet based on the basic four food groups prior to this time. She is allergic to grapes and dislikes spinach intensely. She does not drink alcoholic beverages. At the present time, she is not working outside her home.

Prepare a nutritional care plan.

BIBLIOGRAPHY

BRIGGS, GM AND CALLOWAY, DH: *Bogert's Nutrition and Physical Fitness,* ed 10. WB Saunders, Philadelphia, 1979. Chapter 20, *Nutrition during pregnancy and lactation.*

KRAUSE, MV AND MAHAN, LK: *Food, Nutrition and Diet Therapy,* ed 6. WB Saunders, Philadelphia, 1979. Chapter 13, *Nutrition for pregnancy and lactation.*

RANCILO, N: *When a pregnant woman is diabetic: Postpartal care.* American Journal of Nursing 79(3), March, 1979.

SCHULER, K: *When a pregnant woman is diabetic: Antepartal care.* American Journal of Nursing 79(3), March, 1979.

SUITOR, CW AND HUNTER, MF: *Nutrition: Principles and Application in Health Promotion.* JB Lippincott, Philadelphia, 1980. Chapter 7, *Promoting sound eating habits in pregnancy and lactation.*

WIMBERLY, D: *Intrapartal care.* American Journal of Nursing 79(3), March, 1979.

WORTHINGTON-ROBERTS, BS: *Contemporary Developments in Nutrition.* CV Mosby, St Louis, 1981. Chapter 16, *Nutritional issues related to pregnancy.*

26

DIET IN DISEASES OF INFANCY AND CHILDHOOD

OBJECTIVES

Upon completion of this chapter the student should be able to:

- Discuss nutritional needs and problems of premature infants.
- Give the diet therapy and nursing actions appropriate to nutritional care of patients with pyloric stenosis, cleft lip and palate, mental retardation, or a handicap.
- Discuss diet therapy and list appropriate foods for a child with diarrhea or constipation.
- Discuss the etiology, diet therapy, and selection of foods for children with celiac disease, cystic fibrosis of the pancreas, lactose intolerance, galactosemia, phenylketonuria, and marasmus.

The many conditions found in infants and children that are also found in adults are usually treated the same. However, there are some conditions peculiar to infants and children that are discussed in this chapter.

PREMATURE INFANTS

Any infant born too early or weighing less than $5^1/_2$ pounds has special nutrition needs. These infants are prone to hypoglycemia, low body temperatures, and inability to digest and absorb nutrients effectively.

The premature infant is usually given a first feeding within a few hours of birth by tube feeding, TPN, or oral means when the infant can suck. The premature infant requires more water than a full-term infant. The infant's metabolic rate is very high and requires a *high-calorie, high-protein formula* with supplementary calcium, iron, and vitamins. When possible, the mother can contribute breast milk. Diet therapy is always individualized for these infants.

Hypoglycemia can occur in premature infants or in infants born to diabetic mothers. The infant has tremors, a fluctuating temperature, and listlessness, and can go into convulsions and coma.

The more premature and the smaller the newborn, the more likely it is to develop hyperbilirubinemia, an excessive amount of bilirubin in the blood. To overcome this, the infant is exposed to ultraviolet light. This treatment causes dehydration and inability to digest lactose. The infant is placed on lactose-free solutions until the treatment has been discontinued.

Complete the following exercises:

1. The premature or low-birth-weight infant is prone to:

2. Compare the premature infant's need for water with that of a full-term newborn.

3. Symptoms of hypoglycemia in newborn infants can occur within the first hour or two after birth. The signs and symptoms include:

4. Treatment of hyperbilirubinemia with ultraviolet light requires what nutritional considerations?

PYLORIC STENOSIS

Some children are born with a narrowing of the pyloric valve, the outlet of the stomach. The infant with pyloric stenosis will show progressive wasting of tissues, persistent projectile vomiting, constipation, and visible gastric peristalsis. There may be a mass over the pyloric valve. Most cases are discovered in the first few months of life. Pyloric stenosis is fatal unless treated.

The infant is fed thick gruel every four hours or oftener. Medications are given to relax the spasms of the pyloric valve so that small amounts of food can get through. If the baby vomits the first feeding, the baby should be fed again, as the second feeding often will be retained. The infant should be fed slowly, and the environment should be as tension-free as possible. If special feedings do not prove successful, surgery may be necessary.

DIARRHEA

The most common causes of diarrhea are:

1. Contamination or spoiling of food.
2. Too many carbohydrates.
3. Too much fat in the formula.
4. Allergic reactions to specific foods.

The loss of water and nutrients in diarrhea is extremely serious in an infant, and treatment should never be delayed. The child may be given only water at first. Later, other liquids may be added, especially those high in glucose and salts. Often, Coca-Cola concentrate is given to replenish nutrients rapidly without creating bulk, which has a tendency to perpetuate the diarrhea. Cold tea may also be given to infants, as tea has a tendency to cause constipation in infants. Rice water is used, especially when the diarrhea has been started by an improperly balanced formula. Infants on formula can sometimes be helped by giving them skim milk or acidified milk. The older child may respond to raw, peeled apple and a *low-fiber diet* after the acute phase of the diarrhea. In all cases, the diet is gradually restored to normal with bland foods.

CONSTIPATION

The bottle-fed baby has more of a tendency to constipation than the breast-fed baby. Human milk is higher in carbohydrates. Cow's milk formulas may need more sugar added to prevent constipation. Orange juice can also be given to infants to prevent constipation. The older child may have orange juice, diluted prune juice, or pureed fruit.

CELIAC DISEASE

Celiac disease is a chronic functional disorder in which fats are not properly absorbed by the intestines. The patient is weak, underweight, and retarded in growth. The child has a bulging, distended abdomen and passes large, pale, foamy stools with a very foul odor. These stools are caused by unabsorbed fats and fermented carbohydrates. Frequently, the condition is complicated by failure to utilize minerals and vitamins, and the child develops rickets and anemia. It has been found that the symptoms of celiac disease are caused by gluten, a protein substance found in cereals.

The child is placed on a *gluten-free diet.* Foods containing wheat, oats, barley, and rye are excluded. The *banana diet* is recommended by some physicians, and some patients take as many as 18 bananas a day. The celiac patient does not tolerate sweet milk but can take sour milk. Dietary treatment must be continued for at least one and a half years. Then simple carbohydrates and proteins are added gradually.

CYSTIC FIBROSIS OF THE PANCREAS

This is a congenital condition in which there is a deficiency of pancreatic juices necessary for digestion. Symptoms are vomiting, constipation, failure to gain weight, and bulky stools containing a high percentage of protein and fat. Dietary treatment consists of eliminating fats and giving the patient a *high-calorie, high-protein diet* of simple sugars. Special high-protein milk is prescribed. Bananas and banana powder are frequently used also.

LACTOSE INTOLERANCE

Lactose intolerance is a condition in which the individual is unable to digest lactose because the enzyme lactase is missing in the digestive tract. The condition can be congenital and is found in Japanese families, Jews in Israel, American Indians, Mexicans, and black Americans. It also can be secondary to malnutrition, surgery, some drug therapies, and certain diseases.

Symptoms of lactose intolerance include diarrhea, flatulence, distention, and abdominal cramps when milk and milk products are ingested. A lactose tolerance test is usually ordered by the physician if intolerance is suspected.

Diet therapy consists of avoiding milk, milk products and foods that have lactose in them. Study of labels on cake mixes, instant tea and coffee, and other prepared food will often reveal the presence of lactose. Lactose-free milk (Lidalac, Zymil) is available and so are several forms of lactase (Lactaid, Maxilac), which can be added to milk to start the digestion of lactose. The milk should not be used for 24 hours after the addition of the enzyme to allow the change to take place. Aged cheese, buttermilk, and yoghurt can be eaten because aging and fermenting remove some of the lactose.

GALACTOSEMIA

Recent research has shown that some infants are born with metabolic disturbances that must be treated by diet. Galactosemia is one of these. In galactosemia, an enzyme that turns galactose into glucose in the liver is missing. About two weeks after birth, the infant becomes jaundiced and has glycosuria. If galactosemia is not diagnosed and treated, mental and physical retardation occur. Early diagnosis is imperative because most of the nervous system damage occurs in the first weeks of life.

A *galactose-free diet* is prescribed. Milk and all milk products are excluded. The infant is placed on a formula of casein hydrolysate. The diet must be continued throughout life, and the child must be taught to avoid all foods containing or cooked with milk. It will be necessary to read labels carefully to be certain that lactose in some form has not been added to the food.

PHENYLKETONURIA

Phenylketonuria (PKU) is caused by a failure to metabolize the amino acid phenylalanine properly. The urine has a strong odor as phenylalanine products are excreted through the kidneys. There is a lightening of the skin, hair, and eyes. The baby is very irritable. If the condition is not diagnosed with a urine or blood test in the early weeks of life, severe mental retardation occurs.

The treatment is dietary: phenylalanine in the diet is restricted. Because all proteins contain phenylalanine, it is difficult to maintain a diet for the infant that is adequate in calories and protein. Unfortunately, the several low-phenylalanine preparations on the market have a bad taste. These formulas and fruits and vegetables (except for beans, peas, and other legumes) make up the PKU diet. Food exchange lists similar to the exchange lists for diabetic patients are available to aid in planning *low-phenylalanine diets.*

MARASMUS

Severe malnutrition is rare in the United States, but it does occur. The infant is emaciated due to lack of food, not just the lack of one or more nutrients. Infectious diseases, diarrhea, vomiting, and lack of appetite often accompany marasmus. First, fluids and salts are given to the infant. Then skim milk and sugar are given, until the baby can tolerate solid foods. Protein intake is kept high and frequent small feedings are easier to retain.

Complete the following:

1. The infant with pyloric stenosis is fed ______________ every four hours in ______________ amounts. If the infant vomits the feedings, the nurse should:

2. Diarrhea results in loss of ______________________________ and ______________ .

3. Diarrhea is caused by:
   A.

   B.

   C.

4. Several regimens are used to treat diarrhea, and the infant may receive any of the following instead of the regular bottle:

5. The ___________-fed baby has more of a tendency to become constipated. By adding ___________ to an infant's cow's milk formula, constipation may be prevented.

6. The older child can have ______________ , ______________ , or ______________ for constipation.

7. One of the factors causing the symptoms of celiac disease is ___________ . This is a protein substance found in ___________ .

8. To obtain a gluten-free diet, ______________, ______________, ______________, and ______________ should be excluded from the diet.

9. Another diet frequently used for celiac disease is the ______________ diet.

10. The dietary treatment of cystic fibrosis of the pancreas consists of the elimination of ________.

11. Lactose intolerance is more common than formerly believed. Symptoms include:

12. As the parent of a child with lactose intolerance, select the foods from this menu that will insure that the meal will be lactose-free. (You may check the labels at the grocers if you are in doubt.)

Orange juice
Honeydew melon
Cheese omelet
Pancakes with maple syrup
Bacon
Grits
Shredded wheat with skim milk
Cream of wheat with half-and-half
Blueberry muffins with butter
Milk
Chocolate milk
Decaffeinated coffee
Instant tea

13. Mental retardation can be caused by metabolic failures present at birth such as the conditions known as ______________ and ______________.

14. In galactosemia, ________________ is improperly metabolized. The dietary treatment is to give the baby a diet free from ________. The food high in this is ______________.

15. Phenylketonuria is treated by giving the infant a diet low in ________________. This amino acid is found in ______________. The dietary treatment consists of:

CLEFT LIP AND PALATE

The infant with a cleft lip or palate, or both, has difficulty in swallowing, as the milk and food escape through the openings. When the palate is not closed properly, milk goes into the nostrils. There is the possibility the infant will aspirate milk into the lungs. Plastic surgery is performed as soon as feasible in these infants.

Using a special cleft palate nurser or a bulb syringe with a rubber tubing tip, the nurse slowly feeds the infant in an upright position to make swallowing easier. If baby foods are given, small bites should be offered and salty or acid foods should be avoided.

MENTAL RETARDATION

In mental retardation, there is usually an accompanying delay in ability to function physically. Often this is manifested in the inability of the muscles to do what is necessary to eat. It not only affects those movements necessary to bring food and drink to the face, but also the acts of chewing and swallowing sometimes show delayed development. When feeding the mentally retarded, the nurse should take care that the patient is not rushed and can handle the food without choking. When trying to teach patients to feed themselves, finger foods and foods that stick to the spoon are best.

The mentally retarded patient should have a well-balanced diet with caloric content matched to physical activity. For patients that are in constant motion, calories need to be increased. The severely retarded have limited activity and, if not watched closely, become obese.

HANDICAPPED CHILDREN

Handicaps can result from brain damage, developmental problems, or diseases. Some of the problems in providing nourishment for handicapped children include disturbances in ingestion, lack of sufficient energy to eat, and problems with gastrointestinal motility. Patients with cerebral palsy have chewing and swallowing problems due to lack of muscle coordination. The muscles of patients with multiple sclerosis are sometimes too weak for swallowing, and in myasthenia gravis the patient tires so rapidly and severely that swallowing is exhausting. When the handicap involves muscle tone and the patient cannot exercise, constipation occurs.

Hyperactive children require additional calories. When the handicap limits activity, as in paralysis, calories must be adjusted so that obesity does not complicate the condition. The patient should receive all the protective nutrients in a *well-balanced diet.* A *high-residue diet,* chopped or pureed when necessary for ease of ingestion, is given to prevent constipation. Adequate fluids must be included.

Gagging is sometimes a problem with the handicapped child. This can be due to a hyperactive or hypoactive gagging reflex. Pacifiers must never be given to an infant with a hyperactive gagging reflex. For those with a hypoactive gagging reflex, feedings of liquid or pureed foods should be given and the infant fed slowly in an upright position.

When there is facial muscle weakness, nasal congestion, or an inability to use the tongue, sucking becomes difficult. Larger holes in the nipple of the bottle make it easier to suck. The best feeding position for the infant is a flexed one.

The handicapped child whose bite reflex is hypersensitive to hunger, feel, and smell of food, can be a problem to feed. It is difficult to remove the nipple or spoon from the child's mouth. Solid foods are handled better than liquids and the child is progressed from pureed to chopped to solid foods as quickly as possible.

Some handicaps cause problems with chewing. Chewing is a learned reflex and children should be taken through liquid, pureed, chopped, and solid foods at their own rate.

Complete the following:

1. One of the dangers in feeding a child with cleft palate is ________ ____________________ .

2. The infant with cleft palate should be fed ____________ and in an ____________ position.

3. Caloric content of the diet for the mentally retarded should be adjusted to the level of ________________ .

4. The nurse feeding the mentally retarded child should use caution because:

5. The foods most suitable when mentally retarded children try to feed themselves are ________________ and ____________________ .

6. Some of the problems in providing nourishment for the handicapped child include:
   A.

   B.

   C.

7. What adjustments, if any, must be made in the diet based on the basic four food groups for a handicapped child?
   Calories:

   Protein:

   Fats:

   Carbohydrates:

   Minerals:

Vitamins:

Water:

Fiber:

Texture:

8. What are the nutritional and nursing actions necessary in:
Hyperactive gagging reflex:

Hypoactive gagging reflex:

Inability to suck:

Hypersensitive bite reflex:

Inability to chew:

OPTIONAL ACTIVITY TO ENHANCE LEARNING

ACTIVITY 1

Case Study

Johnny H. is 14 months old and has been admitted to the hospital with a diagnosis of celiac disease. His mother stated that he had been having large foamy stools. Johnny is thin, pale, and small for his age. His abdomen is distended and his tongue very red. Johnny was placed on pureed foods when he was six months old. Prior to that time his growth and development were normal. His first foods were pureed squash and pears. Gradually, other foods were added. His mother started him on cereal at bedtime at age 9 months in an attempt to get him to sleep all night. At first, Mrs. H. thought that Johnny was not getting enough to eat, as he cried often and was not gaining weight as her other child had. Because Mrs. H. had a part-time job, Johnny and his sister often had babysitters. Mrs. H. attributed Johnny's diarrhea to germs the babysitters introduced and did not seek medical care until one of the babysitters informed her that she thought Johnny was retarded. Orders were left to start Johnny on multivitamins and a gluten-free diet.

Prepare a nutritional care plan.

BIBLIOGRAPHY

BRIGGS, GM AND CALLOWAY, DH: *Bogert's Nutrition and Physical Fitness,* ed 10. WB Saunders, Philadelphia, 1979. Chapter 21, *Nutrition in infancy and childhood.*

CALIENDO, MA: *Nutrition and Preventitive Health Care.* Macmillan, New York, 1981. Chapter 6, *Nutritional status of vulnerable groups throughout the lifespan.*

CHANEY, MS, ROSS, ML, AND WITSCHI, JC: *Nutrition,* ed 9. Houghton Mifflin, Boston, 1979. Chapter 15, *Nutrition during infancy.* Chapter 16, *Nutrition during childhood, adolescence and the later years.*

CHOI, MW: *Breast milk for infants who can't breast-feed.* American Journal of Nursing 78(5), May, 1978.

GALLENDER, CN AND GALLENDER, D: *Dietary Problems and Diets for the Handicapped.* Charles C Thomas, Springfield, Illinois, 1979.

HALPERN, SL ET AL: *Quick Reference to Clinical Nutrition: A Guide for Physicians.* JB Lippincott, Philadelphia, 1979. Chapter 4, *Nutrition in the infant and young child.*

HOFMANN, L: *The Great American Nutrition Hassle.* Mayfield, Palo Alto, California, 1978. Chapter 8, *A new look at old formulas.*

KRAUSE, MV AND MAHAN, LK: *Food, Nutrition and Diet Therapy,* ed 6. WB Saunders, Philadelphia, 1979. Chapter 15, *Nutrition in childhood and adolescence.* Chapter 37, *Nutritional care for low-birth-weight and high-risk neonate.* Chapter 38, *Nutritional care in diseases of infancy and childhood.* Chapter 39, *Nutritional care for children with inborn errors of metabolism.*

KRETCHMER, N: *Human Nutrition: Readings from Scientific American.* WH Freeman & Company, San Francisco, 1978, p 131. *Lactose and lactase.*

LARTER, N: *Cystic fibrosis.* American Journal of Nursing 81(3), March, 1981.

MCWILLIAMS, M: *Nutrition for the Growing Years,* ed 3. John Wiley & Sons, New York, 1980.

NEWCOMER, AD: *Lactase deficiency.* Contemporary Nutrition 4(4), April, 1979.

REYZER, N: *Diagnosis: PKU.* American Journal of Nursing 78(11), November, 1978.

ROBINSON, CH: *Basic Nutrition and Diet Therapy,* ed 4. Macmillan, New York, 1980. Chapter 14, *Nutrition for growth and development.* Chapter 29, *Malabsorption disorders.*

ROSENBERG, FH: *Lactose intolerance.* American Journal of Nursing 77(5), May, 1977.

SUITOR, CW AND HUNTER, MF: *Nutrition: Principles and Application in Health Promotion.* JB Lippincott, Philadelphia, 1980. Chapter 32, *Alterations in ingestion.* Chapter 33, *Alterations in digestion and/or absorption.*

WORTHINGTON-ROBERTS, BS: *Contemporary Developments in Nutrition.* CV Mosby, St Louis, 1981. Chapter 1, *Carbohydrates in health and disease.* Chapter 19, *Suboptimal nutrition and behavior in children.*

27

DIET IN WEIGHT CONTROL

OBJECTIVES

Upon completion of this chapter the student should be able to:

- Give the causes of underweight and the problems encountered with it.
- Describe nutritional therapy for the underweight person, select an acceptable eating pattern for the individual, and plan a menu to fit that pattern.
- Discuss obesity, and give its causes, diagnosis, and the problems encountered when overweight.
- Describe the nutritional therapy of obesity and its psychologic aspects.
- List some of the dangers in trying to overcome obesity using fad diets and medications.
- Plan a menu designed to cause loss of weight.

One of the more immediate concerns in the United States today is the control of weight because it has such an effect upon physical and psychologic health.

UNDERWEIGHT

Although this condition has not had as much publicity as overweight, underweight is a health problem. When an individual is 15 percent below standard normal weight, there is usually less energy available to the individual, less resistance to infections, and, in a child, retarded growth. Underweight persons have more skin surface in relation to body weight and consequently lose body heat easily, causing them to complain of cold. When small amounts of food have been ingested over a period of time, the stomach cannot take larger meals and this leads the underweight person to continue to eat scantily. Persistent malnutrition depresses the appetite and interferes with functioning of the endocrine glands. Many underweight women have menstrual irregularities or fail to menstruate.

Underweight can be caused by not eating, as in anorexia nervosa, or by not eating the right foods. Often the underweight person dislikes foods that are high in calories, such as fats and sweets. Failure to eat can be due to economic or psychologic factors. It can be secondary to cancer or to diseases that increase the metabolic rate. Everyone is familiar with the weight loss that follows a high fever. Diseases that interfere with normal digestion or absorption of nutrients can also cause weight loss. An example of this would be chronic colitis with its persistent diarrhea.

The underweight person should be examined by a physician to determine the cause of the weight problem and to obtain treatment for the cause. After this is done, a study should be made of the individual's eating habits to determine what will need to be modified in order to help the individual gain weight. Hyperactive people, for example, may be so active they may literally "eat on the run." People who lack an appetite may skip lunch. In all cases, the patient should understand that gaining weight requires a lot of effort over a long period of time.

Food intake should be increased gradually. Care must be taken not to force the individual to take more than can be tolerated, as this causes nausea. Concentrated foods are usually better than bulky foods. Moderate fat intake prevents too early satiety. Protein intake is kept at a high normal and high-calorie carbohydrates are used extensively. Men usually prefer to add extra amounts of food at the usual mealtimes, women prefer concentrated foods, and children like snacks between meals. The addition of 500 calories per day is needed for a 1 pound gain per week.

Complete the following:

1. Being underweight can result in:

2. The underweight person may not have an appetite because:

3. Causes of underweight include:

4. What are the first and second steps in treating underweight?

5. In each of the choices below, circle the food that is more likely to aid in gaining weight.
Bacon or poached filet of bass
Potato salad or salad greens with vinegar and oil dressing
String beans or lima beans
Jello or chocolate pie
Cafe au lait or tea with lemon and 1 teaspoon sugar
Bouillon or cream of tomato soup
Half-and-half cream or artificial creamer
$^1/_2$ cup grits with 1 pat butter or $^1/_2$ cup oatmeal with $^1/_4$ cup cream
Buttered popcorn or an equal amount of carrot sticks
Potato chips or baked potato

6. Powdered milk can be added to whole milk to increase caloric content without adding excessive bulk. What would you add to each of the following to increase caloric content and still have an enjoyable dish?
Buttered toast:
Whole milk:
Vanilla ice cream:
Cereal with sugar and milk:
French fried steak:
Jello:

7. Plan a day's menu for each of the following.
   A 46-year-old woman:

   A 25-year-old man:

   A 10-year-old boy:

OVERWEIGHT

Approximately one third of the people in the United States weigh more than they should. When an individual is 20 percent above standard normal weight, overweight becomes *obesity.*

Getting on the scales is not the only method of determining obesity. X-ray films can show the amount of fat around organs and under skin. Pinching the skin on the back or the arm or on the chest can indicate the amount of fat stored under the skin in the subcutaneous area. Some fat in this area is normal but when the skinfold is too thick, it indicates obesity.

Obesity occurs when more food is ingested than the body can use for growth and energy. This may be due to overeating or, more rarely, to metabolic and glandular problems. When parents are obese, children have a greater chance of being overweight. This can be due to learned eating habits or heredity. Overeating can be due to an emotional problem, habit, or ignorance. Some people eat when they feel anxious. Even physicians are guilty of rewarding children with food for taking injections. Mothers establish habits of overeating by insisting that children eat everything on their plates. To many people, being able to have fattening foods proves that they are now affluent enough to afford expensive foods; this enhances social status for them. Meals that are social affairs encourage overeating.

Obesity due to glandular problems is not as common as that due to overeating. A malfunctioning thyroid, pituitary, or adrenal cortex can lead to obesity, but, even in these conditions, weight loss requires reduction of calories in the diet.

The overweight person should be instructed in the dangers of excessive body fat. Excessive weight causes early fatigue and the heart must work harder. The overweight person is a greater surgical risk. There is a chance of fat embolism and some anesthetics are absorbed by fat tissue to be released at a later time, making the recovery period unstable. Obesity is a predisposing factor in diabetes and arteriosclerosis. Excessive weight bearing increases pain in conditions such as arthritis. Obesity shortens the life span.

Perhaps the most damaging aspect of obesity is psychologic. The obese person feels deeply rejected by others (and often is), developing a poor self-image, which is described in negative, derogatory words. Many authorities feel that the first step in overcoming obesity is to change the self-image. Motivation to change is an individual matter and may require re-education of the patient.

Prevention of obesity begins before birth and continues throughout life. The critical periods are during the last three months of pregnancy for the fetus, the first three years of life, adolescence, and middle age. When a baby is overweight, additional fat cells are produced. The size of the cells can be reduced but the number of cells will always remain constant. Childhood-onset obesity is more common in girls and is more difficult to control. Infants should not be force fed and should be given ample water between feedings. There is some evidence that feeding solids before six months of age can increase the possibility of obesity. Infants should be allowed to exercise freely; leaving the limbs free to move while in the crib is a good beginning.

All too often, adults continue to take in the same amount of food as when they were growing during adolescence. After maturity, the metabolic rate begins to decline. "Middle-age spread" usually begins in the late 20s with the individual gaining two or three pounds per year. It is usually due to the individual maintaining the same level of food intake while failing to maintain the same level of activity. A good example of this is the clerk typist, a former cheerleader, who now sits all day at work and goes home to sit in front of the television. Sporadic vigorous exercise is not as effective as consistent moderate exercise.

Men and women do not add adipose tissue in the same places. Women, who have a tendency to add pounds during pregnancy and after menopause, gain weight first around the lower body: the hips, abdomen, and thighs. Men gain weight in the abdomen and around the chest. Also, men usually find it easier to lose weight than women.

Going on a diet and losing the desired number of pounds is only half the task. To lose and maintain the loss requires behavior modification, teaching patients to change actions and attitudes detrimental to their health. The patients keep a record of when they eat, what they eat, and what causes them to eat. After patients understand why they overeat, they try to change their behavior by giving themselves rewards for achievement of desired behaviors, controlling their environment by removing provocative stimuli, and other behavior modification techniques. Television, the automobile, and ads in papers and magazines make it difficult to remove all stimuli. Many persons find that supervision of their efforts or the support of others attempting to lose weight is necessary for success.

The only way to lose weight safely is with a well-balanced, *low-calorie diet* and exercise to maintain muscle tone. Many people, however, are making money selling fad diets, diet foods, mechanical devices, and drugs. Millions of dollars have been spent on books and articles on weight control. Fads can be dangerous; when substantial weight loss is necessary, it should be done under the supervision of a physician.

Fasting and fad diets can cause ketosis and electrolyte imbalances. Some high-protein liquid diets have caused deaths. Drugs to suppress the appetite can be addicting, and may cause side effects such as hypertension. Drugs that produce bulk can interfere with intestinal motility in some individuals. Saunas and steam cabinets can cause vasodilation and fainting, as well as dehydration.

Intestinal bypass surgery may be performed if the obesity is so severe it interferes with the life-sustaining processes. As stated in Chapter 24, malabsorption can result and the individual can be in dire straits. This surgery is usually a last resort.

Wiring of the jaws has been used in some cases. Because the individual still requires the essential nutrients, care must be taken to exclude liquids that do not supply these. Oral hygiene is a problem when the jaws are wired. Unfortunately, after the wires are removed, there is no guarantee that the individual has learned to eat a proper diet to maintain the weight loss.

The recommended diet is a *low-calorie diet* with the protein kept at a high level. Some fat is necessary in the diet to provide the essential fatty acids and to provide satiety. Some people lose weight better and complain of hunger and fatigue less on small, frequent meals. When the diet provides fewer than 1000 calories per day, mineral and vitamin supplements may be necessary. For each pound of weight loss per week, 500 calories must be deleted from the daily diet.

At first, the weight loss is usually due to loss of water. Later, the body replaces this water and when this happens, weight loss may not occur. This is the period known as "the plateau." The patient should continue water intake as this is a normal process and the next weight loss will be due to fat loss. Occasionally, the physician will suggest restricting sodium intake if water retention is severe.

When treating a child, the whole family and peer situation must be considered. Sometimes the entire family must be re-educated. All family members must understand and follow rules about snacks. Temptation must be eliminated, even to the extent of refusing spending money to the child. It is easier to have the child give up one high-calorie food at a time as the child is brought to understand and appreciate healthful foods.

Complete the following:

1. List two ways to determine whether a person is obese without using a scale.

   A.

   B.

2. Can you think of a condition in which the person apparently has gained weight but in reality has not added adipose tissue?

3. A person who is 10 percent over the standard normal weight is overweight. How far above standard normal weight are the obese?

4. If the normal weight for an individual is 120 pounds, how much would that individual have to weigh to be obese?

5. How does overweight occur?

6. What are some of the factors that lead to overeating?

7. When do you, personally, overeat?

8. People who are obese find it more difficult to get jobs and are at a disadvantage socially. List the dangers of excessive body fat.

9. The critical periods when obesity can develop are ______________ , ______________________________ , ______________________________ , and ______________________ .

10. How can you prevent obesity in infants?

11. "Middle-age spread" is less difficult to control than childhood-onset obesity but it usually occurs so gradually it is overlooked until a number of pounds have been gained. What contributes to the development of "middle-age spread"?

12. John and Mary have each gained 20 pounds since they married. Circle the item(s) of clothing you think they will need in a larger size now.

Shirt	Blouse
Pants	Skirt

13. What is the objective of behavior modification in dieting?

14. How you see yourself (your self-image) is the key to what you will become. If your self-image is a pretty, slender, confident woman, or a handsome, muscular, assured man, you will find that you take actions that will insure that you are as you see yourself. How does this apply to the obese person?

15. For the next 24 hours, keep a record of each time you feel you want to eat or drink anything but water. Write down the situation that stimulated your desire to eat or drink. For example, you are at the movies and someone in back of you brings in a bag of popcorn. The smell and sound of the bag crackling make you hungry.

16. Most physicians feel it is best not to attempt to lose more than two or three pounds per week. What is the safe way to lose weight?

17. What are the dangers in trying to lose weight using fad diets, mechanical devices, or drugs?

18. Why are bypass surgery and jaw wiring procedures not used more often?

19. Why do persons losing weight reach a "plateau" and how should the nurse handle this period?

20. Give two rules in treating a child with obesity.
A.

B.

21. Plan a day's menu for a person on a low-calorie diet.

22. What foods can you add to your menu to provide bulk without appreciably increasing the caloric content?

OPTIONAL ACTIVITY TO ENHANCE LEARNING

ACTIVITY 1

Case Study

Mrs. A. is 5 feet 3 inches tall and weighs 198 pounds. She is a 40-year-old mother of two and works as a secretary to one of the vice presidents of a petroleum company. A part of her duties includes attending meetings with her employer; often these are luncheon or dinner meetings. Her duty hours can be erratic, often extending into the early evening when a business transaction requires it. Mrs. A.'s husband is a supervisor at one of the petroleum plants. He leaves for work at 6 AM. Her children catch a bus at 8 AM. Mrs. A. has breakfast with her husband and then prepares breakfast for the children. She has to be in the office by 9 AM, at which time she takes a cup of hot tea and a sweet roll. Mrs. A. is particularly fond of fried chicken, mashed potatoes, and gravy, frequently purchasing these at a fast food service when she is not required at a meeting. She does not like green peas or steamed carrots, which are often on the menus of the luncheons. She has no known food allergies. In the evenings, the family often has hamburgers and french fries when Mrs. A. is late getting home. There is always ice cream in the freezer. Mrs. A. consulted the physician because she wanted some diet pills. Except for her overweight, her physical examination was normal. While her history was being taken, Mrs. A. constantly fidgeted, moving her watch band, touching her hair, and changing her position. She twice remarked that she was hungry. When asked when she felt hunger, she replied, "Every time I get tired or tense." Mrs. A. was placed on a 1000-calorie diet and asked to return in one week. In the meantime, she was to schedule herself for daily exercise periods. A suggestion was made that she try jogging or swimming.

Prepare a nutritional care plan.

BIBLIOGRAPHY

BRIGGS, GM AND CALLOWAY, DH: *Bogert's Nutrition and Physical Fitness,* ed 10. WB Saunders, Philadelphia, 1979. Chapter 24, *Overweight and underweight.*

CALIENDO, MA: *Nutrition and Preventitive Health Care.* Macmillan, New York, 1981. Chapter 9, *Obesity.*

CISEAUX, A: *Anorexia nervosa: The view from the mirror.* American Journal of Nursing 80(8), August, 1980.

COHEN, RJ: *Binge! ... Not a state of hunger—A state of mind.* Family Health Vol 11, May, 1979.

DANOWSKI, TS: *Sugar and disease.* Contemporary Nutrition 3(12), December, 1978.

THE PRESIDENT'S COUNCIL ON PHYSICAL FITNESS AND SPORTS: *Exercise and Weight Control.* US Government Printing Office, Washington, DC, 1980.

HALPERN, SL ET AL: *Quick Reference to Clinical Nutrition: A Guide for Physicians.* JB Lippincott, Philadelphia, 1979. Chapter 17, *Treatment of obesity.*

HOFMANN, L: *The Great American Nutrition Hassle.* Mayfield, Palo Alto, California, 1978. Chapter 14, *Fight fat with behavior control.*

HUTT, PB AND SLOAN, AE: *Final FDA regulations governing label statements for foods represented as useful in reducing or maintaining caloric intake or body weight.* Nutrition Policy Issues November, 1978.

KORNGUTH, ML: *When your client has a weight problem: Nursing management.* American Journal of Nursing 81(3), March, 1981.

KRAUSE, MV AND MAHAN, LK: *Food, Nutrition and Diet Therapy,* ed 6. WB Saunders, Philadelphia, 1979. Chapter 26, *Nutritional care for patients with diseases of the adrenal cortex and thyroid gland and other diseases of metabolism.* Chapter 27, *Nutritional care in conditions of overweight and underweight.*

LANGFORD, RW: *When your client has a weight problem: Teenagers and obesity.* American Journal of Nursing 81(3), March, 1981.

LEON, GR: *The behavior modification approach to weight reduction.* Contemporary Nutrition 4(8), August, 1979.

LUCAS, AR: *Bulimia and vomiting syndrome.* Contemporary Nutrition 6(4), April, 1981.

MCWILLIAMS, M: *Nutrition for the Growing Years,* ed 3. John Wiley & Sons, New York, 1980. Chapter 11, *Weight control.*

MILLER, BK: *Jejunoileal bypass: A drastic weight control measure.* American Journal of Nursing 81(3), March, 1981.

MOJZIZK, CM AND MARTIN, EW, JR: *Gastric partioning: The latest surgical means to control morbid obesity.* American Journal of Nursing 81(3), March, 1981.

PALOMBO, JD AND BLACKBURN, GL: *Human protein requirements.* Contemporary Nutrition 5(1), January, 1980.

RICHARDSON, TF: *Anorexia nervosa: An overview.* American Journal of Nursing 80(8), August, 1980.

ROBINSON, CH: *Basic Nutrition and Diet Therapy,* ed 4. Macmillan, New York, 1980. Chapter 22, *Problems of weight control.*

WHITE, JH AND SCHROEDER, MA: *When your client has a weight problem: Nursing assessment.* American Journal of Nursing 81(3), March, 1981.

WILLIAMS, SR: *Mowry's Basic Nutrition and Diet Therapy,* ed 6. CV Mosby, St Louis, 1980. Chapter 22, *Obesity.* Chapter 23, *Underweight.*

WORTHINGTON-ROBERTS, BS: *Contemporary Developments in Nutrition.* CV Mosby, St Louis, 1981. Chapter 13, *Obesity: New knowledge and current treatments.*

28

DRUG AND NUTRIENT INTERACTIONS

OBJECTIVES

Upon completion of this chapter the student should be able to:

- State when drug-nutrient interaction is most likely to occur.
- List ways in which drugs affect nutritional status.
- List ways in which nutrients affect drug therapy.
- Describe drug-nutrient interactions of some common drugs.

People today take literally hundreds of different drugs and many conditions that were formerly often fatal can be cured because these drugs are available. However, it is now known that many have side effects and some of these affect nutritional status. Also, it has been found that nutrients can affect drug therapy, either decreasing or increasing its effectiveness. Sometimes nutrients, particularly the vitamins, are given as medications.

Drug interaction with nutrients is more likely if drug therapy is lengthy, the individual's nutritional status is poor, or the condition or disease causes intense physical stress.

Some drugs cause loss of appetite; others increase the appetite. Some change the taste sensation or alter the production of saliva. Nausea and vomiting are induced by many drugs. Absorption of nutrients is affected when diarrhea occurs or when bile production is diminished. Antacids reduce the absorption of iron, and mineral oil reduces the absorption of vitamin K. Some drugs act as antivitamins. Others increase the excretion of nutrients. Antidepressants that are monoamine oxidase (MAO) inhibitors cause headaches and severe hypertension if wine, yoghurt, herring, aged cheese, banana, or chocolate is eaten.

Nutrients affect drug action in the body. Fats aid in absorption of griseofulvin. Pyridoxine potentiates the action of phenobarbitol and can cause oversedation. Protein inhibits the absorption of levodopa. Ascorbic acid can reverse the effects of some anticoagulants. Some drugs should not be taken at mealtimes. Food can interfere with absorption because of its bulk, its nutrient content, or because it slows passage of the drug through the alimentary canal, making it more susceptible to change by digestive enzymes.

Because the area of drug-nutrient interaction is so complex, the nurse should make it a habit to consult a pharmacology text or other drug reference to ascertain nutritional considerations for patients receiving medications.

In the following paragraphs, some drug-nutrient interactions are listed. Some drugs are listed by name; others are given as classes when the interactions are common to them all.

ACETAMINOPHEN (used for fevers and minor pains)

Food with high pectin content delays absorption of acetaminophen.

ACETYLSALICYLIC ACID (aspirin)

Interferes with absorption and utilization of folic acid.
Increases excretion of ascorbic acid.
Causes ascorbic acid and vitamin K deficiency.
Food delays absorption of acetylsalicylic acid.

ACTH (adrenocorticotropic hormone)

Causes deficiency of ascorbic acid.

ALCOHOL (whiskey, wine, beer)

Interferes with the absorption and utilization of vitamins A, B_{12}, thiamin, pyridoxine, and folic acid.
Causes ascorbic acid deficiency.
Increases excretion of zinc, magnesium, calcium.
Depresses the appetite.

AMPHETAMINES (used to depress appetite and to treat hyperactive children)

Cause ascorbic acid deficiency.

Increase sensitivity to bitter taste.
Decrease sensitivity to sweet taste.
Can retard growth.

ANESTHETICS
Alter taste sensations.

ANTACIDS (used to treat hyperacidity of the stomach)
Interfere with absorption and utilization of vitamins D and thiamin, iron, and phosphorus.
Increase excretion of phosphates.
Delay the emptying of the gallbladder and thus the use of bile in digestion.

ANTICONVULSIVES (used to treat epilepsy)
Interfere with the absorption and utilization of folic acid.
Interfere with metabolism of vitamins D and K.
Cause deficiency of ascorbic acid.
May depress the appetite.

ANTIHISTAMINES (used for allergies)
Decrease the appetite.

ANTINEOPLASTICS (used to treat cancers and leukemias)
Interfere with absorption and utilization of niacin, folic acid, and B_{12}.
Interfere with absorption of nutrients when diarrhea occurs.
Increase taste sensitivity to sweets in some cases; alter other taste sensations.
May suppress the appetite.

BICARBONATE
Interferes with the absorption and utilization of iron.

BIGUANIDES (hypoglycemic agents used in diabetes)
Interfere with the absorption and utilization of B_{12}.

CHLORAMPHENICOL (antibiotic)
Interferes with absorption of lactose.
Interferes with protein and vitamin K synthesis.
Increases need for riboflavin, pyridoxine, and B_{12}.

CHLORTHALIDONE (diuretic)
Increases the excretion of zinc.

CHLOROTHIAZIDES (diuretic)

Increase calcium absorption.
Decrease carbohydrate tolerance.
Increase excretion of riboflavin, potassium, zinc, and magnesium.
Increase uric acid, producing symptoms of gout.

CHOLESTYRAMINE (used to reduce cholesterol levels)

Interferes with absorption and utilization of vitamins A, D, E, K, folic acid, and B_{12}, calcium, and iron.
Increases excretion of calcium.
Interferes with the use of bile in digestion.
May depress the appetite.

CLOFIBRATE (used to reduce serum lipids)

Interferes with absorption and utilization of vitamins A and B_{12}, glucose, and iron.
Interferes with metabolism of vitamin E.
Decreases taste sensitivity.

COLCHICINE (used to treat gout)

Interferes with the absorption and utilization of vitamins A and B_{12}, fat, and lactose.
Increases excretion of sodium and potassium.

CORTICOSTEROIDS (used to relieve inflammation)

Interfere with the absorption and utilization of calcium and phosphorus.
Increase vitamin D metabolism.
Increase the blood sugar.
Increase sodium retention.
Increase excretion of ascorbic acid, calcium, potassium, zinc, and nitrogen.
Inhibit protein synthesis.
May increase the appetite.
Cause mobility of fat to produce "moon face" and "buffalo hump."

CYCLOSERINE (used to treat tuberculosis and urinary tract infections)

Interferes with the absorption and utilization of folic acid, calcium, and magnesium.

DIGITALIS (used to treat cardiac conditions)

Interferes with the absorption and utilization of glucose.
Increases the need for thiamin.
May depress the appetite.

Food delays absorption of digitalis.
Potassium deficiency can cause digitalis intoxication.
Elevated serum calcium can lead to irregular heart beat when taking digitalis.

ETHACRYNIC ACID (diuretic)
Increases excretion of potassium, sodium, magnesium, and calcium.

FUROSEMIDE (diuretic)
Decreases carbohydrate tolerance.
Increases excretion of potassium, calcium, magnesium, and zinc.
Increases uric acid, producing symptoms of gout.
Food delays absorption of furosemide.

GLUTETHIMIDE (hypnotic)
Interferes with the absorption and utilization of calcium.
Increases excretion of calcium.

GRISEOFULVIN (used to treat fungus)
Decreases the sensitivity to taste.
Fats increase absorption of griseofulvin.

HYDRALAZINE (used to treat hypertension)
Interferes with the absorption and utilization of pyridoxine.
Binds the trace minerals.

INSULIN
Decreases sensitivity to taste of sweet and salt.

ISONICOTINIC ACID HYDRAZIDE (used to treat tuberculosis)
Interferes with the absorption and utilization of pyridoxine, folic acid, and niacin.
Increases iron absorption.
Increases excretion of pyridoxine.

LAXATIVES
Interfere with the absorption and utilization of vitamins D and K, glucose, and calcium.
Increase excretion of potassium, sodium, calcium, magnesium, and water-soluble vitamins.

LEVODOPA (used to treat Parkinson's disease)
Interferes with the absorption and utilization of pyridoxine.

Increases excretion of sodium and potassium.
Food, especially proteins, interfere with absorption of levodopa.

LITHIUM (used to treat manic-depressive psychiatric conditions)
Causes unpleasant taste sensations.
May increase the appetite.
Food increases the absorption of lithium.

MONOAMINE OXIDASE (MAO) INHIBITORS (antidepressants)
May increase the appetite.
Hypertensive crises may occur if tyramine and tyrosine are ingested.

MERCURIAL DIURETICS
Increase excretion of potassium, thiamin, calcium, and magnesium.

METHOTREXATE (used to treat cancer and leukemias)
Interferes with the absorption and utilization of folic acid, B_{12}, and fat.

MILK OF MAGNESIA (cathartic)
Interferes with the absorption and utilization of fat and phosphorus.

MINERAL OIL
Interferes with the absorption and utilization of vitamins A, D, E, and K, calcium, and phosphorus.

MORPHINE (narcotic)
Interferes with digestion by decreasing gastric and pancreatic secretions and intestinal motility.
Depresses the appetite.

NEOMYCIN (antibiotic)
Interferes with the absorption and utilization of vitamins A, B_{12}, and K, protein, lactose, sucrose, fat, calcium, and iron.
Increases excretion of sodium and potassium.
Interferes with the use of bile in digestion.

ORAL CONTRACEPTIVES
Interfere with the absorption and utilization of ascorbic acid, pyridoxine, and folic acid.
Increase absorption of calcium.
Increase the excretion of zinc.
Alter protein, lipid, and vitamin A metabolism.
Elevate blood glucose slightly.
May stimulate the appetite.

PARA-AMINOSALICYLIC ACID (used to treat tuberculosis)

Interferes with the absorption and utilization of folic acid, B_{12}, and fat.

PENICILLIN (antibiotic)

Increases excretion of potassium.

Food delays absorption of penicillin.

PHENOBARBITAL (sedative)

Interferes with the absorption and utilization of vitamins D and thiamin, folic acid, and calcium.

Increases excretion of ascorbic acid.

Pyridoxine potentiates sedative action of phenobarbital.

PHENYTOIN (used to treat epilepsy)

Interferes with the absorption and utilization of calcium.

Increases excretion of ascorbic acid and vitamin D.

Decreases sensitivity to taste.

May interfere with gastrointestinal motility.

Large doses of folic acid decreases phenytoin effectiveness.

Alcohol causes rapid metabolism of phenytoin.

POTASSIUM CHLORIDE (replacement therapy)

Interferes with the absorption and utilization of B_{12}.

Potassium chloride liquids have an unpleasant taste and may depress the appetite.

SALICYLAZOSULFAPYRIDINE (sulfa drug used for colitis)

Interferes with the absorption and utilization of folic acid.

Food delays the absorption of this drug.

TETRACYCLINE (antibiotic)

Interferes with the absorption and utilization of vitamin K, protein, fat, calcium, iron, and magnesium.

Increases excretion of ascorbic acid, riboflavin, folic acid, niacin, and nitrogen.

Decreases sensitivity to taste.

May depress the appetite.

Food, particularly milk and milk products, delay absorption of tetracycline.

THYROXINE (replacement therapy)

Interferes with the absorption and utilization of riboflavin.

TRANQUILIZERS

Increase sodium retention.
Interfere with gastrointestinal motility.
Decrease sensitivity to taste.
Increase or decrease the appetite.

TRIAMTERENE (diuretic)

Interferes with the absorption and utilization of folic acid.
Increases excretion of calcium.

TRIMETHOPRIM (antibiotic)

Interferes with the absorption and utilization of folic acid.

WARFARIN (anticoagulant)

Causes a deficiency of vitamin K.
Cooking oil interferes with the absorption of warfarin.
Alcohol accelerates metabolism of warfarin.

Actual nutritional deficiencies usually occur only in persons already at risk nutritionally, when drugs are used over a long period, or when a combination of drugs having the same effect on nutrients is given. It is apparent that drug effectiveness often depends upon the diet and the timing of the dose. Some drugs can best be absorbed at mealtime or with certain foods; others are better absorbed when the stomach is empty. Understanding this will aid the nurse in establishing medication schedules.

Complete the following:

1. Drug-nutrient interaction is most likely to occur:

2. List some effects of drugs on nutrition.

3. What foods should be avoided when taking MAO-inhibitor antidepressants?

4. What should the nurse do when the patient has an unfamiliar drug order?

5. Which medications in the list given in this chapter may cause electrolyte imbalance?

6. After studying this chapter, how do you feel about people prescribing vitamins for themselves?

OPTIONAL ACTIVITIES TO ENHANCE LEARNING

ACTIVITY 1

A patient has been admitted with the following orders. Plan the nutrition interventions that may be necessary.

1. Lasix 40 mg., p.o., b.i.d.
2. Dimetane 4 mg., p.o., PRN for hayfever
3. Aspirin gr. XV, p.o., q 4 h
4. Eutonyl 25 mg., p.o., q.d.

ACTIVITY 2

The physician has written the following orders. Plan the nutrition interventions that may be necessary.

1. Griseofulvin 125 mg., p.o., q.i.d
2. Prednisone 10 mg., p.o., b.i.d
3. Phenobarbital gr. 1/2, p.o., t.i.d.
4. $FeSO_4$ gr. X, p.o., b.i.d.

OPTIONAL ACTIVITIES—*Continued*

ACTIVITY 3

Plan the nutrition interventions that may be necessary because of the following orders.

1. Achromycin 250 mg., p.o., q 6 h
2. Lithium 300 mg., p.o., t.i.d.
3. Colace cap. 1 h.s.
4. Brevicon 28-day tablet q.d. starting tomorrow.

(Consult a pharmacology text if the drugs are not familiar to you.)

BIBLIOGRAPHY

AFTERGOOD, L AND ALFIN-SLATER, RB: *Women and nutrition.* Contemporary Nutrition 5(3), March, 1980.

Food/Drug Interaction Guide. Ross Laboratories, Columbus, Ohio.

HALPERN, SL ET AL: *Quick Reference to Clinical Nutrition: A Guide for Physicians.* JB Lippincott, Philadelphia, 1979. Chapter 27, *The nutritional management of alcoholism, drug addiction and acute toxicity syndrome.*

HARTSHORN, EA: *Food and drug interactions.* Journal of the American Dietetic Association Vol 70, January, 1977.

HODGES, RE: *Nutrition in Medical Practice.* WB Saunders, Philadelphia, 1980. Chapter 14, *Drug-nutrient interactions.*

HOFMANN, L: *The Great American Nutrition Hassle.* Mayfield, Palo Alto, California, 1978. Chapter 21, *Liquor's good side: Wine and cognac.* Chapter 22, *Drug-vitamin interrelationships.*

KRAUSE, MV AND MAHAN, LK: *Food, Nutrition and Diet Therapy,* ed 6. WB Saunders, Philadelphia, 1979. Chapter 20, *The interactions between drugs, nutrients and nutritional status.*

LIEBER, CS: *Alcohol-nutrition interaction.* Contemporary Nutrition 3(9), September, 1978.

ROE, DA: *Drugs, diet and nutrition.* Contemporary Nutrition 3(6), June, 1978.

REVIEW QUESTIONS FOR SECTION 2

Circle the letter of the phrase that *best* completes each statement in the exercise below:

1. When required to eat a high-calorie diet, children usually prefer:
   A. Extra portions at mealtimes.
   B. Concentrated foods.
   C. Between meal snacks.

2. To turn a normal diet into a high-protein diet, add:
   A. Dried beans, peas, and gelatin.
   B. Milk, eggs, and meat.
   C. Whole-grain cereals.

3. On a low-residue diet, the patient should avoid:
   A. Refined cereals and fruit juice.
   B. Raw fruits and vegetables.
   C. Eggs and fat-free soups.

4. The purpose of the bland diet is to:
   A. Prevent peristalsis and flow of gastric juices.
   B. Prevent weight loss.
   C. Avoid foods with taste and satiety value.

5. A full liquid diet includes the following foods:
   A. Fruit juice, tea, coffee, and jello.
   B. Milk, oatmeal, and vegetable soup.
   C. Noodle soup, ice cream, and crackers.

6. Mr. G. has a peptic ulcer. His physician has ordered the first stage of the Sippy diet. For lunch, Mr. G. may have:
   A. Strained cream soup and toast.
   B. Pureed liver and fruit juice.
   C. Milk and cream.

7. When Mr. G. hemorrhaged, he was placed on a Meulengracht diet. This abundant pureed diet is given to:
   A. Build up his strength.
   B. Prevent digestion of the blood clot that forms on the site of the hemorrhage.
   C. Satisfy his excessive hunger after the blood loss.

8. After surgery, Mr. G. received a mixture of milk, cream, and gelatin every two hours. This is the:
   A. Fourth stage of the Sippy diet.
   B. First stage of the Meulengracht diet.
   C. First stage of the Andresen diet.

9. Mrs. G. has atonic constipation. Her physician has urged her to follow a:
   A. High-residue diet.
   B. Low-calorie diet.
   C. Low-residue diet.

10. Mrs. L. is constipated as a result of excessive use of cathartics, very coarse foods, and alcohol. Her physician ordered a:
    A. High-residue diet.
    B. Low-calorie diet.
    C. Low-residue diet.

11. Which of the following would be the best choice for a patient with cirrhosis and ascites?
    A. Fried steak, gravy, pickles, and chocolate cake.
    B. Broiled steak, carrot sticks, apple, and baked potato.
    C. Macaroni and cheese, consomme, and crackers.

12. The patient with a gallbladder disease is usually given a:
    A. Low-fat diet.
    B. Low-calorie diet.
    C. High-fiber diet.

13. Four rules for diet therapy for most cardiac patients include:
    A. All of the below. B. All but (3). C. All but (4).
    (1) Do not allow the patient to overeat.
    (2) Serve foods that are easily digested.
    (3) Restrict stimulants.
    (4) Limit the sodium in the diet.

14. Mr. F. is a cardiac patient on a moderately restricted sodium diet. When he goes on a coffee break at work, he should choose:
    A. Coffee with sugar only.
    B. Orange juice.
    C. Fat-free consomme.

15. When patients are placed on a low-cholesterol diet, they should avoid:
    A. Fresh fruit and vegetables.
    B. Milk, butter, and egg yolk.
    C. Steak, potatoes, and onions.

16. For most kidney conditions, the dietary prescription is for a:
    A. Low-cholesterol diet.
    B. Low-residue diet.
    C. Low-sodium diet.

17. The patient with renal calculi on an acid-ash diet may have:
   A. Peaches, plums, and strawberries.
   B. Meat, eggs, and cereals.
   C. Green beans, peas, and lentils.

18. The dietary prescription for hyperthyroidism is a:
   A. High-calorie, high-protein diet.
   B. Low-carbohydrate diet.
   C. Low-cholesterol, low-sodium diet.

19. On which food exchange list is an orange found?
   A. Bread.
   B. Meat.
   C. Fruit.

20. If diabetic patients have a piece of avocado on the menu and do not like avocado, they may substitute:
   A. Bacon.
   B. Half of a banana.
   C. Summer squash.

21. Miss M. is diabetic. When she stops at the snack bar after the movie with her boyfriend, she should order:
   A. A glass of milk.
   B. Coffee.
   C. Orange juice.

22. Miss M. did not eat all of her lunch. She should:
   A. Take orange juice to equal that which she did not eat.
   B. Double her portions at supper.
   C. Do nothing.

23. For breakfast, Miss M. is allowed 1 fat exchange, 2 meat exchanges, 2 bread exchanges, and 1 fruit exchange. The following is a good menu for her:
A. Doughnut, applesauce, and coffee with cream.
B. Half a grapefruit, 2 pieces of toast, 1/2 pat butter, and poached egg on a slice of ham.
C. Half a banana, cereal, whole milk, 2 sausages, and toast with 1/2 teaspoon jelly.

24. The foods that most often cause allergies are:
A. Chocolate, eggs, wheat, and strawberries.
B. Oranges, plums, and duck.
C. Oats, barley, grapes, and limes.

25. Because immobilization of a bone healing from a fracture leads to excessive calcium excretion and possible formation of renal calculi, the dietary prescription is a:
A. High-calcium diet.
B. High-carbohydrate diet.
C. High-protein diet.

26. Which of the following may the tonsillectomy patient have?
A. Jello.
B. Hot tea.
C. Chopped veal.

27. In toxemia of pregnancy, the patient may be given a high-protein diet. The best food for her to choose to increase her protein intake is:
A. Low-sodium milk.
B. Egg yolks.
C. Baby beef.

28. Mrs. J. is having "morning sickness" with her pregnancy. To relieve this her physician suggested to:
A. Take only coffee for breakfast.
B. Eat crackers before arising.
C. Skip breakfast entirely.

29. As soon as Mrs. J. goes into true labor, the physician will order:
   A. Surgical liquids.
   B. Regular diet.
   C. Nothing by mouth.

30. Every four hours or oftener, the infant with pyloric stenosis is fed:
   A. A mixture of half milk and half water.
   B. Thick gruel.
   C. Pureed fruits.

31. To prevent constipation in a child, which of the following can be given?
   A. Orange juice or pureed fruit.
   B. Tea.
   C. Coca-Cola concentrate.

32. Phenylketonuria is a condition in which:
   A. There is a failure to metabolize certain amino acids.
   B. There is a deficiency of nutrients.
   C. Carbohydrates fail to convert to carbon, hydrogen, and oxygen.

Complete the following statements:

33. ________________ is the treatment of a disease by modification of the diet.

34. A high-fiber diet is the same as a ________________ diet.

35. A diet is deficient in minerals and vitamins if there are fewer than ____________ calories.

36. A surgical liquid diet consists of ____________________________, ________________, and ________________.

37. In acute gastroenteritis, on the first day the patient is allowed ________________.

38. In the salt-free diet, it is the ________________ that is restricted.

39. The ________________ diet consists of 800 ml of milk per day given in four equal servings.

40. The Kempner diet for severe hypertension consists of ________________, ________________, and ________________.

41. A patient with uremia with 200 ml of fluid output should receive ________ ml of fluid intake.

42. The goals of diet therapy for the obese person are to cause weight loss and to establish ________________.

43. ________________ is a disease in which the patient has difficulty in metabolizing carbohydrates.

44. A patient with fever should force fluids and eat a ________________ diet to replenish the energy used by the increased metabolism.

45. The dietary treatment of gout is to place the patient on a ________________ diet.

46. The ________________ vitamins are especially important in the treatment of neuritis.

47. Osteoporosis is caused by lack of the mineral ____________.

48. Goiter is caused by a deficiency of ____________.

49. A ________________ diet is usually indicated for a patient with hyperemesis gravidarum.

50. Diarrhea in an infant is serious because it results in a loss of ________________ and ________________.

51. The banana diet is sometimes given to a child with ________________.

52. ________________ is excluded from the diet of an infant with galactosemia.

Circle the letter before the food that is most appropriate for the specified diet.

53. Light diet
    A. Baked potato   B. Fried potato

54. Full liquid diet
    A. Ice cream   B. Sponge cake

55. High-protein diet
    A. Tomatoes and macaroni   B. Macaroni with cheese

56. High-calorie diet
    A. Rice   B. Sweet potatoes

57. High-carbohydrate diet
    A. Egg omelet   B. Mashed potatoes

58. Sippy diet, second stage
    A. Pureed peas   B. Stewed tomatoes

59. Low-residue diet
    A. Farina   B. Whole-wheat bread

60. Kempner diet
A. Rice
B. Baked chicken

61. High-iron diet
A. Fried liver
B. Baked fish

62. Bland diet
A. Fried chicken breast
B. Roast chicken breast

63. Low-fat diet
A. Cheddar cheese
B. Cottage cheese

64. High-fiber diet
A. Guacamole salad
B. Celery and apple salad

65. Low-protein diet
A. Summer squash
B. Baked beans

66. Low-calorie diet
A. Condensed milk
B. Evaporated milk

67. Surgical liquid diet
A. Hot tea
B. Orange juice

68. Low-sodium diet
A. Crackers
B. Toast squares

69. Low-cholesterol diet
A. Deviled eggs
B. Sweet pickled peaches

70. Karell diet
A. Milk
B. Coffee

71. High-sodium diet
    A. Cole slaw   B. Sauerkraut

72. Low-purine diet
    A. Liver   B. Bananas

73. Alkaline-ash diet
    A. Roast with gravy   B. Green beans

74. High-calcium diet
    A. Cottage cheese   B. Liver

SECTION 3

APPENDIX

EXAMPLE OF A NUTRITIONAL CARE PLAN

CASE STUDY

Burton J., 24, was seen in the clinic with numbness and tingling of the lower extremities. Mr. J., an accountant, stated that the sensation had started several months previously and was occurring with increasing frequency. He found that exercise, such as tennis, which he plays once a month, was very fatiguing and caused him to pant for breath. He frequently has headaches that he attributes to looking at rows of figures all day. Mr. J. smokes two packs of cigarettes each day. He eats three hearty meals each day, preferring pork to beef. His breakfast consists of bacon, eggs, coffee, and biscuits with butter and jelly. He thinks he is allergic to oysters. Upon examination, Mr. J. appeared to be a normally developed, slightly obese male adult. He is six feet tall and weighs 221 pounds. Pulses could be detected in both feet but the left foot appears cold to the touch. When questioned, Mr. J. said he normally sat on a hard-back stool with his legs flexed while he worked. Mr. J.'s blood pressure was 140/92. Eye grounds showed some narrowing of blood vessels. CBC was normal but blood lipids and cholesterol were severely elevated. The diagnosis was hyperlipidemia and arteriosclerosis. Mr. J. was put on a low-fat, low-cholesterol, low-calorie diet and asked to return in two weeks for further testing.

NUTRITIONAL CARE PLAN

Patient: Burton J. *Sex:* M *Age:* 24 *Occupation:* Accountant

Diagnosis: Hyperlipidemia; arteriosclerosis

Nutritional History:

Diet Pattern: 3 hearty meals per day.
Caloric Intake: Excessive for energy output.
Foods Frequently Eaten: Pork, bacon, eggs, biscuits, butter, jelly, coffee.
Food Dislikes: None noted.
Food Allergies: Oysters, possibly

Dietary Prescription: Low-fat, low-cholesterol, low-calorie diet.

Foods To Be Included: Lean meat, egg white, and low-calorie, bulky fruits and vegetables low in fat.

Foods To Be Excluded: Sweets such as desserts, egg yolk, fat meats, sauces, gravies, cream, brains, kidneys, heart, butter, milk, and milk products.

Nutritional Problem	*Objective/ Evaluation*	*Rationale*	*Intervention*
1. Elevated blood lipids and cholesterol.	He will reduce these by choosing foods low in fat and cholesterol.	Dietary intake of fat and cholesterol increases the blood level.	Give him a diet to follow. On each visit find out which foods he is eating.
2. Obesity	He will reduce his caloric intake and will lose weight.	Regardless of cause of obesity, reduction in caloric intake is necessary for weight loss.	Give him a list of low-calorie foods. Help him plan a meal pattern, consistent with his life style, that will help him overcome objections to a lower caloric intake. Weigh him regularly and encourage exercise.

3. Lack of knowledge about diet.	He will demonstrate understanding of the diet by choosing the proper foods.	It is necessary for him to understand his diet and why he is on it.	Teach him to select foods and to prepare them. Explain role of fats and cholesterol in maintaining healthy blood vessels. Question him to see what he has learned at each visit.

DIABETIC FOOD EXCHANGE LIST*

GENERAL INFORMATION

Use a standard measuring cup or measuring spoons to measure the portion.

Vegetables are prepared without fat. (A fat exchange may be used in the preparation of food if allowed in the diet.)

Fruits are unsweetened if canned or frozen.

Meats are baked, broiled, or boiled unless a fat exchange is allowed.

Foods may not be thickened with flour or cornstarch unless a bread exchange is used.

Seasonings that do not contain sugar may be used as desired.

MILK EXCHANGE

Each serving contains 8 grams protein, trace of fat, 12 grams carbohydrate, and 80 calories. Milk contains saturated fat.

Nonfat fortified milk:

Skim or nonfat milk	1 cup
Powdered (nonfat dry, before adding liquid)	1/3 cup
Canned, evaporated skim milk	1/2 cup

*Adapted from Exchange Lists for Meal Planning, American Diabetic Association and American Dietetic Association, 1976.

Buttermilk, made from skim milk .... 1 cup
Yoghurt, made from skim milk (plain, unflavored) .... 1 cup

Low-fat fortified milk:

1 percent fat fortified milk (omit ½ fat exchange) .... 1 cup
2 percent fat fortified milk (omit 1 fat exchange) .... 1 cup
Yoghurt, made from 2 percent fortified milk (plain, unflavored) (omit 1 fat exchange) .... 1 cup

Whole milk (omit 2 fat exchanges):

Whole milk .... 1 cup
Canned, evaporated whole milk .... ½ cup
Buttermilk, made from whole milk .... 1 cup
Yoghurt, made from whole milk (plain, unflavored) .... 1 cup

VEGETABLE EXCHANGE

Each serving contains 2 grams protein, 5 grams carbohydrate, and 25 calories. All are nonfat. One exchange is ½ cup.

Asparagus
Bean sprouts
Beets
Broccoli
Brussels sprouts
Cabbage
Carrots
Cauliflower
Celery
Cucumber
Eggplant
Green pepper
Greens:
  Beet
  Chard
  Collards
  Dandelion
  Kale
Greens:
  Mustard
  Spinach
  Turnips
Mushrooms
Okra
Onions
Rhubarb
Rutabaga
Sauerkraut
String beans, green or yellow
Summer squash
Tomatoes
Tomato juice
Turnip
Vegetable juice cocktail
Zucchini

The following vegetables may be used ad lib when raw:

Chicory
Chinese cabbage
Endive
Escarole
Lettuce
Parsley
Radishes
Watercress

FRUIT EXCHANGE

Each serving contains 10 grams carbohydrate and 40 calories. All are nonfat.

Apple	1 small
Apple juice	1/3 cup
Applesauce (unsweetened)	1/2 cup
Apricots, fresh	2 medium
Apricots, dried	4 halves
Banana	1/2 small
Berries:	
Blackberries	1/2 cup
Blueberries	1/2 cup
Raspberries	1/2 cup
Strawberries	3/4 cup
Cherries	10 large
Cider	1/3 cup
Dates	2
Figs, fresh	1
Figs, dried	1
Grapefruit	1/2
Grapefruit juice	1/2 cup
Grapes	12
Grape juice	1/4 cup
Mango	1/2 small
Melons:	
Cantaloupe	1/4 small
Honeydew	1/8 medium
Watermelon	1 cup
Nectarine	1 small
Orange	1 small
Orange juice	1/2 cup
Papaya	3/4 cup
Peach	1 medium
Pear	1 small
Persimmon, common native	1 medium
Pineapple	1/2 cup
Pineapple juice	1/3 cup
Plums	2 medium
Prunes	2 medium
Prune juice	1/4 cup
Raisins	2 tablespoons
Tangerine	1 medium

BREAD EXCHANGE

Each serving contains 2 grams protein, 15 grams carbohydrate, and 70 calories. All foods are low-fat except those in the list of prepared foods.

Breads:

White (including French and Italian)	1 slice
Whole wheat	1 slice
Rye or pumpernickel	1 slice
Raisin	1 slice
Bagel, small	1/2
English muffin, small	1/2
Plain roll, bread	1
Frankfurter roll	1/2
Hamburger bun	1/2
Dried bread crumbs	3 tablespoons
Tortilla, 6″	1

Cereals:

Bran flakes	1/2 cup
Other ready-to-eat unsweetened cereals	3/4 cup
Puffed cereal (unfrosted)	1 cup
Cereals (cooked)	1/2 cup
Grits (cooked)	1/2 cup
Rice or barley (cooked)	1/2 cup
Pasta (cooked) (Spaghetti, noodle, and macaroni)	1/2 cup
Popcorn (popped, no fat added)	3 cups
Cornmeal, dry	2 tablespoons
Flour	2 1/2 tablespoons
Wheat germ	1/4 cup

Crackers:

Arrowroot	3
Graham, 2 1/2″ square	2
Matzo, 4″ × 6″	1/2
Oyster	20
Pretzels, 3 1/8″ long by 1/8″ diameter	25
Rye wafers, 2″ × 3 1/2″	3
Saltines	6
Soda, 2 1/2″ square	4

Dried beans, peas and lentils:

Beans, peas and lentils (dried and cooked)	1/2 cup
Baked beans, no pork (canned)	1/4 cup

Starchy vegetables:

Corn	1/3 cup
Corn on the cob	1 small

Lima beans .... ½ cup
Parsnips .... ⅔ cup
Peas, green (canned or frozen) .... ½ cup
Potato, white .... 1 small
mashed .... ½ cup
Pumpkin .... ¾ cup
Winter squash, acorn or butternut .... ½ cup
Yam or sweet potato .... ¼ cup

Prepared foods:

Biscuit, 2″ diameter (omit 1 fat exchange) 1
Cornbread, 2″ × 2″ × 1″ (omit 1 fat exchange) 1
Corn muffin, 2″ diameter (omit 1 fat exchange) 1
Crackers, round butter type (omit 1 fat exchange) 5
Muffin, plain, small (omit 1 fat exchange) 1
Potatoes, french fried, 2″ to 3½″ (omit 1 fat exchange) 8
Potato or corn chips (omit 2 fat exchanges) 15
Pancake, 5″ × ½″ (omit 1 fat exchange) 1
Waffle, 5″ × ½″ (omit 1 fat exchange) 1

MEAT EXCHANGE

Each serving contains 7 grams protein, 3 grams fat, and 55 calories.

Lean meat (All on this list are low in saturated fats.)

Beef: Baby beef (very lean), chipped beef, chuck, flank steak, tenderloin, plate ribs, plate skirt steak, round (bottom, top), all cuts of rump, spare ribs, tripe .... 1 oz.
Lamb: Leg, rib, sirloin, loin (roasts and chops), shank, shoulder .... 1 oz.
Pork: Leg, whole rump, center, shank, ham, smoked (center slices) .... 1 oz.
Veal: Leg, loin, rib, shank, shoulder, cutlets .... 1 oz.
Poultry: Meat without skin of chicken, turkey, cornish hen, guinea hen, pheasant .... 1 oz.
Fish
Any fresh or frozen .... 1 oz.
Canned salmon, tuna, mackerel, crab, or lobster .... ¼ cup
Clams, oysters, scallops, shrimp .... 5 or 1 oz.
Sardines (drained) 3
Cheeses containing less than 5 percent butterfat .... 1 oz.
Cottage cheese, dry and 2 percent butterfat .... ¼ cup
Dried beans and peas (omit 1 bread exchange) .... ½ cup

Medium-fat meat (For each exchange omit 1/2 fat exchange. Peanut butter is the only food in this list low in saturated fats.)

- Beef: Ground (15 percent fat), corned beef (canned), rib eye, round (ground commercial) .... 1 oz.
- Pork: Loin (all cuts tenderloin), shoulder arm (picnic), shoulder blade, Boston butt, Canadian bacon, boiled ham .... 1 oz.
- Liver, heart, kidneys, sweetbreads (these are high in cholesterol) .... 1 oz.
- Cottage cheese, creamed .... 1/4 cup
- Cheese, mozzarella, ricotta, farmer's cheese, neufchatel, parmesan .... 3 tablespoons
- Egg (high in cholesterol) 1
- Peanut butter (omit 2 additional fat exchanges) .... 2 tablespoons

High-fat meat (For each exchange omit 1 fat exchange. No foods on this list are low in saturated fats.)

- Beef: Brisket, corned beef (brisket), ground beef (more than 20 percent fat), hamburger (commercial), chuck (ground commercial), roasts (ribs), steaks (club and rib) .... 1 oz.
- Lamb: Breast .... 1 oz.
- Pork: Spare ribs, loin (back ribs), pork (ground), country style ham, deviled ham .... 1 oz.
- Veal: Breast .... 1 oz.
- Poultry: Capon, duck (domestic), goose .... 1 oz.
- Cheese: Cheddar types .... 1 oz.
- Cold cuts .... 4 1/2″ × 1/8″
- Frankfurter .... 1 small

FAT EXCHANGE

Each serving contains 5 grams fat and 45 calories.

Low in saturated fats:

- Margarine, soft, tub or stick .... 1 teaspoon
- Avocado (4″ diameter) 1/8
- Oil: Corn, cottonseed, safflower, soy, sunflower .... 1 teaspoon
- Oil, olive .... 1 teaspoon
- Oil, peanut .... 1 teaspoon
- Olives .... 5 small
- Almonds .... 10 whole
- Pecans .... 2 large, whole
- Peanuts:
  - Spanish .... 20 whole
  - Virginia .... 10 whole

Walnuts	6 small
Nuts, others	6 small
Saturated fats:	
Margarine, regular, stick	1 teaspoon
Butter	1 teaspoon
Bacon fat	1 teaspoon
Bacon, crisp	1 strip
Cream, light	2 tablespoons
Cream, sour	2 tablespoons
Cream, heavy	1 tablespoon
Cream cheese	1 tablespoon
French dressing	1 tablespoon
Italian dressing	1 tablespoon
Lard	1 teaspoon
Mayonnaise	1 teaspoon
Salad dressing, mayonnaise-type	2 teaspoons
Salt pork	3/4″ cube

FOODS ALLOWED AS DESIRED

Coffee
Tea
Clear broth
Bouillon, without fat
Gelatin, unsweetened
Rennet tablets
Celery seasoning
Cinnamon
Cranberries, without sugar
Garlic
Lemon
Mint
Mustard
Nutmeg
Onion seasoning
Parsley seasoning
Pepper, black or red
Noncaloric sweeteners
Vinegar
Pickles (sour or unsweetened dill)

FOOD VALUES*

In the following table, percentage of water and the grams of protein, fat, and carbohydrate are shown in the nearest whole numbers. Where protein, fat, or carbohydrate content is less than one gram, the nearest tenth of a gram is given.

Dashes (—) indicate that the nutrient is probably present but the exact amount is not known, or one or more factors cause the amount to vary.

Traces (Tr) indicate that the amount of nutrient present in less than 0.01 of the unit of measure used on that nutrient.

Few canned and pre-prepared foods are listed as the nutrition labels required by law on these foods give the necessary information on most of the nutrients included in this table.

---

*Adapted from *Nutritive Value of American Foods in Common Units.* US Department of Agriculture, Agriculture Handbook No. 456, US Government Printing Office, Washington, DC, November, 1975.

FOOD VALUES—EDIBLE PARTS*

FOODS - Edible portions unless otherwise indicated	*Household Measure*	*Weight, g*	*Water, %*	*Energy, Calories*	*Protein, g*	*Fat, g*	*Carbohydrate, g*	*Calcium, mg*	*Phosphorus, mg*	*Iron, mg*	*Sodium, mg*	*Potassium, mg*	*Vitamin A, IU*	*Thiamin, mg*	*Riboflavin, mg*	*Niacin, mg*	*Ascorbic Acid, mg*
Apple, raw, fruit with skin, quarters or finely chopped pieces	1 cup	125	84	73	0.3	0.8	18	9	13	0.4	1	138	110	0.04	0.03	0.1	5
Apple brown betty	1 cup	215	65	325	3	8	64	39	47	1.3	329	215	220	0.13	0.09	0.9	2
Apple juice	1 cup	248	88	117	0.2	Tr	30	15	22	1.5	2	250	—	0.02	0.05	0.2	2
Applesauce	1 cup	244	89	100	0.5	0.5	26	10	12	1.2	5	190	100	0.05	0.02	0.1	2
Apricot, canned, solid and liquid, water packed without artificial sweetener, halved	1 cup	246	89	93	2	0.2	24	30	39	0.7	2	605	4500	0.05	0.05	1	10
Apricot nectar, canned or bottled, approximately 40% fruit	1 cup	251	85	143	0.8	0.3	37	23	30	0.5	Tr	379	2380	0.03	0.03	0.5	8
Asparagus, drained solid, cut spears	1 cup	235	93	49	6	1	8	45	125	5	555	390	1880	0.14	0.24	2	35
Avocado, raw, cubed	1 cup	150	74	251	3	25	10	15	63	0.9	6	906	440	0.17	0.30	2.4	21
Bacon, cooked, broiled or fried, drained, sliced	2 slices	15	8	86	4	8	0.5	2	34	0.6	153	35	0	0.08	0.05	0.8	—
Bacon, Canadian style, broiled or fried, sliced	1 slice	21	50	58	6.7	4	0.1	3	46	0.9	537	91	0	0.19	0.04	1.1	—
Banana, raw, sliced	1 cup	150	76	128	2	0.3	33	12	39	1.1	2	555	290	0.08	0.09	1.1	15
Beans, mature seeds, dry, white, cooked, drained, navy, pea	1 cup	190	69	224	15	1	40	95	281	5.1	13	790	0	0.27	0.13	1.3	0
Beans, canned, solid and liquid, with pork and tomato sauce	1 cup	255	71	311	16	7	49	138	235	4.6	1181	536	330	0.20	0.08	1.5	5
Beans, red kidney, cooked, drained	1 cup	185	69	218	14	1	40	70	259	4.4	6	629	10	0.20	0.11	1.3	—

Beans, lima, cooked, drained	1 cup	170	71	189	13	1	34	80	206	4.3	2	717	480	0.31	0.17	2.2	29
Beans, snap, green, cooked, drained	1 cup	125	92	31	2	0.3	7	63	46	0.8	5	189	680	0.09	0.11	0.6	15
Beef, boneless, for stew, lean with fat, cooked, drained	1 cup	140	49	458	36	36	0	15	196	4.6	64	291	60	0.07	0.28	5.6	—
Beef, chuck rib roast or steaks, choice grade, lean with fat, cooked, chopped	1 cup	140	40	598	31	51	0	14	154	4.1	55	251	100	0.06	0.24	4.9	—
Beef, chuck rib roast or steaks, choice grade, lean with fat, cooked, ground	1 cup	110	40	470	25	40	0	11	121	3.2	43	197	80	0.05	0.19	3.9	—
Beef, chuck roast, choice grade, lean with fat, cooked, drained, chopped	1 cup	140	53	405	388	27	0	17	188	4.8	66	303	50	0.07	0.29	5.9	—
Beef, flank steak, choice grade, cooked, drained, 2 1/2″ × 2 1/2″ × 3/4″	1 piece	85	61	167	26	6	0	12	128	3.2	45	207	10	0.05	0.20	3.9	—
Beef, T-bone steak, choice grade, cooked, broiled, lean with fat	1 lb	454	36	2146	89	196	0	36	753	11.8	217	991	340	0.25	0.73	18.6	—
Beef, round steak, choice grade, cooked, broiled, lean with fat, 4 1/8″ × 2 1/4″ × 1/2″	1 piece	85	55	222	24	13	0	10	213	3	60	272	20	0.07	0.19	4.8	—
Beef, rump roast, choice grade, lean with fat, cooked, chopped	1 cup	140	48	486	33	38	0	14	276	4.3	81	370	70	0.09	0.25	6	—
Beef, ground, lean, cooked, pattie, approximately 3″ diameter, 5/8″ thick, 10% fat	1 pattie	85	60	186	23	10	0	10	196	3	57	261	20	0.08	0.20	5.1	—
Beef, ground lean, cooked, pattie, approximately 3″ diameter, 5/8″ thick, 21% fat	1 pattie	82	54	235	20	17	0	9	159	2.6	49	221	30	0.07	0.17	4.4	—

FOOD VALUES—EDIBLE PARTS—*Continued*

FOODS - Edible portions unless otherwise indicated	*Household Measure*	*Weight, g*	*Water, %*	*Energy, Calories*	*Protein, g*	*Fat, g*	*Carbohydrate, g*	*Calcium, mg*	*Phosphorus, mg*	*Iron, mg*	*Sodium, mg*	*Potassium, mg*	*Vitamin A, IU*	*Thiamin, mg*	*Riboflavin, mg*	*Niacin, mg*	*Ascorbic Acid, mg*
Beef, corned, boneless, cooked	1 lb	454	44	1687	104	138	0	41	422	13.2	4277	272	—	0.09	0.82	6.8	0
Beef, dried, chipped, cooked, creamed	1 cup	245	72	377	20	25	17	257	343	2	1754	375	880	0.15	0.47	1.5	1
Beets, red, cooked, drained, peeled, diced	1 cup	170	91	54	2	0.2	12	24	39	0.9	73	354	30	0.05	0.07	0.5	10
Beverages																	
Alcohol																	
Beer (4.5% alcohol by volume, 3.6% by weight), can or bottle, 12 fl oz	1 container	360	92	151	1	0	14	18	108	Tr	25	90	—	0.01	0.11	2.2	—
Gin, rum, vodka, whiskey, 86 proof (36% alcohol by weight), jigger (1½ fl oz)	1 jigger	42	64	105	—	—	Tr	—	—	—	Tr	1	—	—	—	—	—
Wine, table (12.2% alcohol by volume, 9.9% by weight), wine glass (serving portion 3½ fl oz, or 103 ml)	1 glass	102	86	87	0.1	0	4.3	9	10	0.4	5	94	—	Tr	0.01	0.1	—
Carbonated, non-alcoholic																	
Cola type, bottle or can, 12 fl oz	1 container	369	90	144	0	0	37	—	—	—	—	—	0	0	0	0	0
Fruit flavors (citrus, cherry, grape, strawberry, Tom Collins mixer, others)	1 container	372	88	171	0	0	45	—	—	—	—	—	0	0	0	0	0

(10–13% sugar) bottle or can, 12 fl oz																	
Root beer, bottle or can, 12 fl oz	1 container	370	90	152	0	0	39	—	—	—	—	—	0	0	0	0	0
Special dietary drinks with artificial sweetener (less than 1 cal per oz), bottle or can, 12 fl oz	1 container	355	100	—	0	0	—	—	—	—	—	—	0	0	0	0	0
Biscuits, baking powder, baked from home recipe, made with enriched flour, biscuit 2″ diameter, 1¼″ high	1 biscuit	28	27	103	2	5	13	34	49	0.4	175	33	Tr	0.06	0.06	0.5	Tr
Blackberries, including dewberries, boysenberries, youngberries, raw	1 cup	144	85	84	2	1	19	46	27	1.3	1	245	290	0.04	0.06	0.6	80
Blueberries, raw, cup	1 cup	145	83	90	1	0.7	22	22	19	1.5	1	117	150	0.04	0.09	0.7	20
Boston brown bread, canned, piece 3¼″ diameter ½″ thick	1 piece	45	45	95	3	0.6	21	41	72	0.9	113	131	0	0.05	0.03	0.5	0
Bouillon, cubes, instant, cube size approximately ½″	1 cube	4	4	5	0.8	0.1	0.2	—	—	—	960	4	—	—	—	—	—
Bran flakes, (40% bran), added sugar, salt, iron, vitamins	1 cup	35	3	106	4	0.6	28	19	125	12.4	207	137	1650	0.41	0.49	4.1	12
Bran flakes with raisins, added sugar, salt, iron, vitamins	1 cup	50	7	144	4	0.7	40	28	146	17.7	212	154	2350	0.58	0.71	5.8	18
Brazil nuts, shelled, cup, approximately 32 large kernels	1 cup	140	5	916	20	94	15	260	970	4.8	1	1001	Tr	1.34	0.17	2.2	—
Breads																	
French, bread and rolls, enriched, piece, 5″ × 2½″ × 1″	1 slice	35	31	102	3	1	19	15	30	0.8	203	32	Tr	0.10	0.08	0.9	Tr
Vienna, bread, enriched, piece, 4¾″ × 4″ × ½″	1 slice	25	31	73	2	0.8	14	11	21	0.6	145	23	Tr	0.07	0.06	0.6	Tr

FOOD VALUES—EDIBLE PARTS—*Continued*

FOODS - Edible portions unless otherwise indicated	*Household Measure*	*Weight, g*	*Water, %*	*Energy, Calories*	*Protein, g*	*Fat, g*	*Carbohydrate, g*	*Calcium, mg*	*Phosphorus, mg*	*Iron, mg*	*Sodium, mg*	*Potassium, mg*	*Vitamin A, IU*	*Thiamin, mg*	*Riboflavin, mg*	*Niacin, mg*	*Ascorbic Acid, mg*
Roll, hoagie or submarine, 11½″ × 3″ × 2½″	1 roll	135	31	392	12	4	75	58	115	3	783	122	Tr	0.38	0.30	3.4	Tr
Italian, enriched, slice 3¼″ × 2½″ × ½″	1 slice	10	32	28	1	0.1	7	2	8	0.2	59	7	0	0.03	0.02	0.3	0
Raisin, slice, 3¾″ × 3⅝″ × ½″	1 slice	25	35	66	2	0.7	13	18	22	0.3	91	58	Tr	0.01	0.02	0.2	Tr
Rye, American (⅔ wheat flour, ⅓ rye flour) fresh slice, 4¾″ × 3¾″ × 7/16″	1 slice	25	36	61	2	0.3	13	19	37	0.4	139	36	0	0.05	0.02	0.4	0
Pumpernickel, regular size slice, 5″ × 4″ × ⅜″	1 slice	32	34	79	3	0.4	17	27	73	0.8	182	145	0	0.07	0.04	0.4	0
White, enriched, fresh, slice																	
Regular, 4⅜″ × 4″ × 9/16″	1 slice	28	36	76	2	0.9	14	24	27	0.7	142	29	Tr	0.07	0.06	0.7	Tr
Thin, 4″ × 3⅞″ × ½″	1 slice	24	36	65	2	0.8	12	20	23	0.6	122	25	Tr	0.06	0.05	0.6	Tr
Bread crumbs	1 cup	45	36	122	4	1	23	38	44	1.1	228	47	Tr	0.11	0.09	1.1	Tr
Whole wheat, firm crumb type, fresh, slice, rounded top 4″ × 4″ × 7/16″	1 slice	25	36	61	3	0.8	12	25	57	0.8	132	68	Tr	0.06	0.03	0.7	Tr
Broccoli, stalks (head and bud clusters, stem and leaves), cooked, drained, cut into ½″ pieces	1 cup	155	91	40	5	0.5	7	136	96	1.2	16	414	3180	0.14	0.31	1.2	140

Brussels sprouts, cooked, drained	1 cup, 7–8 sprouts	155	88	56	7	0.6	10	50	112	1.7	16	423	810	0.12	0.22	1.2	135
Butter																	
Regular, 4 sticks per pound, pat 1″ sq. × 1/3″	1 pat	5	16	36	Tr	4	Tr	1	1	0	49	1	170	—	—	—	0
Whipped, 6 sticks or 2 8 oz containers	1 cup, 2 sticks	151	16	1081	2	122	0.6	30	24	0	1490	35	5000	—	—	—	0
Buttermilk, cultured	1 cup	245	91	88	9	0.2	13	296	233	0.1	319	343	10	0.10	0.44	0.2	2
Cabbage, common varieties, raw, shredded coarsely or sliced	1 cup	70	92	17	0.9	0.1	4	34	20	0.3	14	163	90	0.04	0.04	0.2	33
Cakes																	
Angel food, tube cake, piece 2 1/2″ arc	1 piece	60	32	161	4	1	36	5	13	0.1	170	53	0	0.01	0.08	0.1	0
Boston cream pie, piece 3 1/8″ arc	1 piece	103	35	311	5	10	51	69	104	0.5	192	92	220	0.03	0.11	0.2	Tr
Chocolate, without icing, 2″ × 2″ × 2″	1 piece	39	25	143	2	7	21	29	53	0.4	115	55	60	0.01	0.04	0.1	Tr
Chocolate, with chocolate icing, 2 3/8″ arc, 2 layers	1 piece	99	22	365	5	16	55	69	130	1	233	152	160	0.02	0.10	0.2	Tr
Fruit cake, dark, loaf, slice, 1/4″ × 2″ × 1 1/2″	1 slice	15	18	57	0.7	2	9	11	17	0.4	24	74	20	0.02	0.02	0.1	Tr
Gingerbread, piece 3″ × 3″ × 2″	1 piece	117	31	371	5	13	61	80	76	2.7	277	531	110	0.14	0.13	1.1	0
Plain cake, without icing, piece 3″ × 3″ × 2″	1 piece	86	25	313	4	12	48	55	88	0.3	258	68	150	0.02	0.08	0.2	Tr
Plain cake, with boiled white icing, piece 3″ × 3″ × 2″	1 piece	114	23	401	4	12	71	56	88	0.3	299	73	150	0.02	0.08	0.2	Tr
Pound cake, old fashioned, slice 3 1/2″ × 3″ × 1/2″	1 slice	30	17	142	2	9	14	6	24	0.2	33	18	80	0.01	0.03	0.1	0
Candy																	
Butterscotch	1 oz	28	2	113	Tr	1	27	5	2	0.4	19	1	40	0	Tr	Tr	0
Caramel, plain or chocolate	1 oz	28	8	113	1	3	22	42	35	0.4	64	54	Tr	0.01	0.05	0.1	Tr
Fudge, chocolate	1 oz	28	6	122	1	5	21	29	31	0.4	65	55	Tr	0.01	0.04	0.1	0

FOOD VALUES—EDIBLE PARTS—*Continued*

FOODS - Edible portions unless otherwise indicated	*Household Measure*	*Weight, g*	*Water, %*	*Energy, Calories*	*Protein, g*	*Fat, g*	*Carbohydrate, g*	*Calcium, mg*	*Phosphorus, mg*	*Iron, mg*	*Sodium, mg*	*Potassium, mg*	*Vitamin A, IU*	*Thiamin, mg*	*Riboflavin, mg*	*Niacin, mg*	*Ascorbic Acid, mg*
Mints, round, miniature, 3/4″ × 3/8″	1	2	6	10	Tr	0.3	2	1	1	Tr	4	2	Tr	Tr	Tr	Tr	Tr
Jelly beans, approximately 10 to an oz	1 oz	28	6	104	Tr	0.1	26	3	1	0.3	3	Tr	0	0	Tr	Tr	0
Carrots, raw, grated or shredded	1 cup	110	88	46	1	0.2	11	41	40	0.8	52	375	12100	0.07	0.06	0.7	9
Carrots, cooked, drained, sliced	1 cup	155	91	48	1	0.3	11	51	48	0.9	51	344	16280	0.08	0.08	0.8	9
Cauliflower, raw, chopped	1 cup	115	91	31	3	0.2	6	29	64	1.3	15	339	70	0.13	0.12	0.8	90
Cauliflower, cooked, drained	1 cup	125	93	28	3	0.3	5	26	53	0.9	11	258	80	0.11	0.10	0.8	69
Celery, raw, stalk, chopped	1 cup	120	94	20	1	0.1	5	47	34	0.4	151	409	320	0.04	0.04	0.4	11
Cheeses																	
Blue or Roquefort type, not packed	1 cup	135	40	497	29	41	3	425	458	0.7	—	—	1670	0.04	0.82	1.6	0
Cheddar, prepackaged, slice, 2 5/8″ diameter, 1/4″ thick, 1/14th of a piece	1 slice	24	37	96	6	8	0.5	180	115	0.2	168	20	310	0.01	0.11	Tr	0
Cottage cheese, small curds	1 cup	210	78	223	29	9	6	197	319	0.6	481	179	360	0.06	0.53	0.2	0
Cream cheese, regular	1 T	14	51	52	1	5	0.3	9	13	Tr	35	10	220	Tr	0.03	Tr	0
Parmesan, grated	1 T	5	17	23	2	2	0.2	68	46	Tr	44	9	60	Tr	0.04	Tr	0
Swiss, domestic, slice 2″ × 2″ × 1/4″, 1/24th of a piece	1 slice	14	39	52	4	4	0.2	130	79	0.1	99	15	160	Tr	0.06	Tr	0

Pasteurized process, American, slice 2¾″ × 2¼″ × ¼″	1 slice	27	40	100	6	8	0.5	188	208	0.2	307	22	330	0.01	0.11	Tr	0
Cherries, raw, without pits and stems	1 cup	155	84	90	2	0.5	22	34	29	0.6	3	296	1550	0.08	0.09	0.6	16
Chewing gum, candy-coated, ¾″ × ½″ × ¼″	1 piece	2	4	5	—	—	2	—	—	—	—	—	—	0	0	0	0
Chicken																	
All classes, roasted																	
Light meat without skin, chopped	1 cup	140	64	232	44	5	0	15	371	1.8	90	575	80	0.06	0.14	16.2	—
Dark meat without skin, chopped	1 cup	140	64	246	39	9	0	18	321	2.4	120	449	210	0.10	0.32	7.8	—
Fryers, cut-up parts from 2½ pound ready-to-cook fryer																	
Breast without ribs, piece, half breast	1 piece	94	58	160	26	5	1	9	218	1.3	—	—	70	0.04	0.17	11.6	—
Drumstick	1 piece	56	55	88	12	4	0.4	6	89	0.9	—	—	50	0.03	0.15	2.7	—
Thigh	1 piece	65	56	122	15	6	1	7	121	1.2	—	—	100	0.03	0.25	3.5	—
Chicken a la king, made from home recipe	1 cup	245	68	468	27	34	12	127	358	2.5	760	404	1130	0.10	0.42	5.4	12
Clams, raw, meat only, 4 cherrystones, or 5 little necks	4–5 clams	70	80	56	8	0.6	4	48	106	5.3	144	218	—	—	—	—	—
Clams, canned, drained solids	1 cup	160	77	157	25	4	3	—	—	—	—	—	—	—	—	—	—
Cocoa powder with nonfat dry milk	1 oz	28	2	102	5	0.8	20	167	155	0.5	149	227	10	0.04	0.21	0.2	1
Coconut meat, fresh, 2″ × 2″ × ½″	1 piece	45	51	156	2	16	4	6	43	0.8	10	115	0	0.02	0.01	0.2	1
Cod, cooked, broiled with butter or margarine, fillet 5″ × 2½″ × ⅞″	1	65	65	111	19	3	0	20	178	0.7	72	265	120	0.05	0.07	2	—
Coffee, instant, dry powder, regular	1 tsp	0.8	3	1	Tr	Tr	0.3	1	3	Tr	1	26	0	0	Tr	0.2	0
Coleslaw, made with salad dressing	1 cup	120	83	119	1	10	9	52	34	0.5	149	230	180	0.06	0.06	0.4	35

FOOD VALUES—EDIBLE PARTS—*Continued*

FOODS - Edible portions unless otherwise indicated	*Household Measure*	*Weight, g*	*Water, %*	*Energy, Calories*	*Protein, g*	*Fat, g*	*Carbohydrate, g*	*Calcium, mg*	*Phosphorus, mg*	*Iron, mg*	*Sodium, mg*	*Potassium, mg*	*Vitamin A, IU*	*Thiamin, mg*	*Riboflavin, mg*	*Niacin, mg*	*Ascorbic Acid, mg*
Collards, cooked, leaves without stems, small amount of water	1 cup	190	90	63	7	1	10	357	99	1.5	—	498	14820	0.21	0.38	2.3	144
Cookies, prepared and baked from mixes																	
Brownies, with enriched flour, made with incomplete mix, eggs, water, nuts, 1¾″ × 1¾″ × ⅞″	1 piece	20	11	86	1	4	13	9	27	0.4	33	34	20	0.03	0.02	0.1	Tr
Cookies, commercial																	
Butter, thin, rich, 2⅛″ diameter × ¼″	10 cookies	50	5	229	3	9	36	63	47	0.3	209	30	330	0.02	0.03	0.2	0
Chocolate chip, 2¼″ diameter, ⅜″ thick	10 cookies	105	3	495	6	22	73	41	120	1.9	421	141	130	0.04	0.07	0.4	Tr
Coconut bar, 2⅜″ × 1⅝″ × ⅜″	10 cookies	90	4	445	6	22	58	65	108	1.3	133	205	140	0.04	0.05	0.4	0
Fig bar, 1⅝″ × 1⅝″ × ⅜″	4 cookies	56	14	200	2	3	42	44	34	0.6	141	111	60	0.02	0.04	0.2	Tr
Gingersnap, 2″ diameter, ¼″ thick	10 cookies	70	3	294	4	6	56	51	33	1.6	400	323	50	0.03	0.04	0.3	Tr
Sugar wafer type, 1¾″ × 1⅜″ × ⅜″	10 cookies	70	2	331	7	13	47	29	81	0.6	121	123	140	0.05	0.06	2.0	Tr
Vanilla wafer, 1¾″ diameter × ¼″	10 cookies	40	3	185	2	6	30	16	25	0.2	101	29	50	0.01	0.03	0.1	0
Corn, sweet, cooked, kernels	1 cup	165	77	137	5	2	31	5	147	1.0	Tr	272	660	0.18	0.17	2.1	12
Corn, canned, regular pack, creamed style, white and yellow, solid and liquid	1 cup	256	76	210	5	2	51	8	143	1.5	604	248	840	0.08	0.13	2.6	13

Corn, whole kernel, vacuum packed, yellow	1 cup	210	76	174	5	1	43	6	153	1.1	496	204	740	0.06	0.13	2.3	11
Corn fritter, 2″ diameter × 1½″ thick	1 fritter	35	29	132	3	8	14	22	54	0.6	167	47	140	0.06	0.07	0.6	1
Corn, grits, degermed, cooked	1 cup	245	87	125	3	0.2	27	2	25	0.7	502	27	150	0.10	0.07	1.0	0
Corn flakes, plain, added sugar, salt, iron, vitamins	1 cup	25	4	97	2	0.1	21	Tr	9	0.6	251	30	1180	0.29	0.35	2.9	9
Cornbread, southern style, made with whole ground cornmeal, cube (1 cu inch)	1 cube	8	54	17	0.6	0.6	2	10	18	0.1	52	13	10	0.01	0.02	Tr	Tr
Cow peas, including black-eyed peas, immature seeds, cooked, drained	1 cup	165	72	178	14	1	30	40	241	3.5	2	625	580	0.50	0.18	2.3	28
Crab, cooked, flaked	1 cup	125	79	116	22	2	0.6	54	219	1.0	—	—	2710	0.20	0.10	3.5	2
Crab, deviled	1 cup	240	63	451	27	22	32	113	329	2.9	2081	398	—	0.19	0.26	3.6	14
Crackers																	
Graham, chocolate coated, 2½″ × 2″ × ¼″	1 cracker	13	2	62	0.7	3	9	15	27	0.3	53	42	10	0.01	0.04	0.2	0
Plain, 2 squares, 2½″	2 squares	14	6	55	1	1	10	6	21	0.2	95	55	0	0.01	0.03	0.2	0
Saltines, 1⅞″ square, ⅛″ thick	10 crackers	28	4	123	3	3	20	6	26	0.3	312	34	0	Tr	0.01	0.3	0
Soda, regular, 1⅞″, ⅛″ thick	10 crackers	28	4	125	3	4	20	6	25	0.4	312	34	0	Tr	0.01	0.3	0
Cranberries, raw, whole	1 cup	95	88	44	0.4	0.7	10	13	10	0.5	2	78	40	0.03	0.02	0.1	10
Cranberry juice cocktail	1 cup	253	83	164	0.3	0.3	42	13	8	0.8	3	25	Tr	0.03	0.03	0.1	40
Cranberry sauce, sweetened with nutritive sweetener, home prepared, unstrained	1 cup	277	54	493	0.6	0.8	126	19	14	0.6	3	105	60	0.03	0.03	0.3	6
Cream, fluid																	
Half-and-half (cream and milk, 11.7% fat)	1 T	15	80	20	0.5	2	0.7	16	13	Tr	7	19	70	Tr	0.02	Tr	Tr
Light coffee or table (20.6% fat)	1 T	15	72	32	0.5	3	0.6	15	12	Tr	6	18	130	Tr	0.02	Tr	Tr
Light whipping (31.3% fat)	1 T	15	62	45	0.4	5	0.5	13	10	Tr	5	15	190	Tr	0.02	Tr	Tr
Heavy whipping (37.6% fat)	1 T	15	57	53	0.3	6	0.5	11	9	Tr	5	13	230	Tr	0.02	Tr	Tr

FOOD VALUES—EDIBLE PARTS—*Continued*

FOODS - Edible portions unless otherwise indicated	*Household Measure*	*Weight, g*	*Water, %*	*Energy, Calories*	*Protein, g*	*Fat, g*	*Carbohydrate, g*	*Calcium, mg*	*Phosphorus, mg*	*Iron, mg*	*Sodium, mg*	*Potassium, mg*	*Vitamin A, IU*	*Thiamin, mg*	*Riboflavin, mg*	*Niacin, mg*	*Ascorbic Acid, mg*
Cream puff, with custard filling, 3½″ diameter, 2″ high	1 puff	130	58	303	9	18	27	105	148	0.9	108	157	460	0.05	0.22	0.1	Tr
Cucumber, raw, sliced, ⅛″ thick	1 cup	105	95	16	0.9	0.1	4	26	28	1.2	6	168	260	0.03	0.04	0.2	12
Custard, baked	1 cup	265	77	305	14	15	29	297	310	1.1	209	387	930	0.11	0.50	0.3	1
Dandelion greens, cooked, drained	1 cup	105	90	35	2	0.6	7	147	44	1.9	46	244	12290	0.14	0.17	—	19
Dates without pits	10 dates	80	23	219	2	0.4	58	47	50	2.4	1	518	40	0.07	0.08	1.8	0
Doughnuts, cake type, plain, 3¼″ diameter, 1″ high, weight 1½ oz	1 each	42	24	164	2	8	22	17	80	0.6	210	38	30	0.07	0.07	0.5	Tr
Eclairs, with custard filling and chocolate icing, 5″ long, 2″ wide and 1¾″ high	1 each	100	56	239	6	14	23	80	112	0.7	82	122	340	0.04	0.16	0.1	Tr
Eggs																	
Chicken																	
Whole, fresh, large, 24 oz per dozen	1 egg	57	74	82	7	6	0.5	27	103	1.2	61	65	590	0.05	0.15	Tr	0
Whites, fresh	1 cup	243	88	124	27	0.1	2	22	36	0.2	355	338	0	0.01	0.66	0.2	0
Yolks, fresh	1 cup	243	51	846	39	74	2	343	1383	13.4	126	238	8260	0.54	1.07	0.1	0
Fried, large egg	1 egg	46	68	99	6	10	0.1	28	102	1.1	155	64	650	0.05	0.14	Tr	0
Duck, whole fresh	1 egg	80	70	134	9	10	0.5	39	137	2.0	86	91	870	0.13	0.21	0.1	0
Eggplant, cooked, diced	1 cup	200	94	38	2	0.4	8	22	42	1.2	2	300	20	0.10	0.08	1.1	6
Endive, raw	1 cup	50	93	10	0.9	0.1	2	41	27	0.9	7	147	1650	0.04	0.07	0.3	5
Farina, cooked	1 cup	245	90	103	3	0.2	21	10	29	Tr	353	22	0	0.10	0.07	1.0	0
Fats, cooking (vegetable fat, mixed fat, shortening)	1 T	13	0	111	0	13	0	0	0	0	0	0	—	0	0	0	0

Figs, raw, whole, medium	1 fig	50	77	40	0.6	0.2	10	18	11	0.3	1	97	40	0.03	0.03	0.2	1
Filberts or hazelnuts, shelled, chopped	1 cup	115	6	729	15	72	19	240	388	3.9	2	810	—	0.53	—	1.0	Tr
Fishcakes, fried, 3″ diameter, 5/8″ thick	1 cake	60	66	103	9	5	6	—	—	—	—	—	—	—	—	—	—
Fish sticks, breaded, cooked, 4″ × 1″ × 1/2″	1 stick	28	66	50	5	3	2	3	47	0.1	—	—	0	0.01	0.02	0.5	—
Flounder, baked with butter or margarine, fillet, 6″ long, 2 1/2″ wide, 1/4″ thick	1 fillet	57	58	115	17	5	0	13	196	0.8	135	335	—	0.04	0.05	1.4	1
Fruit cocktail, syrup pack, heavy	1 cup	255	80	194	1	0.3	50	23	31	1.0	13	411	360	0.05	0.03	1.0	5
Gizzards																	
Chicken, cooked, chopped, diced	1 cup	145	68	215	39	5	1	13	103	4.5	83	306	—	0.03	0.30	7.4	—
Turkey, cooked, chopped, diced	1 cup	145	63	284	39	13	2	—	—	—	74	216	—	0.04	0.20	8.4	—
Goose, cooked, flesh only, 3 1/2″ long, 3″ wide × 1/4″ thick	2 1/2 pieces	85	55	198	29	8	0	12	235	1.4	105	514	—	0.09	0.14	7.9	—
Grapefruit, pink, red, or white, half	1/2	184	88	40	0.5	0.1	10	16	16	0.4	1	132	80	0.04	0.02	0.2	37
Grapefruit juice, red, pink, or white	1 cup	246	90	96	1	0.2	23	22	37	0.5	2	399	200	0.10	0.05	0.5	93
Grapes, raw, American type	1 cup	153	82	70	1	1	16	16	12	0.4	3	160	100	0.05	0.03	0.3	4
Grape juice, canned or bottled	1 cup	253	83	167	0.5	Tr	42	28	30	0.8	5	293	—	0.10	0.05	0.5	Tr
Haddock, fried, fillet, 6 3/8″ long, 2 1/2″ wide, 5/8″ thick	1 fillet	110	66	182	22	7	6	44	272	1.3	193	383	—	0.04	0.08	3.5	2
Halibut, broiled, with butter or margarine, fillet, 6 1/2″ long, 2″ wide, 5/8″ thick	1 fillet	125	67	214	12	9	0	20	310	1.0	168	656	850	0.06	0.09	10.4	—
Heart																	
Beef, lean, cooked, braised, chopped	1 cup	145	61	273	45	8	1	9	262	8.6	151	336	40	0.36	1.77	11.0	1

FOOD VALUES—EDIBLE PARTS—*Continued*

FOODS - Edible portions unless otherwise indicated	*Household Measure*	*Weight, g*	*Water, %*	*Energy, Calories*	*Protein, g*	*Fat, g*	*Carbohydrate, g*	*Calcium, mg*	*Phosphorus, mg*	*Iron, mg*	*Sodium, mg*	*Potassium, mg*	*Vitamin A, IU*	*Thiamin, mg*	*Riboflavin, mg*	*Niacin, mg*	*Ascorbic Acid, mg*
Hog, cooked, braised, chopped	1 cup	145	61	283	45	10	0.4	6	175	7.1	94	186	60	0.29	2.49	9.7	1
Lamb, cooked, chopped	1 cup	145	54	377	43	21	2	20	335	—	—	—	150	0.30	1.49	9.3	Tr
Herring, smoked, kippered, fillet, 7″ long, 2¼″ wide, ¼″ thick	1 fillet	65	61	137	14	8	0	43	165	0.9	—	—	20	—	0.18	2.1	—
Honey, strained	1 T	21	17	64	0.1	0	17	1	1	0.1	1	11	0	Tr	0.01	0.1	Tr
Ice cream, regular, 10% fat, hardened	1 cup	133	63	257	6	14	28	194	153	0.1	84	241	590	0.05	0.28	0.1	1
Ice cream, soft serve	1 cup	173	63	334	8	18	36	253	199	0.1	109	313	760	0.07	0.36	0.2	2
Ice milk, hardened, 5.1% fat	1 cup	131	67	199	6	7	29	204	162	0.1	89	255	280	0.07	0.29	0.1	1
Ices, water, lime	1 cup	193	67	247	0.8	Tr	63	Tr	Tr	Tr	Tr	6	Tr	Tr	Tr	Tr	2
Jams and preserves, sweetened with regular amount nutritive sweetener	1 T	20	29	54	0.1	Tr	14	4	2	0.2	2	18	Tr	Tr	0.01	Tr	Tr
Jellies, sweetened with regular amount nutritive sweetener	1 T	18	29	49	Tr	Tr	13	4	1	0.3	3	14	Tr	Tr	0.01	Tr	1
Kale, cooked, leaves without stems	1 cup	130	91	40	4	0.7	7	157	62	1.3	27	251	10660	0.08	0.20	0.9	49
Kohlrabi, cooked, diced	1 cup	165	92	40	3	0.2	9	54	68	0.5	10	429	30	0.10	0.05	0.3	71
Lamb, cooked, roasted																	
Leg, lean with fat, chopped	1 cup	140	54	391	35	27	0	15	291	2.4	87	396	—	0.21	0.38	7.7	—
Loin chop, lean with fat, cut 3 to a pound	3.4 oz	95	47	341	21	28	0	9	163	1.2	51	234	—	0.11	0.22	4.8	—
Lard	1 T	13	0	117	0	13	0	0	0	0	0	0	0	0	0	0	0

Lemon, raw, wedge, 1 5/8″ arc	1 piece	28	90	5	0.2	0.1	2	5	3	0.1	Tr	26	Tr	0.01	Tr	Tr	10
Lemon juice, raw	1 T	15	91	4	0.1	Tr	1	1	2	Tr	Tr	21	Tr	Tr	Tr	Tr	7
Lemon juice, canned, unsweetened	1 T	15	92	3	0.1	Tr	1	1	2	Tr	Tr	21	Tr	Tr	Tr	Tr	6
Lettuce, raw																	
Butterhead variety, chopped	1 cup	55	95	8	0.7	0.1	1	19	14	1.1	5	145	530	0.03	0.03	0.2	4
Crisphead, such as Iceberg, chopped	1 cup	75	96	10	0.7	0.1	2	15	17	0.4	7	131	250	0.05	0.05	0.2	5
Looseleaf, chopped	1 cup	55	94	10	0.7	0.2	2	37	14	0.8	5	145	1050	0.03	0.04	0.2	10
Lime juice, raw	1 T	15	90	4	Tr	Tr	1	1	2	Tr	Tr	16	Tr	Tr	Tr	Tr	5
Liver, cooked																	
Beef, slice, 6 1/2″ long, 2 3/8″ wide, by 3/8″	1 slice	85	56	195	22	9	5	9	405	7.5	156	323	45390	0.22	3.56	14.0	23
Chicken, chopped	1 cup	140	65	231	37	6	4	15	223	11.9	85	211	17220	0.24	3.77	16.4	22
Hog, slice, 6 1/2″ × 2 3/8″ × 3/8″	1 slice	85	54	205	25	10	2	13	458	24.7	94	336	12670	0.29	3.71	19.0	19
Lobster, northern, cooked, cubed	1 cup	145	77	138	27	2	0.4	94	278	1.2	305	261	—	0.15	0.10	—	—
Macaroni, cooked, enriched	1 cup	140	73	155	5	0.6	32	11	70	1.3	1	85	0	0.20	0.11	1.5	0
Mackerel, Atlantic, broiled with butter or margarine, fillet, 8 1/2″ × 2 1/2″ × 1/2″	1 fillet	105	62	248	23	17	0	6	294	1.3	—	—	560	0.16	0.28	8.0	—
Margarine, regular type, 1″ square 1/3″ high	1	5	16	36	Tr	5	Tr	1	1	0	49	1	170	—	—	—	0
Margarine, whipped type	1 tsp	3	16	23	Tr	3	Tr	1	1	0	32	1	100	—	—	—	0
Marmalade, sweetened with regular amount of nutritive sweetener, citrus	1 T	20	29	51	0.1	Tr	14	7	2	0.1	3	7	—	Tr	Tr	Tr	1
Milk, cow																	
Whole	1 cup	244	87	159	9	9	12	288	227	0.1	122	351	350	0.07	0.41	0.2	2
Skimmed	1 cup	245	91	88	9	0.2	13	296	233	0.1	127	355	10	0.09	0.44	0.2	2
Low fat, 2% nonfat milk solid added	1 cup	246	87	145	10	5	15	352	276	0.1	150	431	200	0.10	0.52	0.2	2
Milk, canned																	
Evaporated, unsweetened	1 cup	252	74	345	18	20	24	635	517	0.3	297	764	810	0.10	0.86	0.5	3
Condensed, sweetened	1 cup	306	27	982	25	27	166	802	630	0.3	343	961	1100	0.24	1.16	0.6	3
Malted, beverage	1 cup	235	78	244	11	10	28	317	287	0.7	214	470	590	0.14	0.49	0.2	2

FOOD VALUES—EDIBLE PARTS—*Continued*

FOODS - Edible portions unless otherwise indicated	*Household Measure*	*Weight, g*	*Water, %*	*Energy, Calories*	*Protein, g*	*Fat, g*	*Carbohydrate, g*	*Calcium, mg*	*Phosphorus, mg*	*Iron, mg*	*Sodium, mg*	*Potassium, mg*	*Vitamin A, IU*	*Thiamin, mg*	*Riboflavin, mg*	*Niacin, mg*	*Ascorbic Acid, mg*
Milk, goat, fluid	1 cup	244	88	163	8	10	11	315	259	0.2	83	439	390	0.10	0.27	0.7	2
Milk, human	1 fl oz	31	85	24	0.3	1	3	10	4	Tr	5	16	70	Tr	0.01	0.1	2
Molasses, cane, second extraction	1 T	20	24	46	—	—	12	58	14	1.2	7	213	—	—	0.02	0.2	—
Mushrooms, raw, diced or sliced	1 cup	70	90	20	2	0.2	3	4	81	0.6	11	290	Tr	0.07	0.32	2.9	2
Muskmelon, raw																	
Cantaloupe, cubed or diced	1 cup	160	91	48	1	0.2	12	22	26	0.6	19	402	5440	0.06	0.05	1.0	53
Casaba, cubed or diced	1 cup	170	92	46	2	Tr	11	24	27	0.7	20	427	50	0.07	0.05	1.0	22
Honeydew, cubed or diced	1 cup	170	91	56	1	0.5	13	24	27	0.7	20	427	70	0.07	0.05	1.0	39
Mustard greens, cooked, drained	1 cup	140	93	32	3	0.6	6	193	45	2.5	25	308	8120	0.11	0.20	0.8	67
Mustard, prepared, yellow	1 tsp	5	80	4	0.2	0.2	0.3	4	4	0.1	63	7	—	—	—	—	—
Noodles, egg, enriched, cooked	1 cup	160	71	200	7	2	37	16	94	1.4	3	70	110	0.22	0.13	1.9	0
Noodles, chow mein, canned	1 cup	45	1	220	6	11	26	—	—	—	—	—	—	—	—	—	—
Oatmeal, cooked	1 cup	240	87	132	5	2	23	22	137	1.4	523	146	0	0.19	0.05	0.2	0
Ocean perch, cooked, fried	1 lb	454	59	1030	86	60	31	150	1025	5.9	694	1288	—	0.45	0.50	8.2	—
Oils, salad or cooking																	
Corn, cottonseed, safflower, sesame, soybean oils, soybean-cottonseed oil blends	1 T	14	0	120	0	14	0	0	0	0	0	0	—	0	0	0	0
Olive or peanut oil	1 T	14	0	119	0	14	0	0	0	0	0	0	—	0	0	0	0

Okra, cooked, drained	1 cup	160	91	46	3	0.5	10	147	66	0.8	3	278	780	0.21	0.29	1.4	32
Olives, pickled, canned or bottled																	
Whole, large	10 olives	46	78	45	0.5	5	0.5	24	7	0.6	926	21	120	—	—	—	—
Ripe, sliced	1 cup	135	80	174	2	19	4	113	22	2.2	1098	46	80	Tr	Tr	—	—
Onions, raw, mature, dry, chopped	1 cup	170	89	65	3	0.2	15	46	61	0.9	17	267	70	0.05	0.07	0.3	17
Onions, cooked, boiled, drained	1 cup	210	92	61	3	0.2	14	50	61	0.8	15	231	80	0.06	0.06	0.4	15
Onions, young, green, raw, chopped	1 cup	100	89	36	2	0.2	8	51	39	1.0	5	231	2000	0.05	0.05	0.4	32
Orange, all commercial varieties, raw, peeled, whole fruit, 2⅝″ diameter	1	180	86	64	1	0.3	16	54	26	0.5	1	263	260	0.13	0.05	0.5	66
Orange juice, raw	1 cup	248	88	112	2	0.5	26	27	42	0.5	2	496	500	0.22	0.07	1.0	124
Orange juice, canned, unsweetened	1 cup	249	87	120	2	0.5	28	25	45	1.0	2	496	500	0.17	0.05	0.7	100
Oysters, raw, meat only	1 cup	240	85	158	20	4	8	226	343	13.2	175	290	740	0.34	0.43	6.0	—
Oysters, fried, oz is approximately 2½ select oysters	1 oz	28	55	68	2	4	5	43	68	2.3	58	58	120	0.05	0.08	0.9	—
Pancake, enriched flour, baked from home recipe, cake 6″ diameter, ½″ thick	1	73	50	169	5	5	25	74	101	0.9	310	90	90	0.12	0.16	0.9	Tr
Pancake and waffle mixes, pancakes baked from mixes, cake, 6″ diameter, ½″ thick	1	73	51	164	5	5	24	157	190	0.9	412	112	180	0.11	0.18	0.6	Tr
Papaya, raw, cubed	1 cup	140	89	55	0.8	0.1	14	28	22	0.4	4	328	2450	0.06	0.6	0.4	78
Parsley, common garden, plain and curled leaf, raw, chopped	1 T	4	85	2	0.1	Tr	0.3	7	2	0.2	2	25	300	Tr	0.01	Tr	6
Parsnips, pared, without tops, boiled, drained, diced	1 cup	155	82	102	2	0.8	23	70	96	0.9	12	587	50	0.11	0.12	0.2	16
Peach, raw, diced	1 cup	185	89	70	1	0.2	18	17	35	0.9	2	374	2460	0.04	0.09	1.9	13
Peach nectar, canned	1 cup	249	87	120	0.5	Tr	31	10	27	0.5	2	194	1070	0.02	0.05	1.0	Tr
Peanuts, roasted, shelled, chopped	1 cup	144	2	838	38	70	30	104	586	3.2	7	1009	—	0.46	0.19	24.6	0

FOODS - Edible portions unless otherwise indicated	*Household Measure*	*Weight, g*	*Water, %*	*Energy, Calories*	*Protein, g*	*Fat, g*	*Carbohydrate, g*	*Calcium, mg*	*Phosphorus, mg*	*Iron, mg*	*Sodium, mg*	*Potassium, mg*	*Vitamin A, IU*	*Thiamin, mg*	*Riboflavin, mg*	*Niacin, mg*	*Ascorbic Acid, mg*
Peanut butter, made with moderate amount of fat, nutritive sweetener, salt	1 T	16	2	94	4	8	3	9	61	0.3	97	100	—	0.02	0.02	2.4	0
Pears, raw, cubed	1 cup	165	83	101	1	0.7	25	13	18	0.5	3	215	30	0.03	0.07	0.2	7
Pear nectar	1 cup	250	86	130	0.8	0.5	33	8	13	0.3	3	98	Tr	Tr	0.05	Tr	Tr
Peas, green, immature, cooked, drained	1 cup	160	82	114	9	0.6	19	37	158	2.9	2	314	860	0.45	0.18	3.7	32
Peas, canned, Early June, solids and liquids	1 cup	249	83	164	9	0.7	31	50	164	4.2	588	239	1120	0.22	0.12	2.2	22
Peas, mature seeds, dry, cooked, split without seed coat	1 cup	200	70	230	16	0.6	42	22	178	3.4	26	592	80	0.30	0.18	1.8	—
Pecans, shelled, chopped	1 cup	118	4	811	11	84	17	86	341	2.8	Tr	712	150	1.01	0.15	1.1	2
Peppers, sweet garden variety, immature, green, chopped, raw	1 cup	150	93	33	2	0.3	7	14	33	1.1	20	320	630	0.12	0.12	0.8	192
Peppers, mature, red, raw, chopped	1 cup	150	91	47	2	0.5	11	20	45	0.9	—	—	6680	0.12	0.12	0.8	306
Pickles																	
Dill, sliced	1 cup	155	93	17	1	0.3	3	40	33	1.6	2213	310	160	Tr	0.03	Tr	9
Sour, 4″ long, 1 3/4″ diameter	1 pickle	135	95	14	0.7	0.3	3	23	20	4.3	1827	—	140	Tr	0.03	Tr	9
Sweet, whole, gherkin, 3″ long, 1″ diameter	1 pickle	35	61	51	0.2	0.1	13	4	6	0.4	—	—	30	Tr	0.01	Tr	2
Relish, sweet, finely cut	1 T	15	63	21	0.1	0.1	5	3	2	0.1	107	—	—	—	—	—	—
Pie, baked, 1/8 of a pie																	
Apple	1 piece	118	48	302	3	13	45	9	26	0.4	355	94	40	0.02	0.02	0.5	1
Banana custard	1 piece	114	54	252	5	11	35	75	93	0.6	221	231	290	0.05	0.15	0.3	1

Blackberry	1 piece	118	51	287	3	13	41	22	31	0.6	316	118	110	0.02	0.02	0.4	5
Blueberry	1 piece	118	51	286	3	13	41	13	27	0.7	316	77	40	0.02	0.02	0.4	4
Cherry	1 piece	118	47	308	3	13	45	17	30	0.4	359	124	520	0.02	0.02	0.6	Tr
Chocolate meringue	1 piece	114	48	287	6	14	38	79	112	0.8	292	158	220	0.03	0.14	0.2	Tr
Coconut custard	1 piece	114	55	268	7	14	28	107	132	0.8	282	186	260	0.07	0.22	0.3	0
Custard	1 piece	114	58	249	7	13	27	109	129	0.7	327	156	260	0.06	0.18	0.3	0
Lemon meringue	1 piece	105	47	268	4	11	40	15	51	0.5	296	53	180	0.03	0.08	0.2	3
Mince	1 piece	118	43	320	3	14	49	33	45	1.2	529	210	Tr	0.08	0.05	0.5	1
Pumpkin	1 piece	114	59	241	5	13	28	58	79	0.6	244	182	2810	0.03	0.11	0.6	Tr
Rhubarb	1 piece	118	47	299	3	13	45	76	31	0.8	319	188	60	0.02	0.05	0.4	4
Pigs feet, pickled	2 oz	57	67	113	10	8	0	—	—	—	—	—	—	—	—	—	—
Pineapple, raw, diced	1 cup	155	85	81	0.6	0.3	21	26	12	0.8	2	226	110	0.14	0.05	0.3	26
Pineapple juice, canned, unsweetened	1 cup	250	86	138	1	0.3	34	38	23	0.8	3	373	130	0.13	0.05	0.5	23
Pizza, frozen with cheese, commercial, baked, 10″ diameter, slice 1″ arc	1 piece	13	45	31	1	0.9	5	20	20	0.1	82	14	60	0.01	0.02	0.1	1
Plums, raw, Damson, pitted, halves	1 cup	170	81	112	0.9	Tr	30	31	29	0.9	3	508	510	0.14	0.03	0.9	—
Popcorn, popped, oil and salt added	1 cup	9	3	41	0.9	2	5	1	19	0.2	175	—	—	—	0.01	0.2	0
Popovers, made from home recipe, with enriched flour, 2¾″ diameter at top, 2″ diameter at bottom, height at center 4″	1	40	55	90	4	4	10	38	56	0.6	88	60	130	0.06	0.10	0.4	Tr
Pork, fresh, retail cuts																	
Ham, cooked (baked or roasted), lean with fat (74% lean, 26% fat), chopped	1 cup	140	46	524	32	42	0	14	330	4.2	79	361	0	0.71	0.32	6.4	—
Loin or loin chops, cooked (baked or roasted), lean, chopped or diced	1 cup	140	46	507	34	40	0	15	358	4.5	84	384	0	1.29	0.36	7.8	—
Boston butt, cooked, lean with fat, chopped	1 cup	140	48	494	32	40	0	14	321	4.1	77	353	0	0.70	0.32	6.2	—
Pork, cured, retail cuts																	
Ham, baked, lean with fat (84% lean, 16% fat), chopped	1 cup	140	54	405	29	31	0	13	241	3.6	1049	328	0	0.66	0.25	5.0	—

FOOD VALUES—EDIBLE PARTS—*Continued*

FOODS - Edible portions unless otherwise indicated	*Household Measure*	*Weight, g*	*Water, %*	*Energy, Calories*	*Protein, g*	*Fat, g*	*Carbohydrate, g*	*Calcium, mg*	*Phosphorus, mg*	*Iron, mg*	*Sodium, mg*	*Potassium, mg*	*Vitamin A, IU*	*Thiamin, mg*	*Riboflavin, mg*	*Niacin, mg*	*Ascorbic Acid, mg*
Potato, baked in skin, 2 1/3″ diameter, 4 3/4″ long	1	202	75	145	4	0.2	33	14	101	1.1	6	782	Tr	0.15	0.07	2.7	31
Potatoes, boiled in skin, diced	1 cup	155	80	118	3	0.2	27	11	82	0.9	5	631	Tr	0.14	0.06	2.3	25
Potatoes, French fries, strips, 3 1/2″ to 4″ long	10	78	45	214	3	10	28	12	87	1.0	5	665	Tr	0.10	0.06	2.4	16
Potatoes, hash browns, after holding overnight	1 cup	155	54	355	5	18	45	19	122	1.4	446	736	Tr	0.12	0.18	3.3	14
Potatoes, mashed, milk and table fat added	1 cup	210	80	197	4	9	26	50	101	0.8	695	525	360	0.17	0.11	2.1	19
Potatoes, scalloped and au gratin with cheese	1 cup	245	71	355	13	19	33	311	299	1.2	1095	750	780	0.15	0.29	2.2	25
Potato chips, 1 3/4″ × 2 1/2″ × 2/32″	10 chips	20	2	114	1	8	10	8	28	0.4	—	226	Tr	0.04	0.01	1.0	3
Potato salad, from home recipe, made with cooked salad dressing, seasonings	1 cup	250	76	248	7	7	41	80	160	1.5	1320	798	350	0.20	0.18	2.8	28
Pretzel, twisted, Dutch, 2 3/4″ × 2 5/8″ × 5/8″	1	16	5	62	2	0.7	12	4	21	0.2	269	21	0	Tr	Tr	0.1	0
Prunes, dehydrated, nugget type, pieces, uncooked	1 cup	100	3	344	3	0.5	91	90	107	4.4	11	940	2170	0.12	0.22	2.1	4
Prunes, dehydrated, nugget type, cooked, fruit and liquid with added sugar	1 cup	280	51	504	3	0.6	132	87	104	4.2	11	921	2130	0.08	0.20	2.0	3
Prune juice, canned or bottled	1 cup	256	80	197	1	0.3	49	36	51	10.5	5	602	—	0.03	0.03	1.0	5

Puddings, with starch base, prepared from home recipe																
Chocolate	1 cup	260	66	385	8	12	67	250	255	1.3	146	445	390	0.05	0.36	0.3	1
Vanilla	1 cup	255	76	283	9	10	41	298	232	Tr	166	352	410	0.08	0.41	0.3	2
Puddings, mixes, and puddings made from mixes, made with milk, cooked	1 cup	260	70	322	9	8	59	265	247	0.8	335	354	340	0.05	0.39	0.3	2
Puddings, mixes, made with milk, without cooking	1 cup	260	69	325	8	7	63	374	237	1.3	322	335	340	0.08	0.39	0.3	2
Pumpkin, canned	1 cup	245	90	81	3	0.7	19	61	64	1.0	5	588	15680	0.07	0.12	1.5	12
Rabbit, domesticated, flesh only, cooked, stewed, chopped	1 cup	140	60	302	41	14	0	29	363	2.1	57	515	—	0.07	0.10	15.8	—
Radishes, whole, large, 1½″ diameter	10	90	95	14	0.8	0.1	3	24	25	0.8	15	261	10	0.02	0.02	0.2	21
Raisins, seedless, unbleached, whole, uncooked	1 cup	145	18	419	4	0.3	112	90	146	5.1	39	1106	30	0.16	0.12	0.7	1
Raspberries, raw, red	1 cup	123	84	70	2	0.6	17	27	27	1.1	1	207	160	0.04	0.11	1.1	31
Rhubarb, cooked, added sugar, diced	1 cup	270	63	381	1	0.3	97	211	41	1.6	5	548	220	0.05	0.14	0.8	16
Rice, brown, cooked	1 cup	195	70	232	5	1	50	23	142	1.0	550	137	0	0.18	0.04	2.7	0
Rice, white, enriched, cooked	1 cup	205	83	223	4	0.2	40	21	57	1.8	767	57	0	0.23	0.02	2.1	0
Rice, precooked, instant, long grain	1 cup	165	73	180	4	Tr	40	5	31	1.3	450	—	0	0.21	—	1.7	0
Rice, presweetened, puffed, added honey, cocoa, salt, vitamins, iron	1 cup	35	2	140	2	1	30	7	29	1.2	148	33	1650	0.41	0.49	4.1	12
Rice pudding with raisins	1 cup	265	66	387	10	8	71	260	249	1.1	188	469	290	0.08	0.37	0.5	Tr
Rolls and buns, commercial, ready to serve																
Danish pastry, plain, 3⅛″ arc or ⅛ package	1	41	22	179	3	10	19	21	46	0.4	156	48	130	0.03	0.06	0.3	Tr

FOOD VALUES—EDIBLE PARTS—*Continued*

FOODS - Edible portions unless otherwise indicated	*Household Measure*	*Weight, g*	*Water, %*	*Energy, Calories*	*Protein, g*	*Fat, g*	*Carbohydrate, g*	*Calcium, mg*	*Phosphorus, mg*	*Iron, mg*	*Sodium, mg*	*Potassium, mg*	*Vitamin A, IU*	*Thiamin, mg*	*Riboflavin, mg*	*Niacin, mg*	*Ascorbic Acid, mg*
Hard rolls, enriched, round, 3¾″ diameter by 2″ high	1 roll	50	25	156	5	2	30	24	46	1.2	313	49	Tr	0.13	0.12	1.4	Tr
Partially baked, brown-and-serve, enriched, 12 oz package, 12 rolls, browned	1 roll	26	27	84	2	2	14	20	23	0.5	136	25	Tr	0.07	0.06	0.6	Tr
Rusk, ⅜″ diameter, ½″ thick	1 rusk	9	5	38	1	0.8	6	2	11	0.1	22	0.4	20	0.01	0.02	0.1	Tr
Rutabagas, cooked, cubed or sliced	1 cup	170	90	60	2	0.2	14	100	53	0.5	7	284	940	0.10	0.10	1.4	44
Salad dressings, commercial																	
Blue and Roquefort cheese, regular	1 T	15	32	76	0.7	8	1	12	11	Tr	164	6	30	Tr	0.02	Tr	Tr
French, regular	1 T	16	39	66	0.1	6	3	2	2	0.1	219	13	—	—	—	—	—
Italian, regular	1 T	15	28	83	Tr	9	1	2	1	Tr	314	2	Tr	Tr	Tr	Tr	—
Mayonnaise	1 T	14	15	101	0.2	11	0.3	3	4	0.1	84	5	40	Tr	0.01	Tr	—
Salad dressing, regular	1 T	15	41	65	0.2	6	2	2	4	Tr	88	1	30	Tr	Tr	Tr	—
Thousand island, regular	1 T	16	32	80	0.1	8	3	2	3	0.1	112	18	50	Tr	Tr	Tr	Tr
Salmon, canned, solid and liquid, net weight 7¾ oz	1 can	220	64	447	48	27	0	—	—	—	—	—	—	—	—	—	—
Salmon, broiled or baked, steak, with butter or margarine, 6¾″ × 2½″ × 1″ thick	1	145	63	232	35	9	0	—	528	1.5	148	565	200	0.20	0.08	12.5	—

Salsify, cooked, boiled, drained, stored	1 cup	135	81	94	4	0.8	20	57	72	1.8	236	359	10	0.04	0.05	0.3	9
Salt, table	1 tsp	6	0.2	0	0	0	0	14	—	Tr	2132	Tr	0	0	0	0	0
Sandwich spread, with chopped pickle, regular	1 T	15	45	57	0.1	5	2	2	3	0.1	94	14	40	Tr	Tr	Tr	1
Sardines, Atlantic, canned in oil, solid and liquid, can, net weight 3¾ oz	1 can	106	50	330	22	26	0.6	375	460	3.7	541	594	190	0.02	0.17	4.7	—
Sauerkraut, canned, solid and liquid	1 cup	235	93	42	2	0.5	9	85	42	1.2	1755	329	120	0.07	0.09	0.5	33
Sauerkraut juice, canned	1 cup	242	95	24	2	Tr	6	90	34	2.7	1905	—	—	0.07	0.10	0.5	44
Sausage, cold cuts, and luncheon meats																	
Bologna, including kinds made with and without binders, and meat byproducts or variety meats, slice, 4″ diameter, ⅛″ thick	1	22	56	67	3	6	0.2	2	28	0.4	286	51	—	0.04	0.05	0.6	—
Braunschweiger (smoked liverwurst) slice, 3⅛″ diameter, ¼″ thick	1	28	53	90	4	8	0.7	3	69	1.7	—	—	1850	0.05	0.41	2.3	—
Brown-and-serve sausage, browned, yield from 1 pattie (from 8 oz package of 8–9 patties)	1	23	40	97	4	9	0.6	—	—	—	—	—	—	—	—	—	—
Brown-and-serve sausage, browned, yield from 1 link (from 8 oz package of 10–11 links)	1	17	40	72	3	6	0.5	—	—	—	—	—	—	—	—	—	—
Cervelat, dry, slice, 1½″ diameter, ⅛″ thick	4	12	29	54	3	5	0.2	2	35	0.3	—	—	0	0.03	0.03	0.7	—
Country style sausage	1 lb	454	50	1565	69	141	0	41	762	10.4	—	—	—	1.0	0.86	14.1	—
Deviled ham, canned	1 T	13	51	46	2	4	0	1	12	0.3	—	—	0	0.02	0.01	0.2	—

FOOD VALUES—EDIBLE PARTS—*Continued*

FOODS - Edible portions unless otherwise indicated	*Household Measure*	*Weight, g*	*Water, %*	*Energy, Calories*	*Protein, g*	*Fat, g*	*Carbohydrate, g*	*Calcium, mg*	*Phosphorus, mg*	*Iron, mg*	*Sodium, mg*	*Potassium, mg*	*Vitamin A, IU*	*Thiamin, mg*	*Riboflavin, mg*	*Niacin, mg*	*Ascorbic Acid, mg*
Frankfurter, hot dog, weiner, including kind made with and without binders and meat byproducts or variety meats, chilled or refrigerated, 5″ long, 7/8″ diameter	1	57	56	176	7	16	1	4	76	1.1	627	125	—	0.09	0.11	1.5	—
Headcheese, slice 4″ × 4″ × 3/32″	1 slice	28	59	76	4	4	6	3	49	0.7	—	—	0	0.01	0.03	0.3	—
Knockwurst, link, 4″ long, 1 1/8″ diameter	1 link	68	58	189	10	16	2	5	105	1.4	—	—	—	0.12	0.14	1.8	—
Luncheon meat																	
Boiled ham, slice, 6 1/4″ × 4″ × 1/16″	1 slice	28	59	66	5	5	0	3	47	0.8	—	—	0	0.12	0.04	0.7	—
Potted meat, includes potted beef, chicken, turkey	1 T	13	61	32	2	3	0	—	—	—	—	—	—	Tr	0.03	0.2	—
Salami, slice, 1 3/4″ diameter, 1/8″ thick	1 slice	5	30	23	1	2	0.1	1	14	0.2	—	—	—	0.02	0.01	0.3	—
Scrapple, slice, 2 3/4″ × 2 1/8″ × 1/4″	1 slice	25	61	54	2	3	4	1	16	0.3	—	—	—	0.05	0.02	0.5	—
Souse, slice, 3 7/8″ × 3 7/8″ × 1/8″	1 slice	28	70	51	4	4	3	—	—	—	—	—	0	—	—	—	—
Thuringer cervelat (summer sausage) slice, 4 3/8″ diameter, 1/8″ thick	1 slice	28	49	87	5	7	0.5	3	61	0.8	—	—	—	0.03	0.07	1.2	—

Vienna sausage, canned, 2″ long, 7/8″ diameter	1	16	63	38	2	3	Tr	1	24	0.3	—	—	—	0.01	0.02	0.4	—
Scallops, bay and sea, cooked, steamed	1 lb	454	73	508	105	6	—	522	1533	13.6	1202	2159	—	—	—	—	—
Shrimp, French fried	1 lb	454	57	1021	92	49	45	327	866	9.1	844	1039	—	0.18	0.36	12.2	—
Syrups																	
Maple	1 T	18	33	50	—	—	13	20	2	0.2	2	35	—	—	—	—	0
Sorghum	1 T	21	23	53	—	—	14	35	5	2.6	—	—	—	—	0.02	Tr	—
Table blends, chiefly corn, light and dark	1 T	21	24	59	0	0	15	9	3	0.8	14	1	0	0	0	0	0
Soybeans, mature, cooked	1 cup	180	71	234	20	10	19	131	322	4.9	4	972	50	0.38	0.16	1.1	0
Soy sauce	1 T	18	63	12	1	0.2	2	15	19	0.9	1319	66	0	Tr	0.05	0.1	0
Spaghetti, enriched, regular, thin, vermicelli, cooked, firm stage	1 cup	130	64	192	7	0.7	39	14	85	1.4	1	103	0	0.23	0.13	1.8	0
Spinach, raw, chopped	1 cup	55	91	14	2	0.2	2	51	28	1.7	39	259	4460	0.06	0.11	0.3	28
Spinach, cooked, drained, leaves	1 cup	180	92	41	5	0.5	7	167	68	4.0	90	583	14580	0.13	0.25	0.9	50
Squash																	
Summer, all varieties, cooked, drained, cubed or diced	1 cup	210	96	29	2	0.2	7	53	53	0.8	2	296	820	0.11	0.17	1.7	21
Winter, all varieties, cooked, baked, mashed	1 cup	205	81	129	4	0.8	32	57	98	1.6	2	945	8610	0.10	0.27	1.4	27
Winter, all varieties, cooked, boiled, mashed	1 cup	245	89	93	3	0.7	23	49	78	1.2	2	632	8580	0.10	0.25	1.0	20
Strawberries, raw, whole berries	1 cup	149	90	55	1	0.7	13	31	31	1.5	1	244	90	0.04	0.10	0.9	88
Sugars																	
Beet or cane																	
Brown, packed	1 cup	220	2	821	0	0	212	187	42	7.5	66	757	0	0.02	0.07	0.4	0
Granulated	1 tsp	4	0.5	15	0	0	4	0	0	Tr	Tr	Tr	0	0	0	0	0
Powdered, confectioners	1 T	8	0.5	31	0	0	8	0	0	Tr	Tr	Tr	0	0	0	0	0
Sunflower seeds, kernels, dry, hulled	1 cup	145	5	812	35	67	29	174	1214	10.3	44	1334	70	2.84	0.33	7.8	—

FOOD VALUES—EDIBLE PARTS—*Continued*

FOODS - Edible portions unless otherwise indicated	*Household Measure*	*Weight, g*	*Water, %*	*Energy, Calories*	*Protein, g*	*Fat, g*	*Carbohydrate, g*	*Calcium, mg*	*Phosphorus, mg*	*Iron, mg*	*Sodium, mg*	*Potassium, mg*	*Vitamin A, IU*	*Thiamin, mg*	*Riboflavin, mg*	*Niacin, mg*	*Ascorbic Acid, mg*
Sweet potato, cooked, baked in skin, 5″ long, 2″ diameter	1	146	64	161	2	0.6	37	46	66	1.0	14	342	9230	0.10	0.08	0.8	25
Sweet potatoes, canned, solids and liquids, regular pack in syrup, mashed	1 cup	255	72	275	5	0.5	64	64	105	2.0	122	510	19890	0.13	0.10	1.5	36
Tangerine, raw, whole fruit, 2³/₈″ diameter	1	116	87	39	0.7	0.2	10	34	15	0.3	2	108	360	0.05	0.02	0.1	27
Tapioca, dry, pearl and granulated, quick cooking	1 T	8	13	30	0.1	Tr	7	1	2	Tr	Tr	2	0	0	0	0	0
Tapioca cream pudding	1 cup	165	72	221	8	8	28	173	180	0.7	257	223	480	0.07	0.30	0.2	2
Tartar sauce, regular	1 T	14	34	74	0.2	8	0.6	3	4	0.1	99	11	30	Tr	Tr	Tr	Tr
Tomato, ripe, raw, 3″ diameter	1	200	94	39	2	0.4	8	23	48	0.9	5	429	1580	0.11	0.07	1.2	40
Tomatoes, cooked, boiled	1 cup	241	94	51	2	0.5	10	14	46	1.2	313	523	2170	0.12	1.07	1.7	41
Tomato catsup	1 T	15	69	16	0.3	0.1	4	3	8	0.1	156	54	210	0.01	0.01	0.2	2
Tomato chili sauce	1 T	15	68	16	0.4	Tr	4	3	8	0.1	201	56	210	0.01	0.01	0.2	2
Tomato juice, canned or bottled	1 cup	243	94	46	2	0.2	10	17	44	2.2	486	552	1940	0.12	0.07	1.9	39
Tongue																	
Beef, cooked, braised, slice, 3″ long, 3″ wide, ¹/₈″ thick	1 slice	20	61	49	4	3	0.1	1	23	0.4	12	33	—	0.01	0.06	0.7	—
Lamb, cooked, braised, slice, 3″ × 2″ × ¹/₈″ thick	1 slice	20	60	51	4	4	0.1	—	20	—	—	—	—	—	—	—	—
Tuna, canned, in oil, drained solids	1 cup	160	61	315	46	13	0	13	374	3.0	—	—	130	0.08	0.19	19.0	—

Tuna, canned, water packed, solid pack, can $3^{1}/_{2}$ oz	1 can	99	70	126	28	0.8	0	16	188	1.6	41	276	—	—	0.10	13.2	—
Turkey, cooked, all classes, roasted, without skin, chopped or diced	1 cup	140	61	266	44	9	0	11	351	2.5	182	514	—	0.07	0.25	10.8	—
Turkey, light meat without skin, chopped	1 cup	140	62	246	46	6	0	—	—	1.7	115	575	—	0.07	0.20	15.5	—
Turkey, dark meat without skin, chopped	1 cup	140	61	284	42	11	0	—	—	3.2	139	557	—	0.06	0.32	5.9	—
Turkey giblets, some gizzard fat, simmered, chopped	1 cup	145	61	338	30	22	2	—	—	—	—	—	—	—	3.94	—	—
Turnips, cooked, drained, cubed	1 cup	155	94	36	1	0.3	8	54	37	0.6	53	291	Tr	0.06	0.08	0.5	34
Turnip greens, leaves with stems, cooked, drained	1 cup	145	93	29	3	0.3	5	267	54	1.6	—	—	9140	0.22	0.35	0.9	100
Veal																	
Chuck cuts and boneless veal for stew, braised, pot-roasted, or stewed, drained, chopped	1 cup	140	59	329	39	18	0	17	211	4.9	68	313	—	0.13	0.41	9.0	—
Loin cuts, cooked, braised or broiled, chopped	1 cup	140	59	328	37	19	0	15	315	4.5	91	414	—	0.10	0.35	7.6	—
Round with rump (roasts or leg cutlets), cooked, braised or broiled, chopped	1 cup	140	60	302	38	16	0	15	323	4.5	93	424	—	0.10	0.35	7.6	—
Vegetable juice cocktail, canned	1 cup	242	94	41	2	0.2	9	29	53	1.2	484	535	1690	0.12	0.07	1.9	22
Vinegar, cider	1 T	15	94	2	Tr	0	0.9	1	1	0.1	Tr	15	—	—	—	—	—
Waffle, baked from home recipe, made with enriched flour, round 7″ diameter, $^{5}/_{8}$″ thick	1	75	41	209	7	7	28	85	130	1.3	356	109	250	0.13	0.19	1.0	Tr

FOOD VALUES—EDIBLE PARTS—*Continued*

FOODS - Edible portions unless otherwise indicated	*Household Measure*	*Weight, g*	*Water, %*	*Energy, Calories*	*Protein, g*	*Fat, g*	*Carbohydrate, g*	*Calcium, mg*	*Phosphorus, mg*	*Iron, mg*	*Sodium, mg*	*Potassium, mg*	*Vitamin A, IU*	*Thiamin, mg*	*Riboflavin, mg*	*Niacin, mg*	*Ascorbic Acid, mg*
Waffle, baked from mixes, enriched flour, made with eggs and milk, round, 7″ diameter, 5/8″ thick	1	75	42	206	7	8	27	179	257	1.0	515	146	170	0.11	0.17	0.7	Tr
Walnuts, Persian or English, shelled, chopped	1 cup	120	4	781	18	77	19	119	456	3.7	2	540	40	0.40	0.16	1.1	2
Watercress, leaves including stem, finely chopped	1 cup	125	93	24	3	0.4	4	189	68	2.1	65	353	6130	0.10	0.20	1.1	99
Watermelon, raw, diced	1 cup	160	93	42	0.8	0.3	10	11	16	0.8	2	160	940	0.05	0.05	0.3	11
Wheat products used mainly as ready-to-eat breakfast cereals																	

Wheat flakes, added sugar, salt, iron, vitamins	1 cup	30	4	106	3	0.5	24	12	83	4.0	310	81	1410	0.35	0.42	3.5	11
Wheat puffed, with sugar or sugar and honey and salt, added iron and vitamins	1 cup	35	3	132	2	0.7	31	7	53	1.2	56	61	1650	0.41	0.49	4.1	12
Wheat, shredded, without sugar, salt, or other added ingredients, biscuit $3^3/_4'' \times 2^1/_4'' \times 1$	1	25	7	89	3	0.5	20	11	97	0.9	1	87	0	0.6	0.03	1.1	0
Whitefish, cooked, baked (stuffed)	1 oz	28	63	61	4	4	2	—	70	0.1	55	82	570	0.03	0.03	0.7	Tr
White sauce, medium	1 cup	250	73	405	10	31	22	288	233	0.5	948	348	1150	0.10	0.43	0.5	2
Yeast, bakers, compressed	1 oz	28	71	24	3	0.1	3	4	112	1.4	5	173	Tr	0.20	0.47	3.2	Tr
Yeast, bakers dry	1 oz	28	5	80	11	0.5	11	12	366	4.6	15	566	Tr	0.66	1.53	10.4	Tr
Yoghurt, made from partially skimmed milk	1 cup	245	89	123	8	4	13	294	230	0.1	125	350	170	0.10	0.44	0.2	2
Yoghurt, made from whole milk	1 cup	245	88	152	7	8	12	272	213	0.1	115	323	340	0.07	0.39	0.2	2
Zwieback, $3^1/_2'' \times 1^1/_2'' \times {}^1/_2''$	1 piece	7	5	30	0.7	0.6	5	1	5	Tr	18	11	Tr	Tr	Tr	0.1	0

SOURCES OF EDUCATIONAL MATERIAL

Many drug companies publish materials suitable for use in teaching diet therapy. Contact your local representatives.

Government publications may also be used. To keep informed as to what is available from the government, request that your name be placed on the mailing list to receive all government publications. Contact the Superintendent of Documents in regard to materials from the Departments of Agriculture and Health, and Education and Welfare.

Additional sources are given below.

American Can Company
730 Park Avenue
New York, NY 10017

American Cancer Society
(Contact nearest unit)

American Celiac Society, Inc.
45 Gifford Avenue
Jersey City, NJ 07304

American Dental Association
Bureau of Dental Health Education
211 East Chicago Avenue
Chicago, IL 60611

American Diabetic Association, Inc.
1 West 48th Street
New York, NY 10017

American Dietetic Association
630 North Michigan Avenue
Chicago, IL 60611

American Dry Milk Institute
221 North LaSalle Street
Chicago, IL 60601

American Health Foundation
1370 Avenue of the Americas
New York, NY 10019

American Heart Association
(Contact nearest chapter)

American Home Economics Association
1600 Twentieth St., N.W.
Washington, DC 20009

American Institute of Baking
400 East Ontario Street
Chicago, IL 60611

American Institute of Nutrition
9650 Wisconsin Avenue
Washington, DC 20014

American Medical Association
Council on Foods and Nutrition
535 North Dearborn Street
Chicago, IL 60610

American Public Health Association
1790 Broadway
New York, NY 10019

American Red Cross
(Contact nearest chapter)

The Borden Company
350 Madison Avenue
New York, NY 10017

Campbell Soup Company
Home Economics Department
385 Memorial Avenue
Camden, NJ 08103

Cereal Institute, Inc.
135 South LaSalle Street
Chicago, IL 60603

Cooperative Extension Services of States
(Contact nearest unit)

Cornell University
Division of Nutritional Sciences
Media Services B-10
Martha van Rensselaer Hall
Ithaca, NY 14853

Evaporated Milk Association
228 North LaSalle Street
Chicago, IL 60601

Food and Nutrition Board
National Research Council
2101 Constitution Avenue
Washington, DC 20237

General Foods Corporation
250 North Street
White Plains, NY 10602

General Mills, Inc.
9200 Wayzata Boulevard
Minneapolis, MN 55440

Gerber Products
Department of Nutrition
Fremont, MI 49412

The Heinz Company
Post Office Box 57
Pittsburgh, PA 15212

LaLeche League International, Inc.
9616 Minneapolis Avenue
Franklin Park, IL 60131

National Dairy Council
111 North Canal Street
Chicago, IL 60601

National Kidney Foundation
2 Park Avenue
New York, NY 10016

National Livestock and Meat Board
407 South Dearborn Street
Chicago, IL 60605

The Nutrition Foundation, Inc.
99 Park Avenue
New York, NY 10016

United Fresh Fruit
and Vegetable Association
1019 19th Street, N.W.
Washington, DC 20036

United Ostomy Association, Inc.
(Contact nearest Unit)

Wheat Flour Institute
309 West Jackson
Chicago, IL 60606

Superintendent of Documents
U.S. Government Printing Office
Washington, DC 20402

RECOMMENDED DAILY ALLOWANCES (US RDA)*

	Adults and Children over 4 years	*Children under 4 years*	*Infants under 13 months*	*Pregnant or Lactating Women*
Protein	65 gm†	28 gm†	25 gm†	65 gm†
Vitamin A	5000 IU	2500 IU	1500 IU	8000 IU
Ascorbic acid	60 mg	40 mg	35 mg	60 mg
Thiamin	1.5 mg	0.7 mg	0.5 mg	1.7 mg
Riboflavin	1.7 mg	0.8 mg	0.6 mg	2.0 mg
Niacin	20 mg	9 mg	8 mg	20 mg
Calcium	1 gm	0.8 gm	0.6 gm	1.3 gm
Iron	18 mg	10 mg	15 mg	18 mg
Vitamin D	400 IU	400 IU	400 IU	400 IU
Vitamin E	30 IU	30 IU	30 IU	30 IU
Pyridoxine	2 mg	0.7 mg	0.4 mg	2.5 mg
Folacin	0.4 mg	0.2 mg	0.1 mg	0.8 mg
Vitamin B_{12}	6 mcg	3 mcg	2 mcg	8 mcg
Phosphorus	1 gm	0.8 gm	0.5 gm	1.3 gm
Iodine	150 mcg	70 mcg	45 mcg	150 mcg
Magnesium	400 mg	200 mg	70 mg	450 mg
Zinc	15 mg	8 mg	5 mg	15 mg
Copper	2 mg	1 mg	0.6 mg	2 mg
Biotin	0.3 mg	0.15 mg	0.15 mg	0.3 mg
Pantothenic acid	10 mg	5 mg	3 mg	10 mg

*Adapted from Recommended Dietary Allowances. Food and Nutrition Board, National Academy of Sciences—National Research Council, Washington, DC, 1979.

†If protein efficiency ration of protein is equal to or better than that of casein, US RDA is 45 grams for adults and pregnant or lactating women, 20 grams for children under age 4, and 18 grams for infants.

METRIC CONVERSION TABLE

Metric	*Household*
	WEIGHT
50 grams	1.8 ounces
100 grams	3.5 ounces
250 grams	8.8 ounces
500 grams	1.1 pounds
1 kilogram	2.2 pounds
28 grams	1 ounce
113 grams	4 ounces
227 grams	8 ounces
454 grams	16 ounces (1 pound)
	VOLUME
50 milliliters	0.21 cup
100 milliliters	0.42 cup
150 milliliters	0.63 cup
200 milliliters	0.84 cup
250 milliliters	1.06 cup
1 liter (1000 milliliters)	1.05 quarts
5 milliliters	1 teaspoon (60 drops)
15 milliliters	1 tablespoon (1/2 ounce)
50 milliliters	1/4 cup (2 ounces or 4 tablespoons)
118 milliliters	1/2 cup (4 ounces or 8 tablespoons)
237 milliliters	1 cup (8 ounces or 16 tablespoons)
480 milliliters	1 pint (16 ounces or 2 cups)
0.946 liter	1 quart (32 ounces or 2 pints)
3.79 liters	1 gallon (4 quarts)

FOOD EXCHANGES
FOR PHENYLALANINE-RESTRICTED DIETS*

VEGETABLES

Each serving contains approximately 15 milligrams phenylalanine, 1/2 gram protein, and 10 calories.

	Grams	*Phenylalanine (Mg)*
Asparagus, raw, 1 1/2 spears	25	14
Asparagus, canned, green, 1 1/2 spears	28	17
Beans, snap, green, 4 T	31	11
Beets, solids, 1/4 cup	42	7
Cabbage, raw, 1/3 cup	33	16
Cabbage, cooked, 5 T	50	12
Carrot, raw, 1 small	50	15
Carrots, cooked, 2/3 cup	100	18
Cauliflower, cooked, 3 T	25	18
Cucumber, raw, 1/2 medium	50	12
Eggplant, cooked, 2 T	25	11
Lettuce, 1/2 cup	25	17
Okra, cooked, 2 pods	3	18
Tomato, raw, 1/2 small	50	16
Tomatoes, canned, 1/4 cup	50	14
Tomato juice, 1/4 cup	50	13
Turnip root, white, raw, 6 T	50	9
Turnip root, cooked, 2/3 cup	100	14

Gerber's strained and junior vegetables:

Amount—7 T or 100 gm

Beets	17
Carrots	22
Green beans	63
Sweet potatoes	68

Amount—1 T or 14+ gm

Beets	2
Carrots	3
Green beans	9
Sweet potatoes	10

FOOD EXCHANGES
FOR PHENYLALANINE-RESTRICTED DIETS—*Continued*

FRUITS

Each serving contains approximately 10 milligrams phenylalanine, 0.4 gram protein, and 55 calories.

	Grams	*Phenylalanine (Mg)*
Apple, raw, 1 small	100	10
Applesauce, 2/3 cup	200	10
Apple juice, 1 1/2 cups	423	10
Apricots, raw, 1 1/2 medium	50	6
Apricots, canned, 1 1/2 halves	50	10
Avocado, 2 T	20	9
Banana, 1/4 small	25	11
Dates, dried, 1	10	7
Orange, 1/3 small	33	10
Orange juice, frozen, 3 T or 1 1/2 oz	53	10
Peach, raw, 1/2 medium	50	9
Peaches, canned, 2 medium halves	100	9
Strawberries, raw, 3 large	25	6

Gerber's strained and junior fruits

Amount—7 T or 100 gm

Applesauce	10
Applesauce and apricots	10
Apricots with tapioca	8
Bananas with tapioca	14
Peaches	22
Pears	10
Apple juice	< 3
Orange juice	< 3
Orange and apple juice	3
Orange-apricot juice	3
Orange-pineapple juice	6

Amount—1 T or 14+ gm

Applesauce	1.4
Applesauce and apricot	1.5
Apricots with tapioca	1.2
Bananas with tapioca	2
Peaches	3.1
Pears	1.5

FOOD EXCHANGES
FOR PHENYLALANINE-RESTRICTED DIETS—*Continued*

BREAD AND CEREAL

Each serving contains approximately 18 milligrams phenylalanine, 0.4 gram protein, and 15 calories.

	Grams	Phenylalanine (Mg)
Dry cereals		
Bran flakes, 2 T		20
Bran, Raisin, 2 T		20
Cheerios, 2 T		22
Corn flakes, 3 T		17
Rice flakes, 3 T		19
Rice Krispies, 4 T		19
Rice, Puffed, 8 T		19
Hot cereals		
Cream of Wheat, cooked, 1 T		13
Farina, cooked, 2 T		22
Grits, cooked, 2 T		18
Malt-O-Meal, cooked, 1 T		13
Miscellaneous		
Corn, canned, 1 T	26	14
Macaroni, cooked, tender, 1 T	18	16
Potato, boiled, 1/4 medium	25	21
Rice, brown, cooked, 1 T	24	12
Rice, white, parboiled, cooked, 2 T	22	20
Yams, cooked, 1 T	32	16
Special products		
Anellini, uncooked, 3/4 cup	100	12
Rigatini, uncooked, 1 1/2 cups	100	12
Paygel low protein bread, 1 slice	32	7
Rusks, 1 slice	11.5	4
Taglitelle, uncooked, 1 1/4 cups	100	12

Gerber's baby cereals

Amount—1 T

Barley		15
Mixed		15
Oatmeal		18
Rice		9
Barley with mixed fruit		12

FOOD EXCHANGES FOR PHENYLALANINE-RESTRICTED DIETS—*Continued*

	Grams	*Phenylalanine (Mg)*
Mixed with bananas		12
Oatmeal with bananas		15
Rice with strawberries		8
Cereals in jars		
Mixed with applesauce-bananas		9
Oatmeal with applesauce-bananas		7
Rice with applesauce-bananas		2
Rice with mixed fruit		10

FATS

Each serving contains approximately 4 milligrams phenylalanine, 0.1 gram protein, and 90 calories.

	Grams	*Phenylalanine (Mg)*
Butter, 2 tsp	9	4
Cream, heavy (40% fat), 1 tsp	5	5
Italian dressing, 3 T	14	4
Margarine, 1 T	14	5
Mayonnaise, 1 T	14	5
Tartar sauce, 1/2 T	10	4
Thousand island dressing, 1 T	14	4

FREE FOODS

The following contain little or no protein and may be used as desired, as long as the appetite is not depressed or the child overweight.

- Candies
  - Butterscotch, 1 piece
  - Cream mints, 1 piece
  - Fondant, patties or mints, 1 piece
  - Gum drops, 1 large
  - Hard Candy, 2 pieces
  - Jelly beans, 10
  - Lollipops, 1 medium (2 1/4″ diameter)
- Corn syrup, 1 T
- Danish desserts, 1/2 cup
- Fruit ices, 1/2 cup
- Kool-Aid, 1/2 cup
- Maple syrup, 1 T
- Molasses, 1 T
- Popsicle, 1 twin bar
- Prono, 1/3 cup
- Start liquid, 1/2 cup
- Sugar, granulated, 1 T
- Tang liquid, 1/2 cup

*Adapted from Acosta, P. and Elsas, L.: *Dietary Management of Inherited Metabolic Disease: Phenylketonuria, Galactosemia, Tyrosinemia, Maple Syrup Urine Disease.* ACELMU Publishers, Atlanta, GA, 1976.

IDEAL WEIGHTS FOR ADULTS*

Height†		*Weight‡*					
		Small frame		*Medium frame*		*Large frame*	
Feet and Inches	***Centimeters***	***Pounds***	***Kilograms***	***Pounds***	***Kilograms***	***Pounds***	***Kilograms***
Men							
5′2″	157	112–120	51–55	118–129	54–59	126–141	57–64
5′3″	160	115–123	52–56	121–133	55–60	129–144	59–65
5′4″	163	118–126	54–57	124–136	56–62	132–148	60–67
5′5″	165	121–129	55–59	127–139	58–63	135–152	61–69
5′6″	167	124–133	56–60	130–143	59–65	138–156	63–71
5′7″	170	128–137	58–62	134–147	61–67	142–161	65–73
5′8″	173	132–141	60–64	138–152	63–69	147–166	67–75
5′9″	175	136–145	62–66	142–156	65–71	151–170	69–77
5′10″	178	140–150	64–68	146–160	66–73	155–174	70–79
5′11″	180	144–154	65–70	150–165	68–75	159–179	72–81
6′	183	148–158	67–72	154–170	70–77	164–184	75–84
6′1″	185	152–162	69–74	158–175	72–80	168–189	76–86
6′2″	188	156–167	71–76	162–180	74–82	173–194	79–88
6′3″	191	160–171	73–78	167–185	76–84	178–199	81–90
6′4″	194	164–175	75–80	172–190	78–86	182–204	83–93

Women							
4′10″	147	92–98	42–45	96–107	44–49	104–119	47–54
4′11″	150	94–101	43–46	98–110	45–50	106–122	48–55
5′	152	96–104	44–47	101–113	46–51	109–125	50–57
5′1″	155	99–107	45–49	104–116	47–53	112–128	51–58
5′2″	157	102–110	46–50	107–119	49–54	115–131	52–60
5′3″	160	105–113	48–51	110–122	50–55	118–134	54–61
5′4″	163	108–116	49–53	113–126	51–57	121–138	55–63
5′5″	165	111–119	50–54	116–130	53–59	125–142	57–65
5′6″	167	114–123	52–56	120–135	55–61	129–146	59–66
5′7″	170	118–127	54–58	124–139	56–63	133–150	60–68
5′8″	173	122–131	55–60	128–143	58–65	137–154	62–70
5′9″	175	126–135	57–61	132–147	60–67	141–158	64–72
5′10″	178	130–140	58–64	136–151	62–69	145–163	66–74
5′11″	180	134–144	61–65	140–155	64–70	149–168	68–76
6′	183	138–148	63–67	144–159	65–72	153–173	70–79

*Adapted from Statistical Bulletin, October, 1977, Metropolitan Life Insurance Company. Metric measures are expressed in the nearest whole numbers.

†Heights are measured with men wearing shoes with 1-inch heels and women wearing shoes with 2-inch heels.

‡Weights are measured with both men and women wearing indoor clothing.

GLOSSARY

ADDITIVES—Substances from natural sources or from chemicals, added to foods to preserve them or to make them more appealing in some way.

ADULTERATION—The addition of an impure or weaker, usually cheaper, substance to another; addition of a substance, intentionally or unintentionally to food.

AMINO ACID—Organic compound marked by presence of both an amino (NH_3) and a carboxyl (COOH) radical; the building blocks of which protein is constituted and the end product of protein digestion or hydrolysis. Essential amino acids are necessary for growth or metabolism and are not produced by the body.

AMYLASE—Enzyme that converts starch to simpler carbohydrates.

ANABOLISM—The building up of body tissue as in growth and maintenance.

ANTIVITAMIN—A substance, natural or synthetic, that inhibits the normal functioning of certain vitamins.

ASCORBIC ACID—Vitamin C.

AVITAMINOSIS—Disease due to lack of vitamins in the diet; a deficiency condition.

BASAL METABOLISM—The amount of energy needed for maintenance of life when the body is at complete rest; the amount of metabolic processes that takes place in the body at rest and fasting, and which are necessary to keep the body alive and functioning.

BERIBERI—A deficiency disease due to malnutrition; a deficiency of thiamin in the diet, characterized by polyneuritis, cardiovascular changes, and edema. Endemic in areas where rice, particularly refined rice, is the principal food.

CALORIE—A unit of heat; the amount of heat required to raise the temperature of one kilogram of water one degree Centigrade. The *large or kilogram calorie* is used when writing of human nutrition. The abbreviation is C., Cal., or kcal.

CARBOHYDRATE—One of a group of chemical substances, including sugars, glycogen, starches, and cellulose, that contain only carbon, hydrogen, and oxygen.

CATABOLISM—The opposite of anabolism; all the metabolic processes in which complex substances are converted to simpler substances, usually with the release of energy; the breaking down of body tissues into simpler chemical units known as waste.

CATALYST—An agent that causes chemical reactions without entering into or being altered by the reactions.

CELLULOSE—Plant fiber; a fibrous form of carbohydrate making up the framework of plants and not ordinarily chemically changed and absorbed during digestion.

CRETINISM—Congenital deficiency condition characterized by lack of mental and physical development; thyroid deficiency condition with impaired mental ability.

DEHYDRATE—To lose or deprive the body of water; to become dry.

DEXTROSE—A simple sugar of the monosaccharide group; synonym for glucose.

DIET THERAPY—Treatment through prescription of specific diets.

DIETETICS—Science of applying principles of nutrition to the feeding of individuals or groups; science of the use of foods in health and disease.

DISACCHARIDE—A carbohydrate composed of two monosaccharides; double sugar.

ENRICHED—Made rich or richer; in nutrition, minerals and vitamins removed during processing have been added to the final product.

EREPSIN—Enzyme found in the intestine, which acts upon protein during digestion.

FALSE FATS—Hydrocarbons, like motor oil and mineral oil, that do not digest or provide for heat, energy, or other nutritive functions.

FAT—Chemical substance containing carbon, hydrogen, and oxygen that converts to fatty acids and glycerol during digestion or hydrolysis.

FATTY ACID—Any one of the acids that occurs in natural fats; one of the end products of digestion of fat. Essential fatty acids are those that cannot be synthesized by the body and must be ingested.

FOLACIN—Vitamin essential for formation and maturation of red and white blood cells and other functions. Also known as folic acid and pteroylmonoglutamate.

FOLIC ACID—See folacin.

FOOD—Solid and liquid substances taken into the body through the digestive tract for use in growth, maintenance, and repair of the body; nutritive substances that provide heat, energy, material for tissues, vitamins, and minerals.

FOOD POISONING—Illness caused by bacteria, chemicals, or foods that are poisonous in themselves, such as certain mushrooms.

FORTIFIED—The addition of mineral or vitamins not present in the food before processing so that the end product is more nutritious than the original.

FRUCTOSE—Simple sugar found in fruit, honey, and vegetables; levulose; fruit sugar; one of the monosaccharides.

GALACTOSE—A milk sugar; simple sugar produced by digestion and hydrolysis of the milk sugar, lactose; a monosaccharide that is an isomer of glucose.

GALACTOSEMIA—An inborn error of metabolism, caused by a congenital absence of the enzyme necessary to convert galactose to glucose.

GLUCOSE—Simple sugar; a monosaccharide; the form in which the body absorbs and uses carbohydrates; the end product of digestion and hydrolysis of carbohydrates.

GLYCOGEN—Carbohydrate stored in muscle and liver for future conversion to sugar; polysaccharide commonly called animal starch.

GOITER—An enlargement of the thyroid gland.

HEALTH—A state of complete physical, mental, and social well-being and not merely the absence of disease or infirmity. (World Health Organization)

HOMOGENIZE—To produce a uniform emulsion or suspension of two substances normally not immiscible; homogenized milk has the fat (cream) content uniformly suspended throughout the liquid.

HYDROGENATION—The addition of hydrogen to unsaturated fats to change them to solid saturated fats.

HYPERALIMENTATION—Intravenous feedings that provide excessive calories or even the normal nutritional requirements when the natural digestive processes are interrupted.

HYPERVITAMINOSIS—A condition caused by excessive intake of one or more vitamins.

KERATOSIS—Condition of the skin characterized by horny growth or excessive development of the horny tissues.

LACTASE—Enzyme found in intestinal juice, which converts lactose to glucose and galactose.

LACTOSE—Milk sugar found in all mammalian milk; a disaccharide that yields glucose and galactose upon digestion or hydrolysis.

LACTOSE INTOLERANCE—Condition in which there is a deficiency of lactase. The condition may be congenital or acquired.

LIPASE—Enzyme necessary in the digestion of fats.

LIPID—Any one of a group of fats or fat-like substances, often used as a synonym for fat.

MALNUTRITION—Faulty or imperfect nutrition due to a dietary lack or an excess of one or more nutrients; lack of necessary or proper food substances in the body or improper absorption and distribution of them.

MALTASE—Enzyme that converts maltose to glucose in the intestines.

MALTOSE—Sugar found in malt and malt products produced from grains; disaccharide produced by digestion or hydrolysis of starch.

MARAMUS—Extreme wasting; condition occurring in infants after acute diseases.

MELENA—Stools resembling tar, caused by the action of digestive juices upon blood.

MENADIONE—Vitamin K.

METABOLISM—The total of the physical and chemical changes that occur within the body; all energy and material transformations that occur within living cells.

MICROGRAM—One-millionth of a gram; one-thousandth of a milligram.

MISLABEL—The contents of the container are not as listed on the container.

MONOSACCHARIDE—Simple sugar that cannot be further broken down by digestion or hydrolysis.

NIACIN—Nicotinic acid; one of the B complex vitamins; the anti-pellegra vitamin.

NICOTINIC ACID—See niacin.

NUTRIENT—Substance that nourishes the body; food that supplies the body with necessary elements.

NUTRITION—Combination of processes by which the body receives and uses food for growth, development, and maintenance.

NUTRITIONAL DEFICIENCY—Condition in which the body is not supplied with sufficient amounts of one or more nutrients. Deficiencies can be *primary* due to lack of supply or *secondary* when there is interference with digestion, absorption, or utilization of nutrients or when there is an increased need for a nutrient.

NUTRITIONAL STATUS—The condition of the body as a result of its receiving and using nutrients; the body's condition resulting from the nutrients ingested.

OBESITY—Abnormal amount of fat on the body; exogenous obesity is caused by excessive intake of food; endogenous obesity is caused by some abnormality within the body.

OSTEOMALACIA—Softening of the bones.

OSTEOPOROSIS—Porous condition of the bones.

PANTOTHENIC ACID—One of the B complex vitamins.

PASTEURIZATION—The process of heating a fluid at a moderate temperature for a period of time to destroy bacteria. Milk is pasteurized by heating to 62°C for 30 minutes.

PELLEGRA—Deficiency condition caused by the lack of or failure to utilize niacin.

PEPSIN—Enzyme in gastric juices, which converts protein into peptones and proteoses.

PHENYLALANINE—An essential amino acid.

PHENYLKETONURIA (PKU)—Condition caused by recessive hereditary trait in which phenylalanine is not metabolized properly and mental retardation results. PKU is characterized by phenylpyruvic acid in the urine.

POLYDIPSIA—Excessive thirst.

POLYOLS—Polyalcohols; derivatives of sugar, which require little insulin to metabolize.

POLYPHAGIA—Eating excessive amounts.

POLYSACCHARIDES—Complex carbohydrates such as starches, cellulose, and glycogen; one of a group of which upon digestion or hydrolysis yields more than two molecules of simple sugars.

POLYUNSATURATED FATS—Fats in which carbon atoms are joined by double and triple bonds; fats that can take on hydrogen during hydrogenation.

POLYURIA—Excessive urination; passing large amounts of urine.

PRECURSOR—One that precedes; the beginning substance; forerunner.

PROTEIN—Complex nitrogenous substances occurring in plants and animals and which are essential to growth and repair of body tissues and which yield amino acids upon digestion or hydrolysis

PTOMAINE POISONING—Poisoning caused by ptomaines. Ptomaines are formed during putrification of organic substances. Ptomaine poisoning occurs only when obviously decayed food is eaten and therefore is extremely rare.

RANCID—Having a sour smell or taste due to partial decomposition of fat.

RENNIN—Enzyme that coagulates milk.

RESTORED—The minerals or vitamins lost during processing of a food that are replaced so that the proportion of minerals or vitamins is the same in the finished product as in the unprocessed food.

RIBOFLAVIN—Vitamin B_2.

RICKETS—Form of osteomalacia in children resulting from calcium or vitamin D deficiency, producing abnormalities in shape or structure of bones.

SATURATED FATS—Fats that contain all the hydrogen possible in their molecules.

SCURVY—A deficiency condition resulting from the lack of vitamin C.

STARCH—Carbohydrates of the polysaccharide group found in plants.

SUCRASE—Enzyme from intestinal juices that acts upon sucrose to convert it to monosaccharides.

SUCROSE—Table sugar from sugar cane, sugar beets, and maple sap; a disaccharide that converts to glucose and fructose when digested or hydrolyzed.

THIAMIN—Vitamin B_1. Also spelled thiamine.

THIRST—Sensation resulting from lack of or need for water. May be due to general dehydration, poor distribution of body fluids, or dry mouth and throat membranes.

TRYPSIN—Enzyme in intestinal juices, which converts partly digested protein to amino acids.

UNSATURATED FATS—Those fatty acids that can take on more hydrogen under certain conditions.

VEGETARIAN DIET—Diet composed of plant food only. If milk and eggs are allowed, the diet is called a *lacto-ovovegetarian diet.*

ANSWERS TO REVIEW QUESTIONS

Section 1

1. C
2. B
3. A
4. A
5. A
6. C
7. B
8. C
9. A
10. A
11. B
12. A
13. C
14. B
15. A
16. A
17. B
18. C
19. C
20. A
21. B
22. A
23. A
24. B
25. B
26. A
27. B
28. C
29. A
30. C
31. Nutritional deficiency or malnutrition
32. 1 pint
33. Two
34. Fortified
35. Metabolism
36. Glycogen
37. Sucrose
38. 4 calories
39. 90 calories
40. Saturated
41. Soybeans
42. 4 calories
43. Calcium
44. Sodium chloride (salt)
45. Vitamin A
46. A, D, E, and K
47. Rickets
48. K
49. Vitamin B_1 (thiamin)
50. All the B vitamins
51. Pellagra
52. Ascorbic acid
53. C
54. 10 percent, 20 percent
55. Kidneys, bowels, skin, and lungs
56. Cellulose
57. Cellulose
58. 1 quart
59. 1½ quarts
60. 1000
61. Doubled
62. Cow's
63. Milk, sugar, and water
64. Before

65. Condensed
66. Meat
67. Cottage cheese
68. Meat
69. B
70. Cooked
71. Low to moderate
72. 20 percent fruit
73. Ripe
74. Meat
75. Smallest amount possible
76. B
77. A
78. Sugar
79. Flavor and color
80. Tomatoes
81. Tomatoes
82. Peas
83. Tomatoes
84. C
85. A
86. A
87. B
88. A

Section 2

1. C
2. B
3. B
4. A
5. A
6. C
7. B
8. C
9. A
10. C
11. B
12. A
13. A
14. B
15. B
16. C
17. B
18. A
19. C
20. A
21. B
22. A
23. B
24. A
25. C
26. C
27. A
28. A
29. B
30. C
31. B
32. A
33. A
34. Diet therapy
35. High-residue
36. 1000
37. Tea, coffee, fat-free broth
38. No food
39. Sodium
40. Karell
41. Rice, fruit, and sugar
42. 200 ml
43. Desirable eating habits
44. Diabetes mellitus
45. High-caloric
46. Low-purine
47. B complex
48. Calcium
49. Iodine
50. Dry
51. Water and nutrients
52. Celiac disease
53. Milk
54. A
55. A
56. B
57. B
58. B
59. A
60. A
61. A
62. A
63. B
64. B
65. B
66. A
67. B
68. A
69. B
70. B
71. A
72. B
73. B
74. B
75. A

INDEX

An italic number indicates a figure.
A "t" following a number indicates a table.